Field Guide
to Wilderness
Medicine

cf also Wilderness medicine
ed. Paul S. auerbach
3ed 1995 Mosby publ 0-8016-7044-6

Field Guide to Wilderness Medicine

PAUL S. AUERBACH, MD, MS, FACEP

Chief Operating Officer, MedAmerica,
Oakland, California;
Clinical Professor of Surgery,
Division of Emergency Medicine,
Stanford University School of Medicine,
Stanford, California

HOWARD J. DONNER, MD

Telluride Medical Center,
Telluride, Colorado

ERIC A. WEISS, MD

Clinical Assistant Professor of Surgery,
Division of Emergency Medicine,
Associate Director of Trauma,
Stanford University School of Medicine,
Stanford, California

Art by Christine Gralapp, MA, CMI

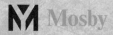 Mosby

St. Louis   Baltimore   Boston   Carlsbad
Chicago   Minneapolis   New York   Philadelphia   Portland
London   Milan   Sydney   Tokyo   Toronto

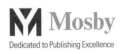

Dedicated to Publishing Excellence

A Times Mirror
Company

Publisher: Laura DeYoung
Managing Editor: Kathryn Falk
Project Manager: Carol Sullivan Weis
Senior Production Editor: Rick Dudley
Designer: Jennifer Marmarinos
Manufacturing Manager: Debbie LaRocca
Cover Photographs: Mountain, Paul S.
Auerbach; *Foliage,* PhotoDisc.

FIRST EDITION

Composition by The Clarinda Company
Lithography/color film by Pinnacle Press, Inc.
Printing/binding by R.R. Donnelly & Sons, Inc.

Mosby, Inc.
11830 Westline Industrial Drive
St. Louis, Missouri 63146

Library of Congress Cataloging in Publication Data

Auerbach, Paul S.
    Field guide to wilderness medicine/Paul S. Auerbach, Howard J.
Donner, Eric A. Weiss; art by Christine Gralapp. — 1st ed.
       p.   cm.
    Includes index.
    "Parent textbook: Wilderness medicine--management of wilderness
and environmental emergencies"—Pref.
    ISBN 0-8151-0926-1
    1. Outdoor medical emergencies—Handbooks, manuals, etc.
I. Donner, Howard J.   II. Weiss, Eric A., M.D.   III. Wilderness
medicine.   IV. Title.
    [DNLM: 1. Emergencies handbooks. 2. Wounds and Injuries—therapy
handbooks.   3. Environment handbooks.   WB 39A917f 1999]
RC88.9.095A938   1999
616.02'5—dc21
DNLM/DLC
for Library of Congress   98-29514
                                                CIP

98 99 00 01 02 / 9 8 7 6 5 4 3 2 1

This book is dedicated to
Sherry Auerbach, Martha Donner,
and Amy Weiss, the persons we love and
who have the impossible task of helping
us balance our lives.

Preface

This first edition of *Field Guide to Wilderness Medicine* was created in response to requests from readers of the parent textbook, *Wilderness Medicine: Management of Wilderness and Environmental Emergencies.* We have attempted to create a collection of clinical information and therapeutics that is appropriate for an expedition physician or physician extender, understanding the limited resources of a field setting.

To complete this effort, I engaged the collaboration of Doctors Howard J. Donner and Eric A. Weiss. These physicians are well known in the wilderness medicine community for their ability to teach their peers in a practical and entertaining manner. In addition, they continue to be true practitioners of medicine in the wilderness and have a keen sense of what works and what doesn't under adverse environmental conditions. Furthermore, they share my enthusiasm for educating persons who need to learn the basics, whether they be physicians or laypersons.

I expect to gather feedback from the practitioners who use this book to care for persons in wilderness settings. Subsequent editions will seek to refine the content and be structured to meet the readers' needs.

Our *Field Guide to Wilderness Medicine* relies significantly upon the collected wisdom from contributors to the textbook. For their generous contributions and unwavering enthusiasm, I am enormously grateful.

Be cautious, be safe, and seek every opportunity to help your fellow man. I hope this field guide makes you more effective as you practice the art of wilderness medicine.

Paul S. Auerbach

Contents

CHAPTER 1

High-Altitude Medicine

DEFINITIONS

High altitude is considered to be 1500 to 3500 m (4950 to 11,500 feet). Onset of illness is marked by decreased exercise performance and increased ventilation at rest. Altitude illness is common with rapid ascent above 2500 m (8200 feet).

Very high altitude ranges from 3500 to 5500 m (11,500 to 18,050 feet). Arterial partial pressure of oxygen (PaO_2) falls below 60 mm Hg, and maximal arterial oxygen saturation (SaO_2) drops below 90%. Extreme hypoxia may occur during exercise or sleep and with altitude sickness.

Extreme altitude is that extending beyond 5500 m. Marked hypoxemia and hypocapnia occur, and acclimatization is impossible. Abrupt ascent to this altitude without supplemental oxygen is extremely dangerous.

DISORDERS
Sleep Disturbances

Sleep disturbances are common at high altitude and are believed to result from cerebral hypoxia.

Signs and Symptoms
1. Increased wakefulness
2. Periodic breathing
3. Frequent arousal
4. Decreased rapid eye movement (REM) sleep, which may be caused by cerebral hypoxia

Periodic Breathing

Signs and Symptoms
Nocturnal hyperpnea followed by apnea, reflecting alternating periods of respiratory alkalosis (hyperpnea)

Treatment for Sleep Disturbances and Periodic Breathing
1. Give acetazolamide 125 mg PO at bedtime.
2. Use hypnotics cautiously because of the potential for respiratory depression.
3. If the disturbed sleep is thought to be unrelated to altitude and a sleep agent is elected, use triazolam 0.125 to 0.25 mg or temazepam 15 mg.

High-Altitude Deterioration

Signs and Symptoms
1. Acclimatization impossible, with victim's condition deteriorating, marked by weight loss, lethargy, weakness, headache, and poor-quality sleep
2. More common in persons with chronic diseases, particularly those associated with hypoxemia

Treatment
The only definitive treatment is descent to a lower altitude.

Acute Mountain Sickness (AMS)

Signs and Symptoms
1. Headache, usually throbbing, bitemporal or occipital, worse at night and with Valsalva's maneuver or stooping over

2. Fatigue, lassitude
3. Dizziness **(ataxia)**
4. Anorexia
5. Nausea
6. "Hangover"
7. Frequent awakening during sleep
8. Periodic breathing and sensation of suffocation
9. Sensation of inner chill
10. Facial pallor
11. Vomiting
12. Dyspnea on exertion
13. Irritability
14. Rales (fever with pulmonary edema)
15. Funduscopic venous tortuosity and dilation
16. Absence of normal-altitude diuresis

Treatment
1. **Do not proceed to a higher sleeping altitude.**
2. Monitor the victim for progression of illness (to pulmonary or cerebral edema).
3. If symptoms worsen despite an additional 24 hours of acclimatization, descend.
4. **Immediately descend if victim has ataxia, altered consciousness, or pulmonary edema.**
5. For mild AMS, halt the ascent and wait for acclimatization to occur (12 hours to 4 days). Administer acetazolamide 125 to 250 mg PO bid.
6. Administer aspirin 650 mg or acetaminophen 650 to 1000 mg for headache.
7. Administer prochlorperazine 5 mg IV for nausea and vomiting.
8. Avoid sedative-hypnotics.
9. Minimize exertion.
10. *Consider* descending 500 to 1000 m (1650 to 3300 feet).
11. *Consider* administering oxygen 0.5 to 1 L/min by mask or nasal cannula during sleep. This is particularly effective for headache.

12. *Consider* administering dexamethasone 4 mg PO or IM q6h, in conjunction with descent, for progressive neurologic symptoms or ataxia.
13. *Consider* undertaking a 2- to 6-hour treatment in a portable hyperbaric bag inflated to 2 psi (equivalent to a descent of 1600 m [5280 feet]) with or without supplemental oxygen.

High-Altitude Cerebral Edema (HACE)

Signs and Symptoms
1. Ataxic gait
2. Severe lassitude
3. Altered consciousness (confusion, drowsiness, stupor, coma)
4. Headache
5. Nausea and vomiting
6. Hallucinations
7. Cranial nerve palsy
8. Hemiparesis or hemiplegia
9. Seizures
10. Focal neurologic deficit
11. Retinal hemorrhages
12. Cyanosis or pallor
13. Hypoxemia associated with concomitant pulmonary edema

Treatment
1. **Immediately descend at least 500 to 1000 m.**
2. Administer dexamethasone 4 to 8 mg IV, IM, or PO, followed by 4 mg q6h.
3. Administer oxygen 2 to 4 L/min by face mask or nasal cannula to maintain SaO_2 greater than 90%. Higher O_2 concentrations may be required.
4. If the victim is comatose, manage the airway and drain the bladder.
5. *Consider* giving furosemide 20 to 40 mg or bumetanide 1 to 2 mg if intravascular volume is thought to be adequate.

6. *Consider* undertaking a 2- to 6-hour treatment in a portable hyperbaric bag inflated to 2 psi (equivalent to a descent of 1600 m) with or without supplemental oxygen.
7. If neurologic symptoms persist despite treatment with oxygen, steroids, and descent, a cerebrovascular accident (CVA, stroke) may be present. Carefully evaluate the situation.

High-Altitude Pulmonary Edema (HAPE)

Signs and Symptoms

1. Decreased exercise performance and increased recovery time
2. Fatigue
3. Weakness
4. Dyspnea on exertion
5. Headache
6. Anorexia
7. Lassitude
8. Dry cough
9. Cyanotic nail beds and lips
10. Tachycardia and tachypnea at rest
11. Audible chest rales
12. Orthopnea
13. Pink or blood-tinged sputum (late finding)
14. Mental changes, ataxia, decreased level of consciousness, coma
15. Hypoxemia on arterial blood gases (ABGs) or oximetry

Treatment

1. **Immediately descend at least 500 to 1000 m.**
2. **Administer oxygen 4 to 6 L/min by face mask (preferred) or nasal cannula to maintain SaO_2 greater than 90%. Higher O_2 concentrations may be required.**
3. Keep the victim warm.
4. *Consider* using pursed-lip breathing or a continuous positive airway pressure (CPAP) mask.

5. *Consider* giving nifedipine 20-mg sustained-release capsule q8h or 10 mg sublingually (PO), the latter dose repeated as necessary to reduce pulmonary arterial pressure without causing persistent hypotension.
6. *Consider* giving furosemide 20 to 40 mg or bumetanide 1 to 2 mg if intravascular volume is felt to be adequate.
7. *Consider* giving morphine sulfate 2 to 15 mg if intravascular volume is believed to be adequate.
8. *Consider* undertaking a 2- to 6-hour treatment in a portable hyperbaric bag inflated to 2 psi (equivalent to a descent of 1600 m) with or without supplemental oxygen.

Prevention
Some evidence suggests that acetazolamide, 125 to 250 mg PO bid or 500-mg sustained-release capsule q24h, prevents HAPE in persons with a history of recurrent episodes. Nifedipine 20-mg sustained-release capsule q8h may also accomplish this.

Peripheral Edema
Signs and Symptoms
Edema of the hands, face, and ankles

Treatment
1. Examine the victim for signs or AMS, HAPE, or HACE.
2. In the absence of AMS, administer a diuretic (furosemide 10 to 20 mg PO).
3. Maintain adequate intravascular hydration.

High-Altitude Flatus Expulsion (HAFE)
Signs and Symptoms
Excessive flatulence of colonic gas

Treatment
1. Administer oral simethicone 80 mg PO prn.
2. Encourage a carbohydrate diet.

High-Altitude Pharyngitis and Bronchitis

Signs and Symptoms
1. Sore throat
2. Chronic cough, dry or productive
3. Dry or cracking nasal passages

Treatment
1. Force hydration.
2. Give nasal saline spray prn.
3. Apply topical nasal ointment (mupirocin or bacitracin).
4. Give lozenges or hard candies.
5. Administer steam inhalation.
6. Give antibiotics if sputum becomes purulent (relatively ineffective).
7. Use an antitussive agent (codeine 30 mg PO q8-12h).

Chronic Mountain Polycythemia

Signs and Symptoms
1. Headache
2. Insomnia
3. Lethargy
4. Plethoric appearance
5. Polycythemia (hemoglobin > 20 g/dl of blood; hematocrit > 60%)

Treatment
1. Descend to a lower altitude.
2. Administer supplemental oxygen during sleep.
3. Perform a phlebotomy.
4. Give medroxyprogesterone acetate 20 to 60 mg/day as a respiratory stimulant.
5. Give acetazolamide 250 mg PO bid as a respiratory stimulant.

Ultraviolet Keratitis ("Snowblindness")

Signs and Symptoms

1. Eye pain
2. Sensation of grittiness in the eyes
3. Sensitivity to light
4. Tearing
5. Conjunctival erythema
6. Chemosis
7. Eyelid swelling

Treatment

1. Remove contact lenses.
2. Give a topical anesthetic for evaluation, but not repetitively (inhibits corneal reepithelialization).
3. Administer aspirin or ibuprofen PO.
4. Use external cold compresses.
5. Instill a mydriatic-cycloplegic agent to reduce ciliary spasm, dilate the pupil, and thereby prevent synechiae.
6. Avoid topical corticosteroids.
7. Patch the affected eye(s) for 24 hours, then reexamine. Do not patch the eye if there is a purulent discharge, facial rash consistent with herpes zoster, or any suggestion of corneal ulcer.
8. If the victim has both eyes affected and must use one eye, patch the more severely affected eye.
9. Encourage the victim to rest.

ACCLIMATIZATION

Acclimatization is the key to successful habitation at high altitude. Beginning at an altitude of 1500 m (4950 feet), the following physiologic changes are noted:

1. Increased ventilation, which decreases alveolar carbon dioxide and increases alveolar oxygen. This is mediated in part by the hypoxic ventilatory response (carotid body), which can be affected positively by respiratory stimulants (progesterone, almitrine) and negatively by alcohol, sedative-hypnotics, and frag-

mented sleep. Acetazolamide is a respiratory stimulant that acts on the central respiratory center.

2. Renal bicarbonate excretion in response to increased ventilation, hypocapnia, and the resulting respiratory alkalosis. Without this correction in pH, the alkalosis would inhibit the central respiratory center and limit ventilation. Ventilation reaches a maximum after 4 to 7 days at the same altitude. Acetazolamide facilitates this process.

3. Hypoxic pulmonary vasoconstriction leads to increased pulmonary artery pressure. This is not completely ameliorated by the administration of oxygen at altitude.

4. Red blood cell mass increases over a period of weeks to months. This may lead to polycythemia. Long-term acclimatization leads to increased plasma volume as well.

How to Acclimatize to Altitude

1. Avoid abrupt ascent to sleeping altitudes above 3000 m (9850 feet).

2. Spend 2 or 3 nights at 2500 to 3000 m (8200 to 9850 feet) before further ascent.

3. Add an extra night of acclimatization for every 600 to 900 m (1980 to 2970 feet) of ascent.

4. Make day trips to a higher altitude with a return to lower altitude for sleep.

5. Avoid alcohol and sedative-hypnotics for the first 2 nights at altitude.

6. Encourage a high-carbohydrate diet.

7. Be aware that mild exercise may be beneficial and extreme exercise deleterious.

8. Administer acetazolamide 125 to 250 mg PO bid starting 24 hours before ascent. An alternative dose is 500-mg sustained-release capsule q24h.

    a. Continue the drug during the ascent and until acclimatization has occurred (generally, for 48 hours at maximum altitude).

   b. **Do not use in the presence of allergy to sulfa derivatives.**

   c. Side effects include peripheral paresthesias, polyuria, nausea, drowsiness, impotence, myopia, and altered (bitter) taste of carbonated beverages.

   d. Dexamethasone 4 mg PO q4h can be used if acetazolamide is contraindicated. It is best reserved for treatment, rather than prophylaxis, of AMS.

CHAPTER 2

Hypothermia

DEFINITION

Accidental hypothermia is the unintentional decline of about 2° C in the normal human core temperature of 37.2° to 37.7° C (approximately 98.6° F) that occurs in the absence of any disease in the preoptic and anterior hypothalamic nuclei. It is both a symptom and a clinical disease entity. Hypothermia occurs in mild, moderate, or severe forms.

GENERAL TREATMENT

Handle all victims of hypothermia carefully to avoid unnecessary jostling or sudden impact. *Rough handling can cause ventricular fibrillation.*

1. Prevent further heat loss; insulate the victim from above and below.
2. Anticipate an irritable myocardium, hypovolemia, and a large temperature gradient between the periphery and the core.
3. Treat hypothermia before treating frostbite.

DISORDERS
Mild Hypothermia

Mild hypothermia is diagnosed when the body temperature is between 37° C (98.6° F) and 33° C (91.4° F).

Signs and Symptoms
1. Shivering
2. Dysarthria
3. Poor judgment, perseveration, or neurosis
4. Amnesia
5. Apathy or moodiness
6. Ataxia
7. Initial hyperreflexia, tachypnea, tachycardia, elevated systemic blood pressure
8. Hunger, nausea, fatigue, dizziness

Treatment
The victim is awake.

1. Gently remove all wet clothing and replace it with dry clothing.
2. Insulate the victim with sleeping bags, cloth pads, bubble wrap, blankets, or other suitable material.
3. If the victim is capable of purposeful swallowing (will not aspirate), encourage the drinking of warm and sweet drinks, warm gelatin (Jell-O), reconstituted fruit beverages, juice, or decaffeinated tea or cocoa. Avoid heavily caffeinated drinks.
4. Be aware that if a mildly hypothermic victim is well hydrated and insulated from further cooling, he or she can walk out to safety.

Moderate Hypothermia
Moderate hypothermia is diagnosed when the body temperature is between 32° C (89.6° F) and 27° C (80.6° F).

Signs and Symptoms
1. Stupor progressing to unconsciousness
2. Loss of shivering reflex
3. Atrial fibrillation and other arrhythmias, bradycardia
4. Poikilothermy
5. Mild to moderate hypotension
6. Diminished respiratory rate and effort, bronchorrhea

7. Pupillary dilation
8. Diminished neurologic reflexes and voluntary motion
9. Decreased ventricular fibrillation threshold
10. Prolonged P-R, QRS, and Q-Tc intervals; J (Osborn) wave
11. Paradoxical undressing

Treatment
The victim is confused, stuporous, or unconscious and *shows obvious signs of life.*

1. Handle gently, and effectively immobilize the victim.
2. Keep the victim horizontal to avoid orthostatic hypotension.
3. *Do not massage or vigorously manipulate the victim's extremities.*
4. Provide oxygenation commensurate with the victim's clinical condition.
   a. Options include simple administration of oxygen by nasal cannula or face mask, bag-valve-mask ventilation, or endotracheal intubation.
   b. If endotracheal intubation is performed, avoid overinflation of the tube cuff with frigid air, which will expand and kink the tube as the air within the cuff warms.
5. Initiate an intravenous (IV) line and administer 250 to 500 ml heated (37° to 41° C [98.6° to 105.8° F]) 5% dextrose in normal saline (NS) solution. If NS solution is unavailable, use any crystalloid, preferably with dextrose. Avoid lactated Ringer's solution because a cold liver cannot metabolize lactate. The fluid can be infused rapidly and warmed by any of the following techniques:
   a. Place the IV bag underneath the victim's back, shoulder, or buttocks.
   b. Tape heat-producing packets to the IV bag.
   c. Use an IV fluid-compressor inflatable cuff.
6. *Consider* treatment of hypoglycemia, specifically, therapy with IV 50% dextrose 25 g.

7. *Consider* treatment of opiate effects, specifically, therapy with IV naloxone 0.8 to 1.6 mg.
8. *Consider* the effects of benzodiazepines, and offer therapy with IV flumazenil 3 mg.
9. **Stabilize the victim's body temperature.**
   a. Remove wet clothing and replace it with dry clothing; insulate the victim from above and below.
   b. Apply external warming using blankets, sleeping bags, or shelter. A warmed-air-circulating heater pack may be used as an adjunct. Be cautious with total nude body-to-body contact in a sleeping bag because this may increase core temperature "after drop." Immersion warming in the field is similarly hazardous.
   c. Apply hot water bottles or padded heat packs in the axillae and groin area and around the neck. Take care not to create thermal burns.
   d. Use inhalation rewarming (with active humidification, if possible).

Severe Hypothermia

Severe hypothermia is diagnosed when the body temperature falls below 26° C (78.8° F).

Signs and Symptoms
1. Absent neurologic reflexes (deep tendon, corneal, oculocephalic)
2. Absent response to pain
3. Pulmonary edema
4. Acid-base abnormalities
5. Coagulopathy, thrombocytopenia
6. Significant hypotension
7. Significant risk for ventricular fibrillation
8. Flat electroencephalogram (EEG)
9. Asystole

Treatment

When the victim is confused, stuporous, or unconscious and shows obvious signs of life, follow the treatment guidelines for moderate hypothermia. When no immediate signs of life are present, do the following:

1. Feel for a pulse (best done at the carotid or femoral arteries). Do this for at least 1 minute.
2. *Unnecessary chest compressions of cardiopulmonary resuscitation (CPR) may initiate ventricular fibrillation and thus may be catastrophic.* If a cardiac monitor is available, use it.
   a. If ventricular fibrillation or apparent asystole is determined, defibrillate one time with 2 watt-sec/kg body weight up to 200 watt-sec. Use benzoin to affix nonadherent electrodes. **Do not defibrillate if electrical complexes are seen on a cardiac monitor.** Defibrillation rarely succeeds below a core temperature of 30° C (86° F). If the victim is in asystole or ventricular fibrillation, begin CPR.
   b. If electrical complexes are seen on a cardiac monitor, assess for a central pulse to determine if true electromechanical dissociation exists. This is a difficult judgment call. The victim may have a low blood pressure that cannot be appreciated by the rescuer, in which case the chest compressions of CPR might initiate ventricular fibrillation.
3. Determine if the victim is breathing.
   a. Because chest rise may be difficult to discern, listen and feel carefully around the nose and mouth. A "vapor trail" is usually absent.
   b. If the victim is not breathing, assist with oxygenation and ventilation by endotracheal intubation or the next best method available.
4. If resuscitation is not successful in the field, continue warming and CPR until the victim arrives at a hospital or you cannot continue because of fatigue or danger to yourself.

5. If the resuscitation is successful, follow the preceding protocol for moderate or severe hypothermia.
6. *Use pneumatic military antishock trousers (MAST) only for temporary stabilization of major pelvic fracture.*

REWARMING OPTIONS
Passive External Rewarming in the Field
1. Cover the victim with dry insulating materials in a warm environment.
2. Block the wind.
3. Keep the victim dry.
4. Use an aluminized (reflective) body cover, such as a "space blanket."

Active External Rewarming in the Field
1. Apply hot water bottles, chemical heat packs, or warmed rocks to areas of high circulation, such as around the neck, in the axillae, and in the groin. Take care to avoid thermal burns. *Insulate the heated objects adequately.*
2. Use a forced-air warming system within a sleeping bag.
3. Immerse the victim in a warm (40° C [104° F]) water bath.
4. Place the hands and feet in warm (40° C) water.
5. **Do not rub or massage cold extremities in an attempt to rewarm them.**

Core Rewarming in the Field
1. Use heated (40° to 45° C [104° to 113° F]), humidified oxygen inhalation.
2. Administer heated (40° to 42° C [104° to 107.6° F]) IV solutions.

CARDIOPULMONARY RESUSCITATION

Handle all victims gently to avoid creating a situation of ventricular fibrillation in the nonarrested heart.

1. Carefully determine the victim's cardiopulmonary status.
   a. Feel for carotid and femoral pulses.
   b. Watch the chest for motion (breathing) for at least 30 seconds.
   c. Listen with the ear close to the victim's nose for breathing for at least 30 seconds.
2. If a hypothermic victim has *any* sign of life, do not begin the chest compressions of CPR, even if a peripheral pulse cannot be appreciated.
3. Manage the airway.
   a. If the victim is breathing at a suboptimal rate, assist with mouth-to-mouth or mouth-to-mask technique.
   b. If endotracheal intubation is available, perform it for standard indications (oxygenation, ventilation, protection of the airway).
4. If the victim is without any sign of life, begin standard CPR.
   a. A single rescuer who is fatigued may continue at slower rates of compression and artificial breathing with some expectation that these may be adequate because of the protective effects of hypothermia.
   b. Continue CPR until the victim is brought to a hospital, the rescuer is fatigued, or the rescuer is endangered.
5. Do not begin CPR if the victim has suffered obviously fatal injuries.
   a. A serum potassium (K^+) level greater than 10 mEq/L in the presence of hypothermia is a strong prognostic marker for death.
   b. Remember that a victim who appears dead may recover from hypothermia, so if in doubt, begin the resuscitation.

CHAPTER 3

Frostbite and Trench Foot

DEFINITIONS
In *mild frostbite*, there is no tissue loss, whereas in *severe frostbite*, tissue loss occurs. In another classification, severity of frostbite is divided into first, second, and third degrees.

DISORDERS
First-degree Frostbite
Signs and Symptoms
1. Numbness
2. Erythema
3. White or yellowish plaque
4. Edema
5. Occasional blue mottling
6. Skin insensate and firm with equal or diminished pliability

Second-degree Frostbite
Signs and Symptoms
1. Superficial blisters with clear or milky fluid
2. Erythema and edema surrounding blisters (Plate 1)

Third-degree Frostbite

Signs and Symptoms
1. Injury that extends through the skin into muscle and beyond
2. Leads to mummification and bone involvement (Plate 2)

TREATMENT FOR ALL DEGREES OF FROSTBITE

The preferred field treatment is rapid rewarming, as long as the affected tissue can be kept warm enough to avoid refreezing, which may be disastrous.

1. Protect the victim from the environment; provide appropriate shelter.
2. Replace constricting and wet clothing with dry, loose wraps or garments.
3. Do not attempt rewarming during transport unless it will be "rapid" (see next section). Do not attempt partial rewarming.
4. Do not attempt rewarming using the radiant warmth from a campfire or the exhaust from a car heater or tailpipe.
5. If transport will precede rewarming (victim can be brought to definitive medical attention within 2 hours), pad all affected parts as best as possible.
6. During transport:
   a. Prohibit tobacco use.
   b. Prohibit alcohol consumption.
   c. Leave blisters intact.
   d. Elevate the extremities.

Rapid Rewarming Techniques

1. Immerse in gently circulating water warmed to 40° to 42° C (104° to 108° F).
2. Do not use heated tap water unless the temperature can be measured and precisely controlled.
3. Rewarm until the skin is pliable and erythematous at the most distal parts of the frostbitten extremities.

4. Allow active motion, but do not massage injured parts.
5. Manage pain with analgesics.
6. **After thawing is complete, keep the victim and tissues warm. Do not allow refreezing.**

Adjuncts to Field Therapy

1. Apply a padded, sterile (as clean as possible) dressing to all blistered areas.
   a. Do not rupture blisters.
   b. If blisters rupture spontaneously, apply topical aloe vera or antiseptic (mupirocin) ointment.
2. Pad with cotton or soft cloth between fingers and toes.
3. Observe daily for development of new areas of blistering.
4. Elevate the affected parts.
5. Pad all splints.
6. Administer ibuprofen 400 mg PO q12h.
7. If the injury is extensive or blisters are ruptured, administer an oral antibiotic in a dose appropriate for age.

PREVENTION

1. Avoid fatigue and sleep loss.
2. Maintain an adequate diet in the cold.
3. Wear properly fitted, nonconstricting clothing, particularly footgear.
   a. Avoid wrinkles in socks.
   b. Keep footgear dry.
   c. Wear mittens in preference to gloves.
   d. Keep fingernails and toenails properly trimmed.
   e. Carry extra garments.
4. Maintain oxygenation, using supplemental oxygen at altitude.
5. Maintain adequate systemic hydration.
6. Do not overwash skin; allow natural oils to accumulate.
7. Avoid ingested alcohol and inhaled tobacco.

8. Maintain a dry, warm environment.
9. Do not handle cold liquids or metals.

■ TRENCH FOOT (IMMERSION FOOT) ■

Trench foot occurs in response to exposure to nonfreezing cold and wet conditions over a number of days, leading to neurovascular damage without ice crystal formation.

Signs and Symptoms
1. Red skin, which becomes pale and extremely edematous
2. Early numbness, painful paresthesias
3. Leg cramps
4. During the first few hours to days: limb hyperemic with swelling, then diffusely discolored, mottled, and numb
5. After 2 to 7 days: hyperemia predominant, with regional skin temperature variation, edema, blisters, and ulceration

Treatment
1. Keep the affected area dry and warm.
2. Treat as for frostbite, with the exception that rapid rewarming (thawing) is not necessary.

CHAPTER 4

Heat Illness

DEFINITIONS

The term *heat illness* encompasses a spectrum of syndromes ranging from muscle cramps to heatstroke, a life-threatening emergency. Predisposing factors include the following:

1. Environmental temperature exceeding 35° C (95° F) with humidity level greater than 80%
2. Dehydration, as indicated by dark, yellow-colored urine
3. Obesity
4. Cardiovascular disease
5. Fever
6. Hyperactivity
   a. Seizures
   b. Psychosis
   c. Cocaine or amphetamine intoxication
7. Muscular exertion
   a. Hard labor
   b. Strenuous exercise
8. Burns (including sunburn)
9. Drugs
   a. Anticholinergic agents (antihistamines, phenothiazines, antispasmodics)
   b. Beta-adrenergic blockers, angiotensin-converting enzyme (ACE) inhibitors, diuretics

10. Age, whether very young or very old
11. Fatigue or lack of sleep

Heat stress can be predicted by evaluation of the wet-bulb globe temperature (WBGT) index. Whereas a regular thermometer measures the dry-air temperature, a wet-bulb thermometer (WBT) measures the effect of humidity on temperature. The globe thermometer measures the effect of radiant heat. Because the WBGT is complex and 70% of the value is derived from the WBT, a simple alternative in the field is to use a sling psychrometer. This instrument has a thermometer with a wick surrounding the bulb attached to an aluminum frame with a hinged handle. After the wick is moistened, the psychrometer is slung over the head for approximately 2 minutes. Air passing over the wetted thermometer bulb cools the bulb in inverse proportion to the humidity. The WBGT can be used as a guide for recommended activity levels (Table 4-1).

DISORDERS
Heat Edema
Signs and Symptoms
Peripheral edema developing during the first few days in a hot environment

Treatment
Be aware that the edema is usually self-limited and does not require medical therapy.

"Prickly Heat" (Miliaria Rubra)
Signs and Symptoms
1. Erythematous, papular, pruritic rash developing on actively sweating skin
2. In dry climates, rash confined to skin sufficiently occluded by clothing to produce local high humidity
3. Skin that does not sweat effectively, predisposing to heat exhaustion and heatstroke

Table 4-1.

Wet-bulb Globe Temperature (WBGT) and Recommended Activity Levels

WBGT		RECOMMENDATIONS
° C	° F	
15.5	60	No precautions necessary
16.2-21	61-70	No precautions if adequate hydration maintained
22-24	71-75	Unacclimatized: curtail exercise
		Acclimatized: exercise with caution; rest periods and water breaks every 20 to 30 minutes
24.5-26.6	76-80	Unacclimatized: avoid hiking or sports or sun exposure
		Acclimatized: heavy to moderate work with caution
27-30	81-85	Limited brief activity for acclimatized, fit persons only
31	88	Avoid activity and sun exposure

Treatment
1. Cool and dry affected skin.
2. Administer antihistamines (diphenhydramine 25 to 50 mg q4-6h) to relieve itching.
3. Note that desquamation of the affected epidermis and recovery of sweat gland function occurs in 7 to 10 days.

Heat Syncope

Signs and Symptoms
Syncope after prolonged standing in a hot environment

Treatment
1. Perform a secondary assessment after a primary survey to assess for any trauma that may have occurred because of a fall.

2. Place the victim in Trendelenburg's position.
3. Cool the victim and administer oral fluids (at least 1 L over 1 hour) when he or she is awake and alert. A carbohydrate-containing beverage can be absorbed by the body up to 30% faster than plain water. To disinfected water, add a powdered sports drink mix; a 6% or 7% carbohydrate concentration, such as diluted Gatorade (third to half strength), is ideal. Higher carbohydrate concentrations should be avoided because they can produce stomach cramps and delay absorption.
4. Note that colder fluids are more easily absorbed from the stomach.
5. Be aware that unacclimatized individuals working in the heat for 8 hours a day can develop a salt deficit and electrolyte imbalance unless a small amount of salt is added to their drinking water. The ideal concentration is a 0.1% salt solution, which can be prepared by dissolving two 10-grain salt tablets or ¼ tsp of table salt in a quart of water. Crush the salt tablets before attempting to dissolve them. Salt tablets should not be eaten by themselves. They irritate the stomach, produce vomiting, and do not treat the dehydration that is also present.

Heat Cramps

Signs and Symptoms

1. Painful, spasmodic muscle cramps that usually occur in heavily exercised muscles
2. Recurrent cramps that may be precipitated by manipulation of the muscle
3. Onset during exercise or after the work effort

Treatment

1. Administer an oral rehydration solution containing 3.5 g sodium chloride (¼ tsp salt) and 1.5 g potassium chloride in 1 L drinking water.
2. Allow the victim to rest in a cool environment.

Heat Exhaustion

Signs and Symptoms

1. Flulike symptoms (malaise, headache, weakness, nausea, anorexia)
2. Vomiting
3. Orthostatic hypotension
4. Tachycardia
5. Temperature usually less than 38° to 39° C (100.4° to 102.2° F) and often normal
6. Sweating
7. Normal mental status and neurologic examination

Treatment

1. Stop all exertion and move the victim to a cool and shaded environment.
2. Remove restrictive clothing.
3. Administer an oral rehydration solution.
4. Place ice or cold packs on the neck, chest wall, axillae, and groin. (Do not place ice directly against skin.) Be aware that fanning the victim while spraying with tepid water and soaking the victim in cool water are also effective cooling methods.

Heatstroke

Heatstroke is a true medical emergency; if not promptly and effectively treated, the mortality approaches 80%. Environmental heatstroke can be thought of as the end stage of heat exhaustion, when compensatory mechanisms for dissipating heat fail. The transition from heat exhaustion to heatstroke is often noted when a victim shows abnormal mental status and neurologic function.

Signs and Symptoms

1. Elevated temperature, usually above 40.5° C (105° F)
2. Altered neurologic state (confusion, disorientation, bizarre behavior, ataxia, seizures, coma)
3. Tachycardia
4. Hypotension

5. Tachypnea
6. Sweating present or absent

Treatment

1. Provide rapid cooling. The clinical outcome is a function of the magnitude and duration of hyperthermia. The faster cooling is accomplished, the lower the morbidity and mortality.
   a. Place ice or cold packs on the neck, axillae, chest wall, and groin.
   b. Wet with tepid water, and fan rapidly to facilitate evaporative cooling.
   c. Immerse in cool water if available.
2. Protect the airway, and do not give anything by mouth because of the risk of vomiting and aspiration.
3. Administer IV fluid (1 to 2 L normal saline solution).
4. Treat for shock; specifically, administer oxygen if available.
5. Treat seizures and combative behavior with a benzodiazepine (diazepam 2 to 5 mg IV adult dose) or a barbiturate.
6. Suppress shivering by administering a benzodiazepine or chlorpromazine (Thorazine 25 to 50 mg IM or IV).
7. Evacuate the victim immediately to the nearest medical facility. Continue to cool the victim during transport until his or her temperature has fallen to 38° to 39° C (100.4° to 102.2° F).
8. Recheck the temperature at least every 30 minutes.

ACCLIMATIZATION

Physiologic acclimatization to a hot environment is an important adaptive response. It usually requires 8 to 11 days to reach maximum benefit and mandates some amount of daily exercise (approximately 1 to 2 hr/day). With acclimatization, sweating is initiated at lower body temperatures, and the sweat rate may more than double (up to 1 to 3 L/hr or up to 15 L/day). Sodium is conserved in both urine and sweat, in contrast to the unacclimatized state.

Work in the heat mandates constant fluid replenishment. Because net water absorption in the gut is about 20 ml/min or 1200 ml/hr, compensation for high sweat rates requires rest periods with reduced sweat rates and time for hydration. Thirst is a poor indicator of adequate hydration because it is not stimulated until plasma osmolarity rises 1% to 2% above normal.

CHAPTER 5

Burns and Smoke Inhalation

The severity of a burn injury is related to the size and depth of the burn and the part of the body that is burned. Treatment plans, including first aid and the necessity for evacuation, are based on the overall burn size in proportion to the victim's total body surface area (TBSA) (Box 5-1 and Fig. 5-1).

GENERAL TREATMENT

1. Remove all burned clothing from the victim.
2. Assess the airway and perform a primary and secondary survey.
3. Administer 100% oxygen if smoke inhalation is suspected.
4. Treat smaller burns by applying cool water compresses or immersion. Take care to avoid inducing hypothermia. Do not use ice packs except on small burns, and limit application to no longer than 10 minutes.
5. Remove any jewelry from burned or distal parts.
6. For a chemical burn, flush the site with a copious amount of water.

Box 5-1.

Estimation of Total Body Surface Area (TBSA)

RULE OF NINES (ADULTS)
1. Each upper extremity = 9% of TBSA
2. Each lower extremity = 18%
3. Anterior and posterior trunk each = 18%
4. Head and neck = 9%
5. Perineum = 1%

RULE OF NINES (INFANTS)
1. Each upper extremity = 9% of TBSA
2. Each lower extremity = 14%
3. Anterior and posterior trunk each = 18%
4. Head and neck = 18%
5. Perineum = 1%

For each year of age, subtract 1% from the head and neck and add 1% to the lower extremity.

RULE OF PALMS
A victim's palm covers an area roughly equivalent to 1% of TBSA.

DISPOSITION

1. A burn less than 5% TBSA (excluding a deep burn of the face, hand, foot, perineum, or circumferential extremity) can be treated successfully in a wilderness setting if adequate first-aid supplies are available and wound care is performed diligently.
2. A minor burn that involves less than 15% TBSA in the 10- to 50-year-old age-group or less than 10% in a child under 10 years or an adult over 50 years can usually be treated in an outpatient setting.

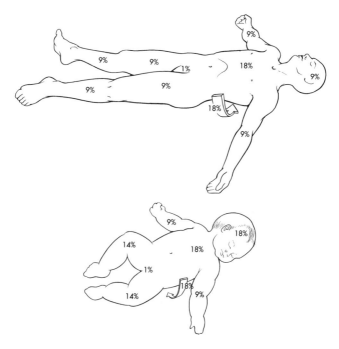

Fig. 5-1. Rule of nines used for estimating burned body surface. **A,** Adult. **B,** Infant.

3. A major burn victim should be immediately evacuated to a burn center. A *major burn* is defined as any of the following:
   a. Partial-thickness burn greater than 25% TBSA in the 10- to 50-year-old age-group or greater than 20% in a child under 10 years or an adult over 50 years
   b. Full-thickness burn greater than 10% TBSA in anyone
   c. Serious burn involving the hand, face, foot, or perineum
   d. Burn complicated by inhalation injury

  e. Electrical burn

  f. Burn in an immunocompromised patient, an infant, or an elderly person

DISORDERS
First-degree Burn (Superficial)
Signs and Symptoms
1. Only involves the epidermis
2. Erythema and pain without blisters
3. Prototype: mild sunburn
4. When over a large surface area: fever, weakness, chills, vomiting

Treatment
1. Cool the burn with wet compresses. (Do not use ice directly on skin.) When the burn is acquired suddenly, immediately apply very cold water to limit extent of tissue damage.
2. Apply aloe vera gel or lotion topically to the burn.
3. Administer ibuprofen, aspirin, or another nonsteroidal antiinflammatory drug (NSAID). Adult dose is ibuprofen 800 mg q8h.
4. For severe sunburn, administer oral prednisone in a rapid taper (80 mg on the first day, 60 mg on the second, 40 mg on the third, 20 mg on the fourth, and 10 mg on the fifth).
5. Be aware that topical corticosteroid creams or ointments have no benefit, and anesthetic sprays with benzocaine may cause sensitivity reactions.

Second-degree Burn
Signs and Symptoms
1. Superficial partial-thickness burn
  a. Involves the upper layer of dermis and creates clear filled blisters
  b. Blisters may not appear until several hours after injury
  c. Skin moist and erythematous, blanches with pressure, and hypersensitive to touch

2. Deep partial-thickness burn
   a. Possible damage to hair follicles and sweat glands
   b. Usually blister formation
   c. Wound surface mottled pink and white immediately after injury
   d. Wound possibly less sensitive to touch than surrounding normal skin
3. Signs of shock (see Chapter 8)

Treatment

1. Remove the victim from the source of the burn.
   a. If clothing is on fire, roll victim on the ground or wrap in a blanket to extinguish the flames.
   b. If the burn is chemical, use large amounts of water to wash the agent(s) off.
   c. If the eyes are involved, copiously irrigate them.
   d. Because phosphorus ignites on contact with air, keep any phosphorus in contact with the victim's skin covered with water.
2. Evaluate the airway for smoke inhalation. If present, administer oxygen by face mask, 5 to 10 L/min, and transport the victim to a medical facility (see Smoke Inhalation).
3. If the victim shows signs of shock, elevate the victim's legs 30 cm (12 inches) off the ground and administer humidified oxygen.
4. Irrigate gently with cool water or saline solution to remove all loose dirt and skin.
5. Peel off or trim any necrotic skin with sharp débridement.
6. Drain large (greater than 2.5 cm [1 inch]), thin, fluid-filled blisters and trim the dead skin if a sterile dressing can be applied.
7. Leave small, thick blisters intact.
8. Apply aloe vera gel or an antibacterial ointment to the burn.
9. Cover the burn with a dressing and change the dressing at least once a day.
   a. Use cool, moist dressings (not ice) if the area is small (less than 10% TBSA).

  b. Use dry, nonadherent dressings if the surface area is large to avoid overcooling the victim.
10. Give oral balanced salt solutions to achieve rehydration if the transport time will be more than 30 minutes, the thermal injuries involve more than 20% TBSA, or there is evidence of burn shock.
  a. Prompt the victim to drink or sip enough fluid to keep the urine clear and copious.
  b. If this is not possible, administer lactated Ringer's or normal saline solution without glucose through a large-bore percutaneous catheter, preferably inserted through unburned skin. The arm is the preferred site. Administer 4 ml/kg body weight/% TBSA/24 hr. Half the calculated 24-hour fluid total is given over the first 8 hours from **the time the burn occurred** (not the time the IV line was established). The second half is infused over the remaining 16 hours. The rate should be adjusted to support the victim's vital signs and maintain a urine output of 1 ml/kg/hr.
  c. Note that fluid resuscitation at the scene may be difficult for children because of the difficulties achieving cannulation with small veins.
11. Avoid chilling the victim by placing a clean sheet under the person and then covering with another clean sheet, followed by clean blankets.
12. Note that antibiotics are only used if the burn becomes infected.
  a. If infection is present, pus, foul odor, cloudy blisters, increased redness and swelling in the normal skin around the burn, and fever greater than 38.3° C (101° F) will be noted.
  b. If an antibiotic is needed, give dicloxacillin, cephalexin, or erythromycin. Be sure to change all dressings daily.

Third-degree Burn (Full Thickness)

Signs and Symptoms

1. Involves all layers of the dermis, may involve muscle and bone, and can heal only by wound contracture or with skin grafting
2. Usually dry, leathery, firm, charred, and depressed when compared with adjoining normal skin, and insensitive to light touch or pinprick
3. Skin possibly waxy and white, with small clotted blood vessels that appear as purple or maroon lines under the surface
4. Can be difficult to differentiate from a deep partial-thickness burn

Treatment

1. Follow the same instructions as for second-degree burn.
2. Be aware that immediate evacuation to a burn center is recommended.

Carbon Monoxide Poisoning

Signs and Symptoms

1. If resulting from a fire: dyspnea, burns of the mouth and nose, singed nasal hairs, sooty sputum, brassy cough
2. Headache, nausea, vomiting, tachypnea, dizziness, loss of manual dexterity
3. Sometimes subtle perceptual and memory abnormalities or frank confusion and lethargy
4. Abnormal skin and nail bed color, with "chocolate cyanosis" or a cherry-red color
5. Bullae
6. Unconsciousness leading to coma
7. Possible cardiac arrest
8. Late complications (after first 48 hours): personality disorders, chronic headaches, seizures, Parkinson's disease (generally after 2 to 40 days)

Treatment
1. Administer 100% oxygen by a non-rebreathing mask.
2. *Consider* initiating evacuation to a hyperbaric chamber for any victim who displays abnormal neurologic signs or symptoms or who is pregnant.

Smoke Inhalation and Thermal Airway Injury

Signs and Symptoms
1. Facial burns
2. Intraoral or pharyngeal burns
3. Singed nasal hairs
4. Soot in the mouth or nose, carbonaceous sputum
5. Hoarseness, inspiratory stridor with a barking sound that seems to originate in the neck, or expiratory wheezing
6. Shortness of breath and coughing that produces carbonaceous black sputum
7. Muffled voice, drooling, difficulty swallowing
8. Swollen tongue
9. Agitation

Treatment
1. Once the injury has occurred, no measures can be taken to limit its progress, so evacuate the victim immediately.
2. Administer humidified oxygen at 5 to 10 L/min by face mask.
3. *Consider* initiating intubation and ventilation if stridor or dyspnea is present. Note that progressive edema can produce complete airway obstruction.
4. Administer a bronchodilator (albuterol 4 to 8 puffs by metered-dose inhaler with a spacer q15-20min prn).

CHAPTER 6

Lightning Injuries

Although the chances of being struck by lightning are minimal, 200 to 400 persons die of strikes in the United States each year. Lightning is the electrical discharge associated with thunderstorms, and an initial stroke can measure 30 million volts, with up to 30 strokes in a lightning flash, which gives lightning its flickering quality. The main stroke measures 6 to 8 cm (about 2 to 3 inches) in diameter, and its temperature has been estimate to range from 8000° to 50,000° C (14,432° to 90,032° F), or 4 times as hot as the surface of the sun. Thunder results from the nearly explosive expansion of the heated and ionized air.

Lightning can cause injury by (1) direct hit, (2) splash as the bolt first hits an object and then jumps to the victim, (3) contact with a conductive material that is hit or splashed by lightning, (4) step voltage where the bolt hits the ground or a nearby object and then flows like a wave in a pond to the victim, or (5) blunt trauma from the explosive force of the positive and negative pressure waves (thunder) it produces.

DISORDERS

Box 6-1 lists the types of injuries that can occur with any of the effects of lightning.

Box 6-1.

Types of Injuries Attributable to Lightning

1. Cardiopulmonary arrest
   a. Immediate cardiac arrest that is brief because of inherent automaticity
   b. Respiratory arrest, caused by paralysis of the medullary respiratory center, that lasts longer and leads to secondary cardiac arrest from hypoxia
2. Neurologic injury
   a. Seizures
   b. Deafness
   c. Confusion or amnesia
   d. Blindness
   e. Extremity paralysis
3. Contusions and fractures
4. Chest pain and muscle aches
5. Tympanic membrane rupture
6. Superficial punctate and feathering burns (Plates 3 and 4)
7. Partial-thickness burns

Signs and Symptoms
1. Generally, a history of lightning strike or near strike
2. Disarray of clothing and belongings
3. Feathering burns
4. Linear or punctate burns with tympanic membrane rupture, confusion, and outdoor location
5. Confusion, amnesia, or lack of consciousness in a person found indoors after or during a thunderstorm
6. Muscle aches and body tingling
7. In more severe cases, skin mottled, extremities paralyzed, pulse difficult to find because muscles of the radial artery are in spasm

Treatment

Note that lightning victims are not "charged" and thus pose no hazard to rescuers.

1. Assess and treat first those victims who appear dead because they may ultimately recover if properly resuscitated.
   a. Assess airway, breathing, and circulation.
   b. Perform CPR if indicated.
   c. If you successfully obtain a pulse with CPR, continue ventilation until spontaneous adequate respirations resume, the victim is pronounced dead, continued resuscitation is deemed not feasible, or you are in danger.
2. Stabilize and splint any fractures.
3. Be aware that the victim may have been thrown a considerable distance by the strike. Initiate and maintain spinal precautions if indicated.
4. Administer oxygen and intravenous fluids if available.
5. Prepare for transport to a medical facility.

PREVENTION

To calculate the approximate distance in miles that you are from a flash of lightning, count in seconds the time from when you see the flash until when you hear the thunder, and divide that number by five.

1. When a thunderstorm threatens, seek shelter in a building or inside a vehicle (not a tent or a convertible automobile). If you are in a car, stay in it. If it is a convertible and there is no other shelter, huddle on the ground at least 45 m (50 yards) away from the vehicle.
2. If you are in a tent, stay as far away from the poles and wet cloth as possible.
3. Do not stand under a tall tree in an open area or on a ridge or hilltop.
4. Move away from open water, and do not stand

near a metal boat. If you are swimming, get out of the water.

5. Move away from tractors and other metal farm equipment. Avoid tall objects, such as ski lifts, boat masts, flagpoles, and power lines.
6. Get off motorcycles, bicycles, and golf carts. Put down golf clubs and fishing poles.
7. Stay away from wire fences, clotheslines, metal pipes, and other metallic paths that could carry lightning to you from some distance.
8. Avoid standing in small, isolated sheds or other small structures in open areas.
9. Once you are indoors, avoid being near windows, open doors, fireplaces, or large metal fixtures.
10. In a forest, seek shelter in a low area under a thick growth of saplings or small trees. Avoid the tallest trees, staying a distance from the tree at least equal to the tree's height. Avoid the entrances to caves.
11. In an open area, go to a low place such as a ravine or valley.
12. If you are totally in the open:
    a. Stay far away from single trees to avoid lightning splashes.
    b. Drop to your knees and bend forward, putting your hands on your knees.
    c. If it is available, place insulating material (e.g., sleeping pad, life jacket, rope) between you and the ground. Do not lie flat on the ground.
13. If your hair stands on end, you hear high-pitched or crackling noises, or you see a blue halo around objects, there is electrical activity around you that typically precedes a lightning strike. If you can, leave the area immediately. If you are unable to do this, crouch down on the balls of your feet and tuck your head down. Do not touch the ground with your hands.

CHAPTER 7

Wilderness Trauma Emergencies: Assessment and Stabilization

PRIMARY SURVEY

Rescuers have nine immediate priorities in managing wilderness trauma, regardless of the injury. The "three ABCs" is a helpful mantra for recalling the nine priorities (Table 7-1).

A1: Assess the Scene

1. Ensure the safety of noninjured members of the party.
2. Assess the scene for further hazards, such as rockfall, avalanche, and dangerous animals, before rendering first-aid care.
3. Avoid approaching the victim from directly above if rockfall or snowslide is possible.
4. Do not allow your sense of urgency to transform an accident into a risky and foolish rescue attempt.

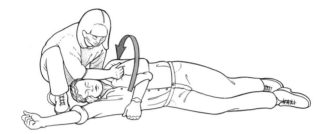

Fig. 7-1.   One-person roll.

Table 7-1.

The Three ABCs of Emergency First Aid	
ABCs	**ACTION**
A1	Assess the scene
A2	Airway
A3	Alert others
B1	Barriers
B2	Breathing
B3	Bleeding
C1	CPR and circulation
C2	Cervical spine
C3	Cover and protect victim from environment

A2: Airway

1. If the victim is unresponsive, immediately determine if he or she is breathing.
   a. If the victim's position prevents adequate assessment of the airway, roll the victim onto the back as a single unit, supporting the head and neck (Fig. 7-1).
   b. Place your ear and cheek close to the victim's mouth and nose to detect air movement, while looking for movement of the chest and abdomen

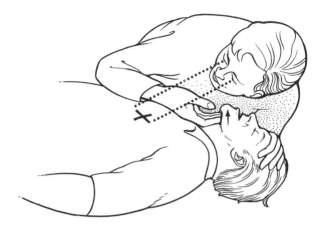

Fig. 7-2. Listening for breathing and watching for movement of chest and abdomen.

(Fig. 7-2). In cold weather, look for a vapor cloud and feel for warm air movement.
2. If no movement of air is detected, clean the mouth out with your fingers and use the chin-lift (Fig. 7-3) or jaw-thrust technique to open the airway.
   a. Perform the jaw thrust by kneeling down with your knees on either side of the victim's head, placing your hands on either side of the victim's mandible, and pushing the base of the jaw up and forward (Fig. 7-4).
   b. Note that the jaw-thrust and chin-lift techniques are labor intensive and tie up your hands. If you are alone, establish a temporary airway by pinning the anterior aspect of the victim's tongue to the lower lip with a safety pin (Fig. 7-5). An alternative to puncturing the lower lip is to pass a string or shoelace through the safety pin and hold traction on the tongue by securing the other

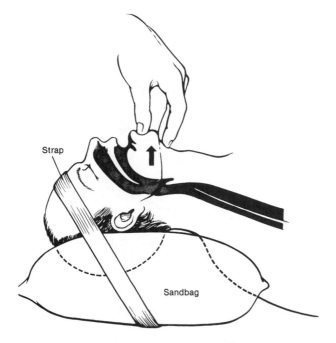

Fig. 7-3. Chin lift. This procedure optimally utilizes two rescuers. One person stabilizes victim's neck. The other person opens victim's airway using thumb to grasp victim's chin just below the lower lip, while fingers of the same hand are placed underneath victim's anterior mandible, and chin is gently lifted.

end to the victim's shirt button or jacket zipper.
3. If an airway cannot be established, cricothyroid-otomy (cricothyrotomy) is indicated.
   a. Cut the barrel of a 3-ml or 1-ml syringe (with the plunger removed) at a 45-degree angle at its midpoint to create an improvised cricothyroid airway device.
   b. After making a vertical 1-cm incision through the skin over the cricothyroid membrane, stabilize the larynx between the fingers and insert the

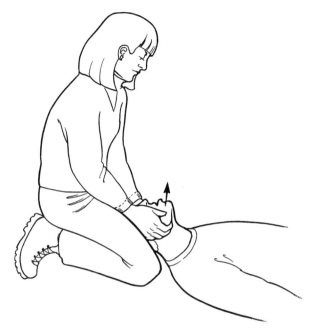

Fig. 7-4. Jaw thrust.

pointed end of the syringe through the membrane while aiming caudally (toward the buttocks) (Fig. 7-6). Note that the proximal phalange of the syringe barrel helps secure the device to the neck and prevents it from being aspirated.

c. Other potential cricothyroid airway devices include small flashlight casings, pen casings, small pill bottles, and large-bore needles and catheters. Several commercial devices are available that are small and lightweight enough to be included in most first-aid kits.

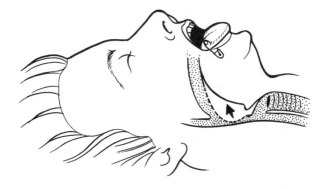

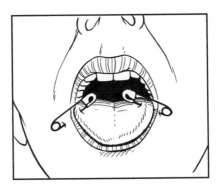

Fig. 7-5. Safely pinning tongue to open airway.

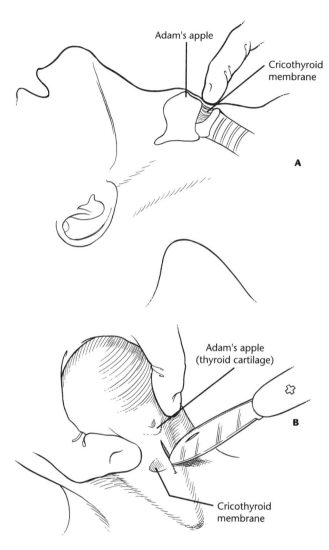

Fig. 7-6. Cricothyroidotomy (cricothyrotomy). **A** to **C,** Locate cricothyroid membrane and make vertical 1-cm incision through skin. **D** and **E,** Cut barrel of syringe cut at 45-degree angle and insert pointed end through membrane.

Continued

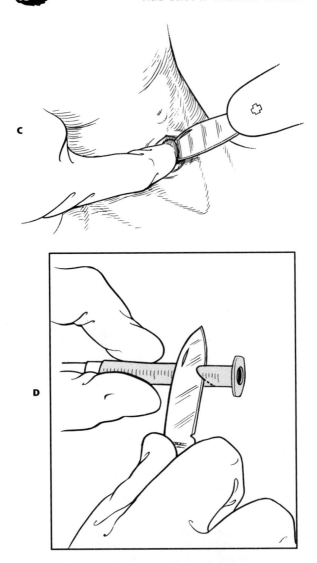

Fig. 7-6, cont'd For legend see p. 47.

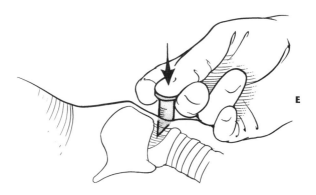

Fig. 7-6, cont'd For legend see p. 47.

A3: Alert Others

Before becoming more involved with the resuscitation, take a moment to alert others about the accident and to call or send someone for help.

B1: Barriers

1. Protect your hands with surgical gloves.
   a. Surgical gloves can leak, so wash hands or wipe them with an antimicrobial-impregnated towelette after removing the gloves.
   b. *Warning:* From 5% to 7% of the population and more than 10% of all medical personnel are allergic to latex. Latex allergies can produce skin rashes, severe anaphylactic reactions, or even death. If you suspect that you might have an allergy to latex, use powder-free nonlatex gloves.
2. Use an effective barrier device when performing mouth-to-mouth rescue breathing (see Fig. 19-1).

B2: Breathing

If the victim is not breathing, initiate ventilation with mouth-to-mouth rescue breathing.

Box 7-1.

How to Apply a Tourniquet

1. Tourniquet material should be wide and flat to prevent crushing tissue. Use a firm bandage, belt, or strap 7.5 to 10 cm (3 to 4 inches) wide that will not stretch. Never use wire, rope, or any material that will cut the skin.
2. Wrap the bandage snugly around the extremity several times as close above the wound as possible, and tie an overhand knot.
3. Place a stick or similar object on the knot, and tie another overhand knot over the stick (Fig. 7-7, *A*).
4. Twist the stick until the bandage becomes tight enough to stop the bleeding. Tie or tape the stick in place to prevent it from unraveling (Fig. 7-7, *B*).
5. Mark the victim with a "TK" where it cannot be missed, and note the time the tourniquet was applied.

If you are more than an hour from medical care, loosen the tourniquet very slowly at the end of 45 minutes, while maintaining direct pressure on the wound. If bleeding is again heavy, retighten the tourniquet. If bleeding is now manageable with direct pressure alone, leave the tourniquet in place but do not tighten it again unless severe bleeding starts.

B3: Bleeding

1. Carefully check the victim for signs of profuse bleeding. Be sure to feel inside any bulky clothing and check underneath the victim for signs of bleeding.
2. Control bleeding with direct pressure.
3. Apply a tourniquet only as a last resort when bleeding cannot be stopped by direct pressure (Box 7-1).

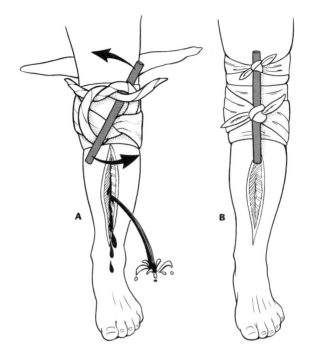

Fig. 7-7. Applying tourniquet.

a. A tourniquet is any band applied around an extremity so tightly that all blood flow distal to the site is cut off.
b. If the tourniquet is left on for more than 3 hours, tissue distal to the tourniquet may die and the extremity may require amputation.

C1: Cardiopulmonary Resuscitation (CPR) and Circulation (see also Chapter 19)

1. If a trauma victim is pulseless and apneic, CPR is not likely to be successful, unless the victim has a tension pneumothorax that can be relieved. A short period of

CPR (10 to 15 minutes, unless the victim is hypothermic) is recommended.
2. If a pulse is present, vital information can be extrapolated from determining where it can be felt.
   a. If a radial artery pulse is palpable, the systolic blood pressure is usually greater than 80 mm Hg.
   b. If the femoral artery pulse is palpable, the blood pressure is above 70 mm Hg.
   c. If the carotid artery pulse is palpable, the blood pressure is above 60 mm Hg.

C2: Cervical Spine

1. Initiate and maintain spine immobilization after trauma if some mechanism is responsible for spinal injury and:
   ✤ The victim is unconscious.
   ✤ The victim complains of midline neck or back pain.
   ✤ The cervical spine is tender to palpation.
   ✤ There are paresthesias or altered sensation in the extremities.
   ✤ There is paralysis or weakness in an extremity not caused by direct trauma.
   ✤ The victim has an altered level of consciousness or is under the influence of drugs or alcohol.
   ✤ The victim has another painful injury, such as a femoral or pelvic fracture, a dislocated shoulder, or broken ribs, that may distract the person from appreciating the pain in the spine.
2. If a cervical spine injury is suspected, immobilize the victim's head and neck and prevent any movement of the torso. (See Box 7-2 for immobilization aids.)
3. Avoid moving the victim with a suspected spinal injury if he or she is in a safe location. The victim will need professional evacuation.

Box 7-2.

Immobilization Aids

CERVICAL COLLAR
1. The cervical collar is always viewed as an adjunct to full spinal immobilization and is never used alone.
2. Properly applied and fitted, the cervical collar is primarily a defense against axial spine loading, particularly in an evacuation that involves tilting the victim's body uphill or downhill.
3. After the collar is placed around the neck, secure plastic bags, stuffed sacks, socks filled with sand or dirt, or rolled-up towels and clothing on either side of the head and neck to prevent any lateral movement.

SAM Splint Cervical Collar (Fig. 7-8)
1. Create a bend in the SAM splint approximately 15 cm (6 inches) from the end of the splint. This bend will form the anterior post.
2. Next, create flares for the mandible.
3. Apply the anterior post underneath the chin and bring the remainder of the splint around the neck. Take up circumferential slack by creating lateral posts.
4. Finally, squeeze the back to create a posterior post, and secure with tape.

Closed Cell Foam System
1. Fold the pad longitudinally into thirds, and center it over the back of the victim's neck.
2. Wrap the pad around the neck and under the chin. If the pad is not long enough, tape or tie on extensions (Fig. 7-9).

Continued

Box 7-2.

Immobilization Aids—cont'd

CERVICAL COLLAR—cont'd
Closed Cell Foam System—cont'd
3. Blankets, beach towels, or a rolled plastic tarp can be used in a similar manner. Avoid small, flexible cervical collars that do not optimally extend the chin-to-chest distance.

Padded Hip Belt
1. Remove the padded hip belt from a large internal- or external-frame backpack, and modify it to function as a cervical collar.
2. Diminish the width by overlapping the belt and securing the excess material with duct tape.

Clothing
1. Use bulky clothing as a collar.
2. Prewrap a wide, elastic ("Ace-type") bandage around a jacket to help compress the material and make it more rigid and supportive.

SPINE BOARDS
Internal-frame Pack/Snow Shovel System
1. Modify an internal-frame backpack by inserting a snow shovel through the center-line attachment points (the shovel's handgrip may need to be removed first).
2. Tape the victim's head to the lightly padded shovel, which serves as a head bed.
3. Use the remainder of the pack suspension system to secure the shoulders and torso as if the victim were wearing the pack.

Box 7-2.

Immobilization Aids—cont'd

SPINE BOARDS—cont'd
Inverted Pack System
1. Make an efficient short board using an inverted internal- or external-frame backpack.
2. Use the padded hip belt as a head bed and the frame as a short board in conjunction with a cervical collar (Fig. 7-10).

Snowshoe System
1. Make a snowshoe into a fairly reliable short board.
2. Be sure to pad the snowshoe first.

C3: Cover and Protect the Victim From Environment

1. If it is cold, place insulating garments or blankets underneath and on top of the victim. Remove and replace any wet clothing.
2. If it is hot, loosen the victim's clothing and create shade.
3. If the victim is in a dangerous area, move to a safer location while maintaining spine immobilization if indicated.

SECONDARY SURVEY

After the primary survey is complete, perform a comprehensive secondary survey. Begin with a physical examination of the head and move in a systematic fashion through a more detailed physical examination of the face, neck, chest, abdomen, pelvis, extremities, and skin.

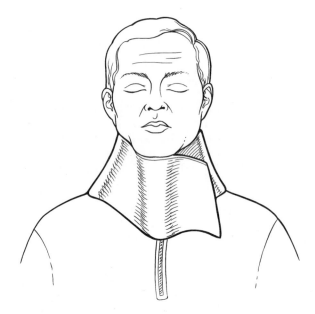

Fig. 7-8.   SAM splint cervical collar.

Head and Face Evaluation

1. Perform and repeat as necessary the Glasgow Coma Scale evaluation (see Appendix A).
2. Perform a more detailed search for focal neurologic signs.
   a. Be aware that sensory defects follow the general dermatome patterns shown in Fig. 7-11.
   b. Changes in reflexes not accompanied by altered mental status do not mandate evacuation unless the victim also has a spinal cord injury.
3. Palpate the scalp thoroughly, looking for tenderness, depressions, and lacerations.
   a. Immediately evacuate any victim with suspected depressed skull fracture, a basilar skull fracture accompanied by penetrating scalp trauma.

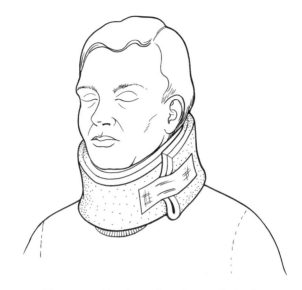

Fig. 7-9. Ensolite pad used as cervical collar.

b. Administer a broad-spectrum antibiotic (cefu-roxime, adult dose 1.5 g IM).
c. Do not remove any impaling foreign bodies pierc-ing the head or neck. Pad these to prevent motion.

Evaluation of the Body

1. Undress the victim sufficiently to perform a proper head-to-toe examination. Keep in mind the weather conditions and appropriate concern for the victim's modesty. Check around the victim's neck or wrist for a medical information bracelet or tag and in the vic-tim's wallet or pack for a medical identification card.
2. Remember to ask the victim to move any injured body part before you move it. If the victim resists be-cause of pain or weakness, you should suspect a frac-ture or spinal cord injury. Never force the victim to move.

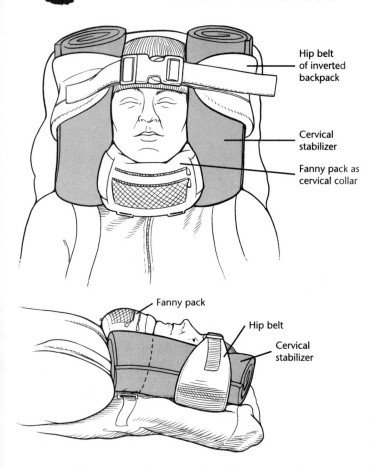

Fig. 7-10.   Inverted pack used as spine board.

3. Examine the victim's skin, looking for sweating; evaluating color; and locating injuries such as bruises, rashes, burns, bites, or lacerations. Check inside the victim's lower eyelids for a pale color, which can indicate anemia or internal hemorrhage. Note any abnormal skin temperature.

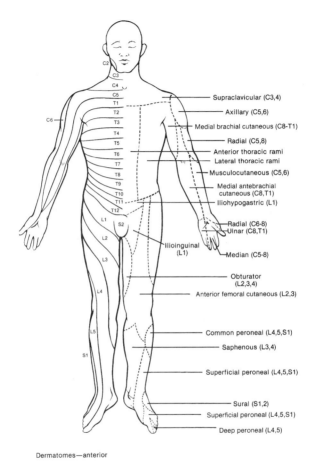

Dermatomes—anterior

Fig. 7-11. Dermatome pattern, the skin area stimulated by spinal cord elements. Sensory deficits follow general dermatome patterns. *Continued*

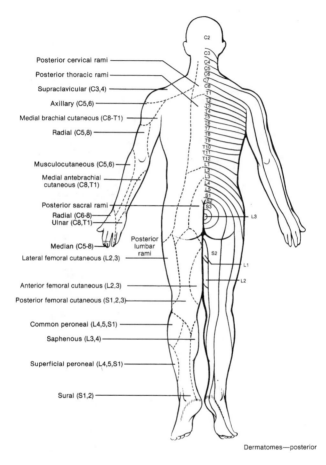

Posterior cervical rami
Posterior thoracic rami
Supraclavicular (C3,4)
Axillary (C5,6)
Medial brachial cutaneous (C8-T1)
Radial (C5,8)
Musculocutaneous (C5,6)
Medial antebrachial cutaneous (C8,T1)
Posterior sacral rami
Radial (C6-8)
Ulnar (C8,T1)
Median (C5-8)
Posterior lumbar rami
Lateral femoral cutaneous (L2,3)
Anterior femoral cutaneous (L2,3)
Posterior femoral cutaneous (S1,2,3)
Common peroneal (L4,5,S1)
Saphenous (L3,4)
Superficial peroneal (L4,5,S1)
Sural (S1,2)

Dermatomes—posterior

Fig. 7-11, cont'd For legend see p. 59.

4. Examine the chest, watching as the victim breathes to see if the chest expands completely and equally on both sides. Examine the chest wall for tenderness and deformities or foreign objects. Auscultate for breath sounds.
5. Gently press all areas of the back and abdomen to find areas of tenderness. Examine the buttocks and genital area.
6. Examine the victim's bony structure. Gently press on the chest, pelvis, arms, and legs to reveal areas of tenderness. Run your fingers down the length of the clavicles and press where they join the sternum. Evaluate the integrity of each rib, and observe for areas of deformation or discoloration.
7. Measure the victim's temperature.
8. Record all findings of your examination.

CHAPTER 8

Shock

DEFINITION

Shock is a life-threatening condition in which blood flow to body tissues is inadequate and cells are deprived of oxygen. Although shock is often categorized into different types, the signs and symptoms are almost always the same, regardless of the cause. Shock is a true emergency that is difficult to treat effectively in the field.

DISORDERS

Box 8-1 outlines the types of shock.

Signs and Symptoms

1. Pale, cool, and diaphoretic skin
2. Decreased pulse pressure when blood loss reaches 15% of total blood volume
3. Tachycardia, tachypnea, anxiety, delayed capillary refill, and decreased urine output when blood loss is 15% to 30% of total blood volume (in neurogenic shock, pulse remains normal or slow)
4. Hypotension, marked tachycardia, and significant changes in mental status related to blood volume loss greater than 40% of total blood volume; confusion, restlessness, combativeness possible

Box 8-1.

Types of Shock

HVPOVOLEMIC SHOCK
1. External bleeding
2. Internal bleeding
   a. Bleeding from a ruptured or lacerated organ
   b. Bleeding from a fractured pelvis or femur
3. Profound dehydration

CARDIOGENIC SHOCK
VASOGENIC SHOCK
NEUROGENIC SHOCK
1. Caused by a spinal cord injury that produces paralysis above the level of the sixth thoracic vertebra (T6)
2. Marked by relative bradycardia, rather than tachycardia, despite concomitant hypotension

ANAPHYLACTIC SHOCK (see Chapter 20)
SEPTIC SHOCK
Produced by toxins from a severe infection

Treatment
1. Keep the victim lying down on his or her back. If the victim experiences shortness of breath because of heart problems, raise the shoulders, or if tolerated, allow to sit up.
2. Elevate the legs *only* if the victim has vasogenic shock or external bleeding that is under control.
   a. You can elevate the legs by simply allowing the victim to recline with the feet uphill.
   b. If the victim has internal bleeding, avoid any unnecessary movement.
   c. With cardiogenic shock, the victim may be more comfortable with the head and shoulders raised slightly.

3. Do not elevate the victim's legs if there is a severe head injury, difficulty breathing, a broken leg, neck or back injury, uncontrolled bleeding, or if doing so causes pain.
4. Keep the victim covered and warm. Take the victim out of harsh weather conditions and insulate from the ground. If you cannot locate sufficient covering for warmth, lie next to the victim and share body heat. Especially try to keep the victim's head, neck, and hands covered.
5. Control remediable causes of bleeding.
6. Loosen restrictive clothing.
7. Splint all fractures. If the femur is fractured, apply and maintain traction (see Chapter 13).
8. Administer IV fluid resuscitation.
   a. This is indicated only for a victim with vasogenic shock, one who is dehydrated, or one in whom hypovolemic shock is caused by bleeding from a wound that has been controlled.
   b. Insert an 18-gauge IV line and administer 1000 ml hetastarch (Hespan) or 3000 ml normal saline or lactated Ringer's solution.
   c. If transportation to a medical center will take longer than 6 hours and the victim suffers shock from external bleeding or vasogenic etiology but is alert, oriented, and not vomiting, administer small, frequent sips of fluid. If this causes vomiting, discontinue the attempt at oral rehydration.
9. Do not administer oral fluids to a victim with suspected intraabdominal or thoracic hemorrhage.
10. Administer high-flow oxygen if available (10 L/min by face mask).
11. For septic shock or penetrating/blunt abdominal trauma, administer an IV antibiotic (ceftriaxone 1 g or cefoxitin 2 g IV over 3 to 5 minutes).
12. For massive soft tissue damage or open fracture, administer a cephalosporin (cefazolin 1 g) IV over 3 to 5 minutes.
13. In a diabetic person, consider a hypoglycemic reaction (see Chapter 21). If the victim is conscious and

can swallow adequately, administer glutose paste or a sugar-sweetened liquid in small sips. Otherwise, do not give the victim anything to eat or drink unless he or she is alert and hungry or thirsty.

14. If the victim appears to be suffering from an allergic reaction to a bite or sting (see Chapter 27), address the cause of that reaction.

15. Because the shock victim cannot be effectively treated in the field, transport him or her to a medical facility as quickly as possible.

CHAPTER 9

Head Injury

Head injury assessment begins with the primary survey, in which life-threatening conditions, such as airway compromise or severe bleeding, are recognized and simultaneous management is begun. For the purposes of wilderness assessment and management, head injuries can be subdivided into three groups: (1) prolonged unconsciousness (more than 5 to 10 minutes), (2) brief loss of consciousness, and (3) no loss of consciousness.

GENERAL TREATMENT

1. Because potential problems include airway compromise from obstruction caused by the tongue, vomit, blood, or broken teeth, make a quick inspection of the victim's mouth as part of the primary survey.
2. Log-roll the victim to clear the mouth without jeopardizing the spine (Fig. 9-1). Be aware that the most common associated serious injury is a broken neck.

DISORDERS
Skull Fracture

Fracture of the skull is not in itself life-threatening, unless associated with underlying brain injury or severe bleeding.

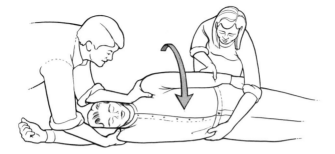

Fig. 9-1. Log-rolling victim to clear mouth without jeopardizing the spine.

Signs and Symptoms
1. Severe headache
2. Deformity, step-off, or crepitus on palpation of scalp
3. Blood or clear fluid draining from ears or nose without direct trauma to those areas
4. Ecchymosis around eyes (raccoon eyes) or behind ears (Battle's sign)
5. In victim with a skull fracture, possible development of seizures, unequal or nonreactive pupils, weakness, or altered level of consciousness from underlying brain injury (Box 9-1).

Treatment
1. Evacuate the victim to a medical facility as soon as possible.
2. Keep the victim with the head slightly uphill or elevated to reduce cerebral edema.
3. *In any person with a serious head injury, immobilize the cervical spine in anticipation of an injury to this area.*

Prolonged Unconsciousness
Signs and Symptoms
Loss of consciousness for more than 5 to 10 minutes, which is a serious warning of significant brain injury

Box 9-1.

Brain Injury Checklist

- ✤ Increasing headache
- ✤ Changing level of consciousness
- ✤ Persistent or projectile vomiting
- ✤ Bleeding from ears or nose (without direct injury to those areas), cerebrospinal fluid rhinorrhea
- ✤ Raccoon eyes or Battle's sign
- ✤ Seizure

Treatment
1. **Be aware that immediate evacuation to a medical center is mandatory.**
2. During transportation, maintain cervical spine precautions and keep the victim's head uphill on sloping terrain.
3. Be prepared to log-roll if the victim vomits.
4. Continually monitor the airway for signs of obstruction and a decreasing respiratory rate.
5. Administer high-flow oxygen, if available, at 10 L/min or by a nonrebreather mask.

Brief Loss of Consciousness
Signs and Symptoms
1. Short-term unconsciousness, in which the victim wakes up after 1 or 2 minutes and gradually regains normal mental status and physical abilities, indicating at least a concussion
2. Confusion or amnesia for the event and repetitive questioning by the victim
3. Headache or nausea

Treatment
1. Be aware that the safest strategy is to evacuate the victim to a medical center for evaluation and observation.

2. Interrupt the victim's normal sleep every 2 to 3 hours briefly to see that the condition has not deteriorated and he or she can be easily aroused.
3. For a victim who is increasingly lethargic, confused, or combative or does not behave normally, immediately evacuate to a medical center.
   a. If the victim develops any signs of brain injury (see Box 9-1), increasing intracranial pressure may have developed. Evacuate immediately.
   b. If the victim has a seizure after a brain injury, even briefly, transport to a medical facility immediately.

No Loss of Consciousness

Signs and Symptoms
Head injury without any loss of consciousness, which is rarely indicative of a serious injury to the brain

Treatment
1. Inspect the scalp for evidence of cuts, which generally bleed copiously, and apply pressure as needed.
2. If the victim appears normal (can answer questions appropriately, including name, location, and date; walks normally; appears to have coordinated movement; has normal muscle strength), no immediate evacuation is required.
3. If the victim develops any signs or symptoms of brain injury (see Box 9-1), evacuate immediately.
4. For a child who has had a head injury, then begins to vomit, refuses to eat, becomes drowsy, appears apathetic, or in any other way seems abnormal, evacuate him or her to a medical facility as soon as possible.

Epidural Hematoma

Signs and Symptoms
1. Victim who wakes up and appears completely normal then becomes drowsy or disoriented or lapses back into unconsciousness (usually within 30 to 60 minutes)

2. Unconscious victim with one pupil significantly larger than the other

Treatment

Because these are indications of bleeding from an artery inside the skull, causing an expanding blood clot (epidural hematoma) that is compressing the brain, evacuate the victim immediately and rush to a medical facility.

CHAPTER 10

Chest Trauma

The common types of chest trauma that may be encountered in wilderness activities are rib fracture, flail chest, pneumothorax/hemothorax, tension pneumothorax, and open ("sucking") chest wound.

DISORDERS
Rib Fracture
Signs and Symptoms
1. Pain in the chest after blunt chest trauma
2. Pain that worsens with inspiration
3. Point tenderness over the fractured rib(s)
4. Crepitus and displacement, occasionally detected on palpation
5. Pain over the fracture site when rescuer pushes on the sternum while the victim lies supine

Treatment
1. Care for any open chest wounds.
   a. Cover the wound quickly, especially if there is air bubbling, to avoid "sucking" chest wounds.
   b. Use a petrolatum-impregnated gauze, heavy cloth, or adhesive tape for the dressing.
2. Treat isolated rib fracture.
   a. Administer an oral analgesic, and instruct the victim to rest.

b. Note that thoracic taping and splinting are not necessary or helpful.

c. Encourage the victim to cough or deep-breathe at least once per hour.

3. Treat multiple rib fractures.

a. Be aware that these are significant because of the potential for serious underlying injuries.

b. Cushion the victim in a position of comfort, and frequently reevaluate the victim's ability to breathe.

c. Do not tape or tightly wrap the ribs because this might prevent complete reexpansion of the lung with inspiration, leading the victim to take only shallow, inadequate breaths and possibly leading to pneumonia. Encourage the victim to take at least one deep breath or give one good cough every hour.

d. Evacuate the victim as soon as possible. If the chest injury is on one side, transport the victim with the injured side down to facilitate lung expansion and oxygenation of the blood within the uninjured side.

Flail Chest

Signs and Symptoms

1. A portion of the chest wall that is mechanically unstable, indicating that a series of three or more ribs is fractured in both the anterior and posterior planes.

2. Unstable segment that paradoxically moves inward during inspiration, thereby inhibiting ventilation

Treatment

1. Immediately evacuate the victim. A small or moderate flail segment can be tolerated for 24 to 48 hours, after which it may need to be managed with mechanical ventilation.

2. Administer an intercostal nerve block to assist in short-term management of pain and pulmonary toilet.

3. Place a bulky pad of dressings, rolled-up extra clothing, or a small pillow gently over the site, or have the
   victim splint the arm against the injury to stabilize
   the flail segment and relieve some of the pain.
   a. Use soft and lightweight materials.
   b. Use large strips of tape to hold the pad in place.
   c. Do not tape entirely around the chest because this
      will restrict breathing efforts.
   d. Do not allow the object to restrict breathing in any
      manner.
4. If the victim is unable to walk, transport him or her
   lying on the back or injured side.
5. If the victim is severely short of breath, assist with
   mouth-to-mouth rescue breathing. Time your breaths
   with those of the victim, and breathe gently to provide added air during the victim's inspirations.

Pneumothorax/Hemothorax

Signs and Symptoms
1. Pain that may be worse with inspiration
2. Tachypnea
3. Unilateral decreased or absent breath sounds
4. Resonance on percussion with a pneumothorax; flat
   or dull on percussion with a hemothorax
5. Tactile fremitus

Treatment
1. Evacuate the victim immediately.
2. Monitor closely for the development of a tension
   pneumothorax.

Tension Pneumothorax

Signs and Symptoms
1. Distended neck veins
2. Tracheal deviation away from the side of the pneumothorax
3. Unilateral, absent or grossly diminished breath
   sounds

Box 10-1.

How to Perform Pleural Decompression

1. Swab the entire chest with povidone-iodine or other antiseptic.
2. If sterile surgical gloves are available, put them on after washing hands.
3. If local anesthesia is available, infiltrate the puncture site down to the rib and over its upper border.
4. Insert a large-bore (14-gauge) intravenous catheter, needle, or any available pointed, sharp object into the chest just above the third rib in the midclavicular line (midway between the top of the shoulder and the nipple in a line with the nipple approximates this location) (Fig. 10-1, *A*). If you hit the rib, move the needle or knife upward slightly until it passes over the top of the rib, thus avoiding the intercostal blood vessels that course along the lower edge of every rib (Fig. 10-1, *B*). The chest wall is 3.75 to 6.25 cm (1½ to 2½ inches) thick, depending on the individual's muscularity and the amount of fat present. A gush of air signals that you have entered the pleural space; do not push the penetrating object in any further. Releasing the tension converts the tension pneumothorax into an open pneumothorax.
5. Leave the needle or catheter in place (Fig. 10-1, *C*) and place the cut-out finger portion of a surgical glove with a slit cut into the end over the external opening to create a unidirectional flutter valve that allows continuous egress of air from the pleural space (Fig. 10-1, *D* to *F*).

4. Hyper-resonant hemithorax to percussion
5. Subcutaneous emphysema
6. Respiratory distress, cyanosis, cardiovascular collapse

Treatment
Use rapid pleural decompression if the victim appears to be decompensating (Box 10-1). Possible complications include infection and profound bleeding from puncture of the heart, lung, major blood vessel, liver, or spleen.

Open ("Sucking") Chest Wound
Signs and Symptoms
A chest wound in which air is sucked into the pleura on inspiration, usually caused by penetrating injury

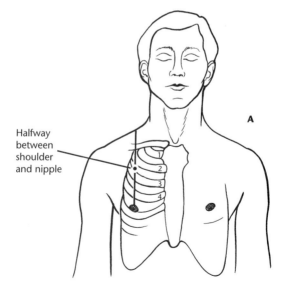

Halfway between shoulder and nipple

Fig. 10-1. Pleural decompression. **A,** Insertion point for pleural decompression. *Continued*

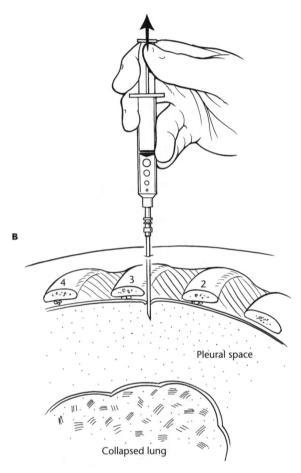

Fig. 10-1, cont'd **B,** "Walk" needle over top of rib to avoid intercostal vessels.

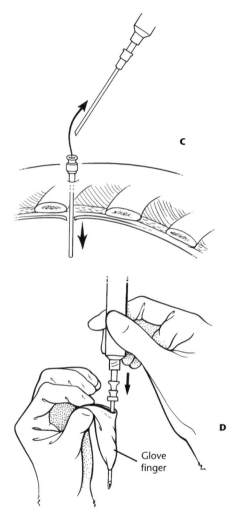

Fig. 10-1, cont'd **C,** Catheter in place. **D,** Finger of glove is attached to needle or cathter to create flutter valve.

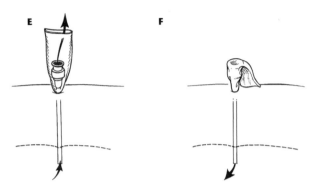

Fig. 10-1, cont'd **E,** Flutter valve allows air to escape. **F,** Flutter valve collapses to prevent air entry.

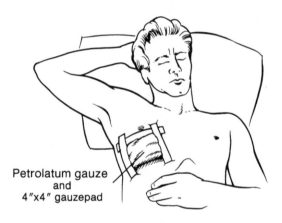

Petrolatum gauze
and
4"x4" gauzepad

Fig. 10-2. Treatment of sucking chest wound. Sealing wound with gel defibrillator pad works best because this pad adheres to wet or dry skin. Petrolatum gauze or plastic wrap also works well.

Treatment

1. Place a petrolatum-impregnated gauze on top of the wound, cover it with a 4-inch × 4-inch gauze pad, and tape it on three sides (Figure 10-2).
2. Allow the untaped fourth side to serve as a relief valve to prevent formation of a tension pneumothorax.
3. If a penetrating object remains impaled in the chest, do not remove it. Place a petrolatum gauze dressing next to the skin around the object, and stabilize it with layers of bulky dressings or pads.
4. A victim with an open chest wound below the nipple line may also have an injury to an intraabdominal organ. (see Chapter 11).

CHAPTER 11

Intraabdominal Injury

Intraabdominal injury may be penetrating or blunt.

■ DISORDERS ■

PENETRATING INJURY
Gunshot Wound
Signs and Symptoms
1. Low caliber: small entrance and no exit wound
2. High caliber, high velocity: relatively innocuous entrance wound, large disfiguring exit wound, extensive internal injuries

Treatment
1. Immediately evacuate the victim.
2. Anticipate and treat for shock (see Chapter 8).
3. Administer a broad-spectrum antibiotic (cefoxitin, adult dose 2 g IM or IV over 3 to 5 minutes).
4. Do not push extruded bowel back into the abdomen. Keep the exteriorized bowel moist and covered at all times.

Stab Wound

Signs and Symptoms

Deep wound laceration caused by knife, piton, ski pole, tree limb, or other sharp object

Treatment

If the wound extends into subcutaneous tissue, consider local wound exploration if adequate light, instruments, and technical skill and knowledge are present, and if the victim is in an extremely remote location. Otherwise, evacuate the victim immediately.

1. Infiltrate the skin and subcutaneous tissue with a local anesthetic.
2. Extend the laceration several centimeters to identify clearly the anterior fascia. Do not probe the wound with any instrument.
3. If thorough exploration of the wound shows no evidence of anterior fascial penetration, and if the victim demonstrates no evidence of peritoneal irritation, close the wound with wound closure strips, staples, or sutures, dress it, and delay the evacuation process. Monitor the victim closely for peritoneal signs over the next 48 hours. If available, administer an antibiotic active against streptococci and staphylococci.
4. Be aware that local wound exploration is contraindicated in a wound that extends above the costal margin, to avoid producing a pneumothorax.

BLUNT INJURY

Signs and Symptoms

1. Signs of shock (tachypnea, tachycardia, delayed capillary refill, weak or thready pulse, cool or clammy skin)
2. Abdominal distention
3. Pain or muscle guarding elicited on palpation
4. Percussion tenderness

5. Pain referred to the left shoulder (ruptured spleen)
6. Gross hematuria

Treatment
1. Immediately evacuate the victim.
2. Anticipate and treat for shock (see Chapter 8).
3. Administer a broad-spectrum antibiotic (cefoxitin, adult dose 2 g IM or IV over 3 to 5 minutes).
4. Do not give anything by mouth.

CHAPTER 12

Maxillofacial Trauma

Maxillofacial trauma covers a wide spectrum, from simple lacerations to massive injuries with extensive bleeding and airway obstruction. In general, the ability to treat these injuries in the wilderness situation is minimal. Among the problems that may be addressed are lacerations, mandibular fracture, midface (LeFort's) fracture, orbital floor fracture, nasal fracture, and epistaxis.

GENERAL TREATMENT

1. Perform a primary survey, paying particular attention to airway compromise from aspiration of blood, avulsed teeth or dental appliance, direct trauma and swelling, or a retrusive tongue secondary to a mobile mandibular fracture (see Fig. 7-5). The most important part of care for maxillofacial trauma is maintenance of a clear airway.
   a. Remove any loose material (teeth, clots, soft tissue, foreign material) from the oropharynx to clear the airway if needed.
   b. Note any deformity or asymmetry of the facial structures, which may indicate underlying bone fracture.
   c. Specifically look for enophthalmos, the sinking of the eye globe, if a blowout fracture of the orbit is suspected.
   d. Look for malocclusion or a step-off in the teeth as an indication of mandibular or maxillary fracture.

e. Observe the position and integrity of the nasal septum. If the septum is bulging on one side into the nasal cavity, it could indicate a septal hematoma. A septal hematoma should be drained in the field by making a small incision into the septum with a safety pin or point of a knife, allowing the blood to drain out.

f. Examine soft tissue injuries, looking for foreign bodies.

g. Test motor and sensory function by checking for sensation on each side of the face and by having the victim wrinkle the forehead, smile, bare the teeth, and close the eyes tightly.

h. Gently palpate the facial structures, noting areas of tenderness, bony defects, crepitus, and false motion.

i. Test dental integrity by grasping the front and bottom anterior teeth and checking for motion.

j. If the patient is unconscious but breathing well and shows no signs of hemorrhaging into the airway, you can use an oropharyngeal or nasopharyngeal airway to ensure airway patency.

2. Anticipate cervical spine trauma and immobilize the spine if indicated. If cervical spine injury is possible and airway protection is required, perform nasotracheal intubation after the cervical spine has been immobilized.

a. Do not perform this maneuver if you believe the victim may have a cribriform plate fracture or laryngeal trauma. In these cases, simply turn the victim to one side on a backboard after immobilization.

b. Percutaneous transtracheal ventilation or extremely careful oral intubation with cervical spine in-line stabilization can also be applied.

3. Control bleeding with direct pressure.

a. For intraoral bleeding, have the patient bite firmly on a gauze pad.

    b. For bleeding from the nose, squeeze and hold the nostrils together, use nasal packing, or deploy a Foley catheter (see Nasal Fracture and Epistaxis).
4. Treat shock, if present.
5. Recover any completely avulsed tissues or organs, irrigate with normal saline solution, and transport in a soaked gauze sponge. Among the tissues that can be avulsed are teeth, the ears, the nose, and areas of soft tissue.

DISORDERS
Lacerations

Facial laceration may be complicated by damage to associated structures that requires specialized medical care.

Signs and Symptoms

1. Lacrimal drainage system: injury confirmed if a probe inserted into the punctum at the medial corner of the lid emerges from the laceration
2. Parotid duct: injury suspected if there is buccal nerve paralysis or leakage from the wound when Stensen's duct is irrigated with saline solution or water
3. Facial nerve: asymmetry when the victim moves the eyebrows, eyelids, and mouth

Treatment

See Chapter 14.

Mandibular Fracture

Signs and Symptoms

1. Inability to occlude the teeth in a normal manner
2. Sublingual hematoma
3. Deformity, crepitus, mandibular mobility
4. Restricted opening or deviation of the jaw when opening
5. Pain elicited by placing one hand over each angle of the jaw and pressing inward

Midface (LeFort's) Fracture

Signs and Symptoms
1. Tenderness, ecchymosis, swelling over fracture site
2. Movement of the entire upper dental arch or face on grasping the alveolar process and anterior teeth between the thumb and forefinger and rocking it back and forth
3. Cerebrospinal fluid rhinorrhea

Treatment for Mandibular or Midface Fracture
1. Elevate the victim's head to reduce bleeding and swelling.
2. Stabilize the site with bandages.
3. Evacuate the victim immediately.
4. Administer antibiotic prophylaxis with phenoxymethyl penicillin (penicillin V, Penapar-VK) 500 mg (clindamycin if penicillin allergic) PO q6h.

Orbital Floor Fracture

Signs and Symptoms
1. Diplopia, worsened with upward gaze
2. Lowering of the globe or decreased upward gaze on the affected side secondary to entrapment of the inferior rectus muscle
3. Decreased facial sensation

Treatment
Evacuate the victim for definitive management.

Nasal Fracture and Epistaxis

Signs and Symptoms
1. Swelling, tenderness, mobility, ecchymosis, or deformity of the nose
2. Evidence of septal hematoma (blue or purplish fluid-filled sac overlying the nasal septum)

Treatment
Treatment of epistaxis depends on whether the source is anterior or posterior.

1. If a septal hematoma is present, make a small incision through the mucosa and perichondrium to allow drainage. Pack the anterior nasal cavity (see below) to prevent reaccumulation of blood.

2. Treat anterior epistaxis.

    a. If bleeding cannot be controlled by firmly pinching the nostrils against the septum for a full 10 minutes, nasal packing may be needed. Insert a piece of cotton or gauze soaked with a vasoconstricting agent, such as oxymetazoline hydrochloride 0.5% (Afrin) or phenylephrine hydrochloride (Neo-Synephrine), into the nose and leave it in place for 5 to 10 minutes. Next, layer-pack petrolatum-impregnated gauze or strips of a nonadherent dressing into the nose so that both ends of the gauze remain outside the nasal cavity to lessen the likelihood that a victim might inadvertently aspirate the packing.

    b. To pack an adult's nasal cavity completely, at least 3 to 4 feet (about 1 m) of ¼-inch material is required to fill the nasal cavity and tamponade the bleeding site. Expandable packing material, such as Weimert Epistaxis packing or the Rhino Rocket, is available commercially. A tampon or balloon tip from a Foley catheter can also be used as improvised packing.

    c. Anterior nasal packing blocks sinus drainage and may predispose the victim to sinusitis. A prophylactic antibiotic (amoxicillin 250 mg q6h) is recommended until the pack is removed in 48 hours.

3. Treat posterior epistaxis.

    a. Use a No. 14 to 16 French Foley catheter with a 30-ml balloon to tamponade the site. The catheter should be lubricated with either petrolatum or a water-based lubricant. Insert the catheter through the nasal cavity into the posterior pharynx. Next, inflate the balloon with 10 to 15 ml of water and gently draw it back into the posterior nasopharynx until resistance is met. Secure the catheter

      firmly to the victim's forehead with several strips
      of tape. Finally, pack the anterior nose in front of
      the catheter balloon with gauze as described ear-
      lier.
  b. Administer a prophylactic antibiotic.
  c. Evacuate the victim.

Foreign Body in Nose

Signs and Symptoms
1. Pain, foul-smelling drainage, sometimes fever
2. Skin extremely sensitive, possibly swollen with accu-
   mulations of mucus and blood

Treatment
A foreign body can be difficult to remove because of the
sensitivity of the tissues involved. Also, irritation in the
nasal area causes swelling that traps the foreign object
inside an accumulation of mucus and blood.

1. Attempt to visualize the object and extract it. Do
   not proceed if you find the object moving deeper
   into the nostril or the victim is in extreme pain.
   Leave the object in place and prepare the victim
   for evacuation.
2. If the victim is a child and develops a fever, administer dicloxacillin 25 mg/kg/day in equally
   divided doses or erythromycin 30 to 50 mg/kg/
   day q8h in equally divided doses.

CHAPTER 13

Orthopedic Injuries

SKELETAL FUNCTION

A victim with a significant extremity injury usually has immediate onset of severe pain and cannot use the extremity. A victim with a fracture or complete ligamentous disruption often reports having heard or felt a pop or snap.

A visible angulated deformity suggests a fracture, and palpable crepitus confirms the diagnosis. Radiographic confirmation can be obtained at the definitive treatment center.

Other than noting the degree and orientation of the limb's position when the victim is found, there is no reason to delay aligning and splinting a fracture.

Making the distinction between a joint injury and an intraarticular or very proximal or distal fracture is difficult even for the experienced practitioner and must wait until the victim arrives at a definitive care facility. Distinguishing a ligamentous injury from a fracture at the wrist or ankle is difficult. Because the initial care of these classes of injuries is identical, differentiation is not required to begin treatment in the field.

JOINT FUNCTION

Begin palpation of the long bones distally and proceed across all joints. Palpable crepitus at the joint level mandates application of a splint. If the victim is able to cooperate, have him or her move every joint through an active range of motion (ROM). This exercise quickly focuses the examination on the injury's location.

When this is not possible, undertake passive ROM of each joint, after palpating the joint for crepitus and swelling. If crepitus, swelling, deformity, or resistance to motion is noted, apply a splint.

If a joint is dislocated, promptly reduce it after completing the neurocirculatory examination. Reduction of the joint generally relieves much of the discomfort (see techniques below). After reduction, assess the stability of the joint by careful, controlled ROM evaluation.

A joint with an associated fracture or interposed soft tissue is frequently unstable after reduction. In such circumstances, take great care while applying the splint to prevent redislocation. Report the details of the reduction maneuver, including orientation of the pull, amount of force involved, degree of victim sedation, and residual instability of the joint, to the definitive care physician.

CIRCULATORY FUNCTION

Injury to the major vessels supplying a limb can occur with penetrating or blunt trauma. A fracture can produce injury to vessels by direct laceration (rarely) or by stretching, which produces intimal flaps. These flaps can immediately occlude the distal blood flow or lead to delay in occlusion. For this reason, repeated examination of circulatory function is mandatory before and during transport.

Assess the color and warmth of the skin of the distal extremity. Distal pallor and asymmetric regional hypothermia may identify a vascular injury.

Pulses palpated in the upper extremity include the brachial, radial, and ulnar. If blood loss and hypothermia make pulses difficult to assess, temperature and color of the distal extremity become keys to diagnosis.

Any suspected major arterial injury mandates immediate evacuation after splinting.

NERVE FUNCTION

Nerve function may be impossible to assess in an unconscious or uncooperative victim. Whenever possible, however, it is important to establish the status of nerve function to the distal extremity after the victim's condition is stabilized.

Periodically compare the initial findings with additional examinations during transport of the victim. Deteriorating neurologic findings guide the speed of evacuation and any ameliorating maneuvers. These decisions may greatly affect the final outcome for the victim.

Carefully document the sensory examination of the peripheral nerves with regard to light touch and pinprick.

Assess muscle function by observing active function and grading the strength of each muscle group against resistance.

GENERAL TREATMENT
Evacuation Decisions

1. Musculoskeletal injuries that warrant immediate evacuation to a definitive care center include any suspected cervical, thoracic, or lumbar spine injury.
2. A victim who has a suspected pelvic injury with posterior instability, significant suspected blood loss, or injury to the sacral plexus should receive immediate emergency evacuation on a backboard.
3. Any open fracture requires definitive débridement and care within 18 hours to prevent the development of deep infection and should prompt emergency evacuation. Administer a broad-spectrum antibiotic, such as cefazolin (Ancef), adult dose 1 to 1.5 g IM or IV q8h, soon after the injury.
4. A victim with a suspected compartment syndrome must be evacuated on an emergency basis.
5. A joint dislocation involving the hip or knee warrants immediate evacuation, even if relocated, because of the associated risk of vascular injury or post-traumatic osteonecrosis of the femoral head.

6. A laceration involving a tendon or nerve warrants urgent evacuation to a center where an experienced surgeon is available.
7. In all but the most remote wilderness expeditions, arrangements should be made to promptly evacuate the victim when treatment or significance of the injury is uncertain.

Special Considerations With Open Fracture

1. An injury that includes disruption of the skin and a broken bone is an open fracture and is at risk for bacterial contamination. Assume that any deep wound over a known fracture represents an open fracture. If soil and foreign body contamination is severe, the victim is at risk for sepsis.
2. If medical care is realistically less than 4 to 6 hours away and the bone (limb) is not severely angulated or malpositioned, treat the injury with a compression dressing, splint, and transport.
3. If the delay will be more than 6 hours before definitive medical care, irrigation of the open wound is beneficial and may help prevent serious soft tissue and bone infection.
   a. The water used for irrigation does not have to be sterile. Clean tap water or disinfected water can greatly diminish the bacterial count.
   b. Use a syringe from the medical kit as an irrigating tool (see Fig. 14-1).
   c. Attach an 18-gauge needle (or irrigation tip) to the syringe.
   d. Irrigate the wound copiously with the pressurized stream of water. For a large wound, more than a liter of water may be necessary.
4. Once the wound has been cleaned and irrigated, cover it with a sterile compression dressing.
5. Realign any angulated or malpositioned fractures and apply the required traction. If 1% to 10% povidone-iodine solution can be applied as a brief

rinse over the visible bone ends, it is less likely that major contamination will occur when the bone fragments slip back into the soft tissue envelope during a reduction maneuver.

6. Administer a broad-spectrum antibiotic, such as cefazolin (Ancef), adult dose 1 to 1.5 g IM or IV q8h, if available, and splint the extremity. If evacuation time exceeds 8 hours, the incidence of osteomyelitis is high.

Special Considerations With Amputation

1. In the wilderness environment, the amputation victim requires immediate evacuation.
2. Control hemorrhage by direct pressure. A tourniquet is virtually never indicated. If a tourniquet is applied as a life-saving measure, be prepared to sacrifice the limb.
3. Without cooling, an amputated part remains potentially viable for only 4 to 6 hours; with cooling, viability may be extended to 18 hours.
4. Cleanse the amputated part with water, wrap it in a moistened sterile gauze or towel, place it in a plastic bag, and transport it on ice or snow, if available. Do not transport it in direct contact with ice or ice water.
5. Make sure the amputated part accompanies the victim throughout the evacuation process.

Special Considerations With Compartment Syndrome

A *compartment syndrome* exists when locally increased tissue pressure compromises circulation and neuromuscular function. In the wilderness setting, this most frequently occurs in association with a fracture or severe contusion. Compartment syndrome also occurs when a victim has been lying for some time across an extremity. The lower leg and forearm are the most common sites for this syndrome because tight fasciae encase the muscle compartments in these regions and because these areas are frequently involved with fractures or severe contusions. A compartment syndrome can also occur in the thigh, hand, foot, and gluteal regions.

Signs and Symptoms

1. Complaints by the conscious victim of severe pain that seems out of proportion to the injury
2. Extremely tight feel to the muscle compartment, with applied pressure increasing the pain
3. In the cooperative victim, decreased sensation to light touch and pinprick in the areas supplied by the nerve or nerves traversing the compartment, usually noted on the dorsum of the foot in the first web space, caused by pressure affecting the deep peroneal nerve in the anterior compartment of the leg
4. Most reliable signs: pain, tightness to palpation, hypoesthesia, and pain on passive stretch
5. Late findings (possibly not seen even with the most severe compartment syndrome): absence of a pulse, presence of pallor, and slow capillary refill

Treatment

1. Expedite emergency evacuation. The victim must be definitively treated in the first 6 to 8 hours after onset of this condition to optimize return of function to the involved limb.
2. Perform an emergency fasciotomy to relieve the pressure, which, untreated, can produce nerve and muscle cell death within 12 hours. Limited fasciotomies can be performed in the field by an experienced surgeon if evacuation will require more than 8 hours.

Special Considerations With Potential Blood Loss From Fracture

1. Keep in mind the potential volume of blood loss resulting from specific closed fractures:
    ✤ Pelvis—6 to 10 units
    ✤ Femur—2 to 4 units

✤ Tibia—1 to 2 units
✤ Humerus—1 to 2 units
2. Be aware that blood loss can be worsened considerably if the skin overlying the fracture is disrupted.

Splinting

Improvisation: General Guidelines

1. When working with a complex improvised system, try to test your creation on an uninjured person (i.e., "work out the bugs") before you use it on the victim.
2. Remember to include improvisation construction materials, including a knife, tape, parachute cord or line, safety pins, wire, and plastic cable ties, in your survival kit.
3. Maintain a creative approach to obtaining improvisational materials. Much of the victim's gear can be harvested to provide necessary items (a backpack can often be dismantled to obtain foam pads, straps, etc.).
4. Practice constructing certain items before you require the skill in an actual rescue setting.

Extremity Splints

1. Splint the fracture before the victim is moved unless the victim's life is in immediate danger. In general, make sure the splint incorporates the joints above and below the fracture. If possible, fashion the splint on the uninjured extremity and then transfer it to the injured one.
2. Skis and poles or canoe and kayak paddles can be used as improvised splints. Airbags used as flotation for kayaks and canoes can be converted into pneumatic splints for arm and ankle injuries. The Minicell or Ethafoam pillars found in most kayaks can be removed and carved into pieces to provide upper and lower extremity splints. A life jacket can be molded into a cylinder splint for knee immobilization or into

a pillow splint for the ankle. The flexible aluminum stays found in internal-frame backpacks can be molded into an upper extremity splint. Other improvised splinting material includes sticks or tree limbs; rolled-up magazines, books, or newspapers; ice axes; tent poles; and dirt-filled garbage bags or fanny packs.

3. Ideally, a splint should immobilize the fractured bone in a functional position. In general, *functional position* means that the leg should be straight or slightly bent at the knee, the ankle and elbow bent at 90 degrees, the wrist straight, and the fingers flexed in a curve as if one were attempting to hold a can of soda or a baseball. "Soda can" position is appropriate for initial management and transport; however, for long-term splinting, apply a hand splint with the metacarpophalangeal joints flexed at 90 degrees and the interphalangeal joints extended. This position places the collateral ligaments at maximum length and helps prevent joint contracture.

4. Secure the splint in place with strips of clothing, belts, pieces of rope or webbing, pack straps, elasticized roller wraps, or gauze bandages.

Ensolite (Closed-cell Foam) Pads

The era of Therm-a-Rest types of inflatable pads has rendered closed-cell foam pads increasingly scarce; however, closed-cell foam remains the ultimate padding for almost any improvised splint or rescue device. Even die-hard Therm-a-Rest fans should carry a small amount of closed-cell foam, which doubles as a lightweight, comfortable seat cushion. Unlike inflatable pads, Ensolite will not puncture and deflate.

1. A Therm-a-Rest pad can be used as padding for a long-bone splint immobilizer (e.g., an improvised universal knee immobilizer).

2. An inflatable pad can also be used to stabilize a pelvic fracture.

a. Wrap the deflated pad around the pelvis.
b. Secure the pad with tape and inflate the pad, thus creating an improvised military antishock trousers (MAST) substitute (see Pelvic Fractures).

SAM Splint

Introduced in 1985, the versatile SAM splint (see Fig. 7-8) has largely filled the niche formerly occupied by military-style ladder splints and wire mesh splints. It is constructed of a thin sheet of malleable aluminum sandwiched between two thin layers of closed-cell foam, weighs approximately 4½ oz, and can be easily rolled into a tight cylinder. Initially the splint has no rigidity, but after structural U-shaped bends are placed along the axis of the splint, it becomes quite rigid.

1. The SAM splint(s) can be used for splinting virtually any long bone in the body (see Fig. 13-9).
2. It can also be used for fabricating an improvised cervical collar (see Fig. 7-8).

Triangular Bandage

One of the most ubiquitous components of first-aid kits and one of the easiest to replace through improvisation is the triangular bandage.

1. Typically used to construct a sling and swath bandage for shoulder and arm immobilization, a good substitute for this bulky item can be made with two or three safety pins. Pinning the shirtsleeve of the injured arm to the chest portion of the shirt effectively immobilizes the extremity against the body (Fig. 13-1, *B*).
2. If the victim is wearing a short-sleeved shirt, fold the bottom of the shirt up and over the arm to create a pouch. This can be pinned to the sleeve and chest section of the shirt to secure the arm (Fig. 13-1, *A*).

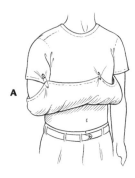 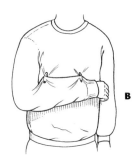

Fig. 13-1. Techniques for pinning arm to shirt as an improvised sling. **A,** With short-sleeved shirt, bottom of shirt is folded up over injured arm and secured to sleeve and upper shirt. **B,** With long-sleeved shirt or jacket, sleeved arm is simply pinned to chest portion of garment.

3. Triangular bandages are also advocated for securing splints and constructing pressure wraps. Common items, such as socks, shirts, belts, pack straps, webbing, shoe laces, fanny packs, and underwear, can easily be substituted.

■ DISORDERS ■

UPPER EXTREMITY FRACTURES
Clavicle

A fracture of the clavicle generally occurs in the middle or lateral third of the bone and is typically associated with a direct blow or fall onto the lateral shoulder.

Signs and Symptoms
1. Complaints of shoulder pain, which may be poorly localized and is exacerbated by arm or shoulder motion
2. Crepitus at the clavicle—confirmation of the diagnosis
3. Although rare, associated pneumothorax, as the cupola of the lung is punctured

4. Shortness of breath and deep pain on inspiration
5. Associated injury to the brachial plexus, axillary artery, or subclavian vessels

Treatment

1. Localize the pain by gentle palpation to identify the area of maximum tenderness.
2. Auscultate the chest for equal breath sounds if a stethoscope is available.
3. Perform a thorough neurocirculatory examination of the adjacent extremity.
4. Examine the skin carefully for disruption because of the subcutaneous location of the bone.
5. If there is a significant open wound, a suspected pneumothorax, or an injury to a nerve or vascular structure, arrange for evacuation.
6. Most clavicular fractures are improved by applying a figure-8 type of support, easily improvised with a shirt or jacket. By pulling the shoulder girdle back, apply longitudinal traction to the clavicle so that the bony fragments are somewhat realigned.
7. In addition, use a sling (also easily improvised) to offer support and some relief, as will judicious use of ice or snow packs, if available, and analgesics. Elevation may provide added relief during rest. Elevate the victim's upper body and head by 10 to 30 degrees when supine.

Humerus

A fracture of the humeral shaft may be produced by a direct blow or torsional force on the arm. This fracture frequently occurs with a fall, rope accident, or skiing accident.

Signs and Symptoms

1. Radial nerve damage
   a. Courses around the posterior aspect of the humerus and is occasionally traumatized when the humeral shaft is injured

   b. Result: numbness over the dorsum of the hand and inability to extend the wrist or fingers

   c. Usually caused by contusion or traction injury to the nerve and not to complete disruption

2. Fracture of the proximal humerus, often caused by a high-velocity fall onto an abducted, externally rotated arm or a direct blow to the anterior shoulder

   a. Difficult to differentiate from a shoulder dislocation in the acute phase

   b. Severe pain around the shoulder and with any arm motion

   c. Anterior fullness in the area of the proximal humerus, suggesting associated anterior humeral head dislocation

3. Fracture of the distal humerus

   a. More frequently extraarticular in children and intraarticular in adults, with the child generally sustaining a supracondylar fracture with an extension moment across the elbow in a fall from a height

   b. Peak age of incidence 4 to 8 years, although this can also occur in an adult

   c. Deformity, swelling, pain, and crepitus

Treatment

1. With radial nerve injury, there is a high incidence of spontaneous recovery of function. However, if the victim complains of arm pain associated with deformity and crepitus, carefully check the sensory and motor function of the radial nerve as part of the overall neurocirculatory examination.

2. When a fracture of the humeral shaft is suspected, firmly apply an appropriate splint of fiberglass, wood, or other improvised material with an elastic bandage on the medial and lateral sides of the humerus. Have the victim use a sling for comfort.

   a. With suspected proximal humeral injury, use the uninjured side as a reference and palpate the ante-

rior aspect of the injured shoulder firmly while rotating the arm.
   (1) Palpable crepitus with arm motion confirms
       the diagnosis.
   (2) It is unlikely that a combined fracture and dis-
       location can be reduced in the field. Treat this
       as a fracture, with splinting of the extremity to
       the torso with a sling or a sling and swath.
   b. Although application of an arm sling is the appro-
      priate field management for a proximal humeral
      fracture, if associated significant distal nerve or
      vascular injury exists, arrange for evacuation.
3. For an adult with pain, crepitus, deformity, and
   swelling after a fall, apply a splint and immobilize
   the arm to the torso. Be sure to apply the splint with
   the elbow at 45 to 90 degrees of flexion, depending
   on the victim's comfort. A splint on the inner and
   outer surface of the arm that is molded to curve
   around the elbow provides very satisfactory stabilization. Arrange for prompt evacuation with an open
   fracture or neurocirculatory deficit.

Radius

Signs and Symptoms
1. Radial shaft fracture: usually a history of a fall with
   angular or axial loading of the forearm
   a. Pain, deformity, and crepitus over the radial shaft
      after a fall or direct blow, with any arm motion ex-
      acerbating the pain
   b. Possibly associated with dislocation of the distal
      radioulnar joint (Galeazzi's fracture); tenderness,
      swelling, and deformity in wrist
   c. If associated with fracture of the ulna:
      (1) Marked forearm instability
      (2) Tenderness, crepitus, and deformity in the el-
          bow and wrist
2. Radial head fracture: generally occurs in a young to
   middle-age adult who falls onto an outstretched
   hand

a. Pain around the elbow with loss of full extension

    b. Tenderness at the radial head on the lateral side of the elbow and pain with passive rotation of the forearm

    c. With a more severe, comminuted radial head fracture: pain and crepitus with attempts at motion; ROM severely limited

    d. Frequently, hemarthrosis of the elbow with effusion

    e. Swelling noted as fullness posterior to the radial head and anterior to the tip of the olecranon

3. Fracture of the distal metaphyseal radius: generally associated with a fall onto the outstretched hand from a significant height

    a. Intraarticular distal radius fracture often associated with fracture of the ulnar styloid

    b. Obvious pain, deformity, and crepitus

Treatment

1. Carefully examine the wrist and elbow, looking for tenderness, swelling, deformity, and crepitus

2. Once a shaft fracture of the radius or radius and ulna is identified, splint the wrist, forearm, and elbow in the position of function.

3. For a radial head fracture, move the elbow through a gentle ROM and then place it in a posterior splint at 90 degrees of flexion with neutral pronation and supination.

    a. On a prolonged expedition when definitive care cannot be reached, remove the splint at 5 days and perform intermittent active ROM exercises, then reapply the splint for comfort.

    b. With a nondisplaced or minimally displaced radial head fracture, early ROM prevents permanent loss of elbow motion.

    c. If hemarthrosis has occurred *and* proper equipment is available *and* you are confident about the

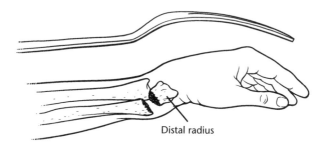

Fig. 13-2. Colles' fracture ("dinner fork deformity").

diagnosis, aspirate the hemarthrosis and instill 5 ml of lidocaine to facilitate pain relief. This must be done under sterile conditions.

4. For a distal radius fracture with significant deformity at the wrist, apply longitudinal traction after appropriate sedation (Fig. 13-2).

   a. Next, apply a splint that immobilizes the wrist and elbow. A U-shaped ("sugar tong") splint, used in conjunction with a sling to limit rotation, is adequate for transport.

   b. With an open fracture, significant neurologic deficits distally, or abnormal circulatory examination, apply the splints promptly and initiate evacuation. Keep the limb elevated above the heart during transport to minimize swelling.

Ulna

Signs and Symptoms

1. Ulnar shaft fracture: when victim attempts to brace a fall with the forearm

   a. Most often associated with fracture of the radial shaft at the same level

   b. When isolated, most often occurs as a result of a direct blow, the so-called nightstick fracture

    c. Can be associated with dislocation of the radial head (Monteggia's fracture), affecting elbow function

    d. Pain, localized swelling, and crepitus

2. Fracture of the proximal ulna (olecranon): result of a fall onto the posterior elbow or from an avulsion after violent asymmetric contraction of the triceps

    a. Inability to extend the elbow actively against gravity if the triceps is dissociated from the forearm with a complete fracture of the olecranon

    b. On initial examination, pain, significant swelling, and ecchymosis, palpable gap in the olecranon, with possible open fracture

    c. With severe trauma, associated with intraarticular fracture of the distal humerus

Treatment

1. For ulnar shaft fracture, apply a long-arm splint in the position of function. If the fracture is open, arrange for prompt evacuation.

2. For fracture of the proximal ulna, after the distal neurocirculatory examination and shoulder and wrist assessment, apply a splint in the position of function. A posterior splint at 90 degrees usually works well. If there is an open fracture, absent pulse, severe swelling, or neurologic deficit, arrange for immediate evacuation.

Wrist and Hand

Signs and Symptoms

1. Wrist fracture: history of significant rotational or high axial loading forces, such as those occurring with a fall onto the hand

    a. Pain at first and later swelling of the wrist

    b. Significant pain with any use of the hand or with rotation of the forearm

    c. Fractures of the carpal bones associated with wrist dislocation

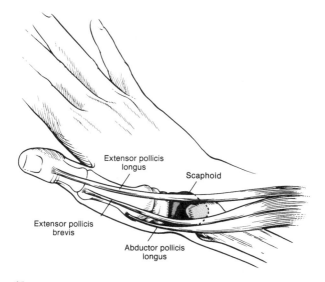

Fig. 13-3. The scaphoid (navicular) bone sits in the "anatomic snuffbox" of the radial aspect of the wrist.

2. Carpal bone fracture: precise diagnosis impossible without radiographs
   a. Scaphoid is the most frequently fractured bone
   b. Diagnosis suspected if the victim's area of maximum tenderness is within the "anatomic snuffbox" (Fig. 13-3)
3. Fracture of the hook of the hamate
   a. Point of maximum tenderness at the base of the hypothenar eminence
   b. History of using the hand to apply great force to an object with a handle, such as an ax or a hammer, and meeting great resistance

Treatment
1. Swelling can become severe. Remove all jewelry as soon as possible to prevent constriction as tissue swells.

2. Make a temporary hand splint with the hand in the position of function, with the wrist straight and the fingers flexed in a curve as if holding a beverage can.
3. Apply a long-term hand splint with the metacarpophalangeal joints flexed 90 degrees and the interphalangeal joints extended. This position places the collateral ligaments at maximum length and prevents later joint contracture.
4. For an open fracture or one accompanied by median nerve dysfunction, arrange for prompt evacuation.
5. For carpal bone fracture/wrist dislocation, reduce the fracture by grasping the hand in a handshake fashion and pulling with axial traction. Apply a short-arm splint.
6. For suspected scaphoid fracture, if appropriate splinting materials are available, apply a thumb spica splint, immobilizing both the radius and the thumb metacarpal.
   a. Encourage the victim to follow up with an orthopedist as soon as practical.
   b. Lack of appropriate immobilization can result in nonunion and chronic pain.
7. For fracture of the hook of the hamate bone, use a short-arm splint, which also suffices for other suspected carpal injuries, until definitive treatment can be obtained.

Metacarpals

Signs and Symptoms
1. Fracture of the metacarpal base or shaft: result of a crush injury or an axial load when a rock or other immovable object is struck; produces tenderness, crepitus, and deformity
2. Fracture of the metacarpal neck: result of the same mechanism as above
   a. Fourth and fifth metacarpals most frequently involved
   b. Occurs at the base of the knuckle and can be associated with significant rotational deformity

3. Fracture of the base of the thumb metacarpal
   a. When an individual falls with an object grasped between the index finger and thumb; a common position with a ski pole
   b. Difficult to differentiate from an ulnar collateral ligament injury because these injuries often occur simultaneously

Treatment
1. For fracture of the metacarpal base or shaft, apply a short-arm splint (e.g., gutter splint, volar splint, U-splint) extending to the proximal interphalangeal (PIP) joint.
2. For possible fracture of the metacarpal neck, check for rotation of the metacarpal by observing the orientation of the fingernails as the metacarpophalangeal and interphalangeal joints are flexed to 90 degrees.
   a. Make sure that the fingernails are parallel to one another and perpendicular to the orientation of the palm.
   b. Ensure that the terminal portions of each digit point to the scaphoid tubercle.
3. For fracture of the metacarpal neck, if malalignment or significant shortening is noted, attempt rotation and reduction with traction on the involved digit.
   a. For a fractured metacarpal shaft or neck, immobilize by applying an aluminum splint (or stick) to the volar surface and taping the involved digit to the next digit with the metacarpophalangeal joint at 45 to 90 degrees.
   b. If splinting material is available, apply a radial or ulnar gutter splint, with the metacarpophalangeal joint at 45 to 90 degrees. Make sure the splint extends to the end of the fingers.
4. For suspected fracture of the base of the thumb metacarpal, when suspected, immobilize the thumb and wrist in a thumb spica splint.

5. For open metacarpal fracture, clean the wound, débride as needed, and give presumptive antibiotic therapy for 48 hours or until definitive care can be obtained.

Phalanx

Signs and Symptoms
1. Fracture usually a result of a crush injury or when a digit is caught in a rope
2. Angular rotational deformity and crepitus
3. Without radiography, intraarticular fracture with subluxation or dislocation difficult to differentiate from interphalangeal joint dislocation

Trauma
1. Reduce the fracture by applying traction and correcting the deformity.
2. Immobilize the fracture by taping the injured digit to a volar splint.
3. Cleanse any nail bed fracture or crush site with soap, then place a sterile dressing and protective volar splint. If the nail bed is lacerated, suture repair may be necessary to preserve future functional nail growth.

UPPER EXTREMITY DISLOCATIONS
Sternoclavicular Joint

Signs and Symptoms
1. Generally injured by a fall onto an abducted shoulder
   a. Direction of dislocation with the medial head of the clavicle anterior to the manubrium of the sternum
   b. Direct blow to the sternum also possibly causative of this injury, along with rib fracture(s)
2. Pain in the sternum region, frequently accompanied by difficulty taking a deep breath
3. With posterior dislocation, significant pressure placed on the esophagus and superior vena cava

    a. Step-off between the sternum and medial head of the clavicle (compared with the uninjured side)

    b. Difficulty swallowing and engorgement of facial veins, similar to that seen with superior vena cava obstruction syndrome

Treatment

1. Attempt reduction as soon as possible.
   a. Place a large roll of clothing or other firm object between the scapulae, and position the victim on a firm surface.
   b. Apply sharp, firm pressure, directed posteriorly, to both shoulders.
   c. Repeat this maneuver several times with a larger object placed between the scapulae if reduction attempts are initially unsuccessful.
   d. After reduction, use a sling.
2. With a posterior dislocation, if the victim transcends into extremis, grasp the midshaft clavicle with a towel clip or pliers and forcefully pull it out of the thoracic cavity. Posterior dislocation mandates evacuation.

Acromioclavicular Joint Separation

Signs and Symptoms

1. Injured by a blow on top of the shoulder
2. First-degree injury: to the capsule between the acromion and the clavicle; no superior migration of the clavicle is seen
3. Second-degree injury: complete capsular disruption, with the coracoclavicular ligaments remaining intact; superior migration of the clavicle relative to the acromion of one half the diameter of the clavicle
4. Third-degree injury: total disruption of the joint capsule and the coracoclavicular ligaments, which allows superior migration of the clavicle of up to 2 cm (about 1 inch) (Fig. 13-4)

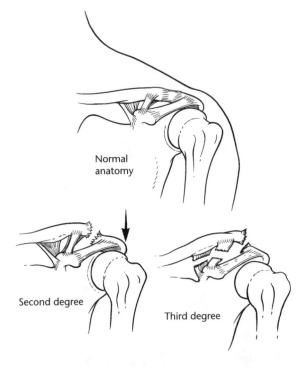

Fig. 13-4.   Acromioclavicular joint injury.

Treatment
1. Because using the arm increases pain, place the arm on the affected side in a sling.
2. As long as the individual can tolerate the discomfort associated with the injury, evacuation is not mandatory.
3. Apply ice packs and administer appropriate analgesics.
4. Elevate the upper torso to provide additional relief during rest.

Glenohumeral Joint (Shoulder) Dislocation

Signs and Symptoms

1. Generally dislocated anteriorly, or anteriorly and inferiorly; mechanism of injury usually a blow to the arm in the abducted and externally rotated position, for example, during "high-bracing" in kayaking or other paddle sports, in which extreme abduction and external rotation occur
2. Recurrent anterior shoulder instability, seen in 30% to 50% of individuals and often easier to reduce than a first-time dislocation
3. Holding the extremity away from the body, unable to bring the arm across the chest
   a. Shoulder that appears square because of anterior, medial, and inferior displacement of the humeral head into a subcoracoid position
   b. No crepitation unless there is an associated fracture
4. With axillary nerve injury, loss of sensation over the mid-deltoid region

Treatment

1. Do a thorough motor, sensory, and circulatory examination of the involved extremity.
2. Carefully assess the axillary and musculocutaneous nerves because they are the nerves most often injured in this dislocation.
3. If within 30 to 60 minutes of definitive medical care, transport the victim with support for the dislocated joint.
4. If skilled individuals are present or if definitive medical care is distant, early reduction of the dislocation can greatly improve the victim's discomfort and enable the victim to function more actively during evacuation (Box 13-1).
   a. The key element is rapid initiation because the longer a shoulder remains dislocated, the more difficult the eventual reduction.

Box 13-1.

Reduction Techniques

STANDING METHOD
- ✤ Have the victim bend forward at the waist while you support the chest with one hand.
- ✤ With the other hand, grasp the victim's wrist and apply steady downward traction and external rotation (Fig. 13-6).
- ✤ While maintaining traction, slowly flex the victim's shoulder by moving it in a cephalad direction until reduction is obtained.
- ✤ If two rescuers are available, one supports the victim at the chest and the other exerts countertraction and flexion at the arm (Fig. 13-7).
- ✤ To help with the reduction, apply scapular manipulation by adducting the inferior tip using thumb pressure and stabilizing the superior aspect of the scapula with the cephalad hand.

SITTING METHOD
- ✤ Perform the reduction with the victim sitting upright with the elbow on the affected side flexed at a 90-degree angle.
- ✤ Form an article of clothing into a 3-foot (90-cm) loop around the proximal forearm.
- ✤ Apply downward traction by placing your foot in the loop, freeing your hands to apply gentle rotation (usually slightly external), while maintaining elbow flexion.
- ✤ Have an assistant stand on the opposite side of the victim and maintain countertraction by placing his or her arms around the victim's chest, with hands in the axilla.

b. Common to all methods of shoulder reduction are the following: relaxation of muscle spasm, reassurance of the victim, and a method of traction to pass the humeral head over the anterior edge of the glenoid.

    c. In some remote settings, it may be easier to apply a method of reduction that can be carried out with the victim either standing or sitting. This requires access to a flat, comfortable area on which to place the victim in the supine or prone position.

5. After any shoulder reduction, remember to monitor circulation and motor-sensory function to the wrist and hand.

6. Narcotic or benzodiazepine premedication may be helpful if muscle spasm has developed, but avoid these in the multiply injured victim.

7. If the shoulder cannot be reduced after three vigorous attempts, arrange for evacuation.

8. After relocation, to prevent a recurrent dislocation, splint the victim's arm across the chest with a sling or swath or by safety-pinning the sleeve of the arm across the chest. If circumstances require further limited use of the arm (e.g., ski pole use, kayak paddling), partially stabilize the shoulder by wrapping an elastic wrap around the torso and upper arm to limit abduction and external rotation (Fig. 13-5).

9. Any victim with a first-time dislocation or severe postreduction pain requires evacuation and formal evaluation.

Posterior Shoulder Dislocation

Signs and Symptoms

1. Occurs in less than 5% of shoulder dislocations; caused by a direct blow to the anterior shoulder or results from marked internal rotation with a grand mal seizure

2. Significant pain and loss of shoulder motion, with external rotation often completely lost

3. Using palpation, can usually detect posterior fullness not appreciated on the uninjured (comparison) side

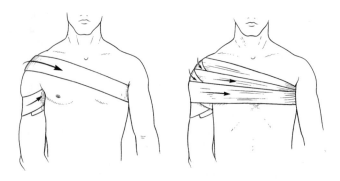

Fig. 13-5. Shoulder harness for support after shoulder dislocation.

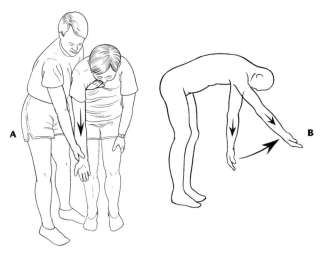

Fig. 13-6. Technique for shoulder relocation with victim standing. **A,** Rescuer supports victim's chest with one hand and pulls down and forward **(B)** with other hand.

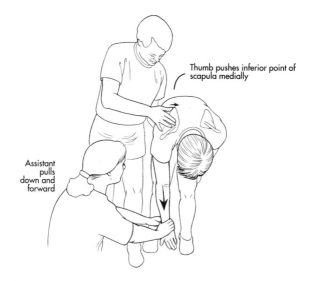

Thumb pushes inferior point of
scapula medially

Assistant
pulls
down and
forward

Fig. 13-7.   If two rescuers are available, scapular rotation to
assist shoulder relocation can be performed while second rescuer pulls arm down and forward. Inferior tip of scapula is
pushed medially.

Treatment
The reduction maneuver, aftercare, and indications for
evacuation are similar to those for anterior dislocation.

Shoulder Fracture/Dislocation
Signs and Symptoms
More common with a high-velocity accident and an
older victim

Treatment
1. Do not reduce suspected fracture/dislocation in the
   field.
2. Treat this injury as a fracture, with splinting of the
   extremity to the torso with a sling or a sling and
   swath.

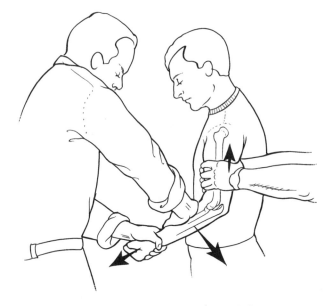

Fig. 13-8. Reduction of dislocated elbow.

Elbow

Signs and Symptoms

1. Occurs with hyperextension or axial loading from a fall onto the outstretched hand; generally posterior and lateral
2. Signs obvious, with posterior deformity at the elbow and foreshortening of the forearm

Treatment

1. After careful examination of the distal sensory, motor, and circulatory status, perform reduction.
   a. With countertraction on the upper arm, apply linear traction with the elbow slightly flexed and the forearm in the original degree of pronation or supination (Fig. 13-8).

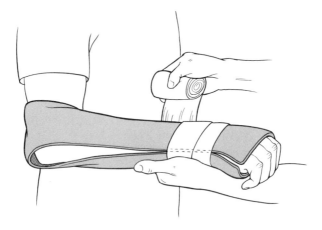

Fig. 13-9. SAM forearm splint intended to also immobilize the elbow.

    b. Be aware that premedication with an opiate or benzodiazepine can be extremely helpful.
    c. Reduction (which can be a very painful maneuver) leads to nearly complete relief of pain and restoration of normal surface anatomy.
2. After reduction, apply a posterior splint with the elbow in 90 degrees of flexion and the forearm in neutral position (Fig. 13-9).
    a. Use a sling for comfort.
    b. If reduction is not successful after three vigorous attempts or if a nerve or vascular injury is suspected, apply a splint to the arm in the most comfortable position and initiate evacuation.

Wrist

Signs and Symptoms
1. Frequently associated with carpal fracture(s)
2. Generally produced by a fall onto the outstretched hand
3. Severe pain, swelling, and deformity within the distal wrist

4. Without x-ray film, difficult to differentiate from a distal radius fracture

Treatment
1. Carefully assess distal neurocirculatory function, emphasizing median nerve function.
2. For wrist dislocation or fracture, perform a reduction maneuver.
3. Grasp the victim's hand as for a handshake, place countertraction on the upper arm, and apply linear traction. Note that significant force is required, and premedication, if available, may be extremely helpful.
4. If reduction is unsuccessful after three vigorous attempts or if there is median nerve dysfunction, arrange for evacuation.
5. Apply a short-arm (U or volar) splint if reduction is successful.
6. Elevate the arm as much as possible until the definitive care center can be reached.

Metacarpophalangeal Joint
Dislocation is rare and usually follows a crush injury or occurs when a hand is caught in a rope. The site is usually dorsal, and it may be difficult to reduce in the field.

Signs and Symptoms
1. Finger shortened, deviated to the ulnar side, and positioned in extension
2. Metacarpal head possibly prominent in the palm
3. The thumb metacarpophalangeal joint typically injured
4. Injury to the ulnar collateral ligament of this joint ("gamekeeper's thumb") a result of a valgus stress, such as when an individual falls holding an object (e.g., pole) in the first web space

Treatment
Metacarpophalangeal joint

1. Be aware that dorsal dislocation may be irreducible if the head of the metacarpal becomes trapped between the volar ligaments. Reduction depends on the degree of disruption of supporting structures, such as the volar plate and collateral ligaments. Thus this dislocation frequently requires open reduction.
2. If reduction of a digital metacarpophalangeal joint dislocation is successful, apply a volar splint with the joint held in 90 degrees of flexion.
3. If reduction is unsuccessful, splint the joint in the position of comfort and arrange for definitive treatment as soon as possible.

Thumb metacarpophalangeal joint

1. Place an ulnar collateral ligament tear in a thumb spica splint. Instability often requires a lateral stress x-ray film for definitive diagnosis and is an indication for surgical repair. Arrange for definitive care within 10 days of the injury.
2. For dorsal dislocation, attempt metacarpophalangeal joint reduction.
   a. Grasp the finger and apply longitudinal traction, moving from the metacarpophalangeal joint extension into flexion ("up and over" the metacarpal head).
   b. Splint the thumb in the position of function (Fig. 13-10).
3. Obtain orthopedic follow-up within 10 days.

Proximal Interphalangeal Joint
PIP joint dislocation is common and occurs with axial loading of a finger.

Signs and Symptoms

1. Dislocation occurring when an individual attempts to catch an object or a finger becomes entangled in a rope or another piece of equipment
2. Dislocation generally dorsal (middle phalanx in relationship to the proximal)

Treatment

1. Be aware that this dislocation is easily reduced with longitudinal traction (Fig. 13-11).
2. Apply a volar splint and tape the finger to the splint in slight flexion.
3. Initiate early motion of the joint to regain full extension.
4. Because the central slip of the extensor mechanism may be ruptured when the dislocation is volar, hy-

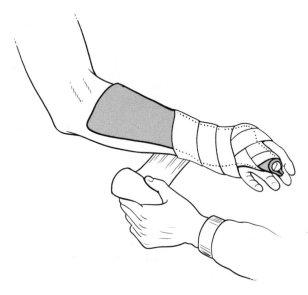

Fig. 13-10.   SAM thumb splint.

perextend the joint slightly as you apply the post-reduction splint.

5. With either volar or distal dislocation, arrange for definitive care as soon as possible.

Distal Interphalangeal Joint

The distal interphalangeal joint is less frequently injured than the PIP joint.

Signs and Symptoms

1. Volar dislocation or subluxation, resulting in disruption of the terminal extensor mechanism

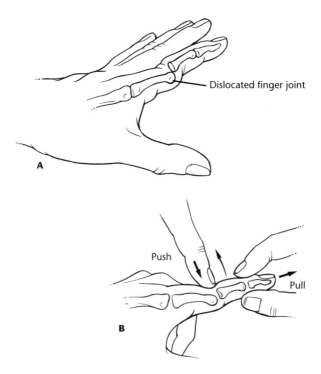

Fig. 13-11. Traction method of joint reduction.

Continued

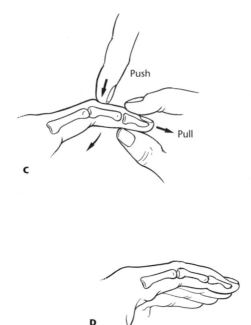

Fig. 13-11, cont'd   For legend see p. 121.

2. Occasionally, when an object is firmly grasped and then pulled away, rupture of the flexor profundus tendon
3. Distal interphalangeal joint dislocation: active extension of the distal interphalangeal joint absent
4. Rupture of the flexor profundus tendon: active flexion of the distal interphalangeal joint absent

Treatment
1. Reduce a distal interphalangeal joint dislocation.
   a. Obtain reduction with traction, then examine the joint for full active extension. If an extension lag is

noted, splint the joint in 15 degrees of hyperextension for 3 weeks.
  b. Be aware that, ultimately, an x-ray examination must be performed to rule out an intraarticular fracture.
2. For rupture of the flexor profundus tendon, splint the digit in flexion and instruct the victim to see an upper extremity surgeon within 10 days.

PELVIC FRACTURES

In the wilderness setting, pelvic fracture is generally associated with a fall from a significant height, a high-velocity ski accident, or vehicular trauma, with the direction of the force directly related to the fracture and having important implications for definitive management. These fractures can be classified as stable or unstable and further as simple, nondisplaced inferior or superior ramus fractures or avulsion fractures and low-velocity (e.g., short-distance fall) lateral compression injuries. Unstable fractures include anteroposterior (AP) compression injuries, vertical shear injuries, and high-velocity lateral compression injuries.

Signs and Symptoms
1. On clinical examination, simple fracture seen as an area of tenderness not associated with detectable instability
2. Posterior ring fracture(s) or dislocation: greater incidence of significant hemorrhage, neurologic injury, and mortality than with other pelvic fractures
3. Diagnosis based on instability of the pelvis associated with posterior pain, swelling, ecchymosis, and motion on examination
4. AP compression injury: anterior instability, along with palpable ramus fracture or gapping of the pubic symphysis
5. Pelvic fracture associated with bladder, prostate, and urethral injury

Treatment
1. To palpate, place hands on each iliac crest. Press outward and then inward to determine whether the pelvis is unstable. An unstable pelvis "gives" with this type of compression or distraction force.
2. The key factor in initial management of a pelvic fracture is the identification of posterior injury to the pelvic ring. If you find this or any unstable pelvic fracture, arrange for immediate evacuation with the victim on a backboard, taking care to minimize leg and torso motion.
3. Be aware that the victim is usually most comfortable with the hips and knees in slight flexion. Pad the victim generously with blankets or sleeping bags.
4. Improvise a MAST garment by wrapping an inflatable mattress around the victim's hips and pelvis, securing it with tape or rolled elastic wrap, and then inflating.
5. Be aware that any unstable pelvic fracture can cause significant hemorrhage. If available, arrange for intravenous fluid volume replacement.

LOWER EXTREMITY FRACTURES
Proximal Femur (Hip)
Most hip fractures occur in the femoral neck or intertrochanteric region.

Signs and Symptoms
1. In the absence of head or spinal cord injury, pain around the proximal thigh
2. Except in the most slender individual, little local reaction in terms of swelling or deformity around the hip region to aid in diagnosis
3. Significant pain from any movement of the affected limb
4. Affected limb often noticeably shortened and externally rotated

Treatment
1. After doing a careful sensory, motor, and circulatory examination, realign the limb and apply a Kendrick, Thomas, or REEL splint, if available.
2. If a manufactured splint is not available, transport the victim on a backboard, with the limbs strapped together or with a tree limb placed between them.
3. Be aware that fracture of the femoral neck is associated with a significant risk of posttraumatic femoral head necrosis. Without a radiograph, this fracture is impossible to distinguish from an intertrochanteric fracture.
4. Because evidence indicates that emergency treatment of a fracture of the femoral neck decreases the risk of posttraumatic necrosis, arrange for rapid evacuation of any victim in whom this injury is suspected.

Femoral Shaft

Fracture of the femoral shaft follows a fall from a significant height or results from a high-velocity injury.

Signs and Symptoms
Crepitus and maximum deformity at mid-thigh

Treatment
1. Be aware that this may be an open injury; split the victim's pants open to complete the examination. If you find an open wound, arrange for rapid evacuation.
2. After completing a neurocirculatory examination, place the limb in a commercial or improvised traction device. Box 13-2 lists general principles of traction; Box 13-3 outlines femoral traction systems and discusses the ankle hitch and rigid support; and Box 13-4 lists traction mechanisms, anchors, method for securing, and padding. A number of commercial traction splints are available, including the Hare, Klippell, Sager, Thomas, Trac 3, REEL, and Kendrick. The Kendrick traction device is the best suited for

Box 13-2.

General Principles of Traction

WHY USE TRACTION?
In the backcountry environment, traction is essential for two fundamental reasons:
1. A general inability to provide IV volume expansion
2. Prolonged transport time to definitive care

One primary purpose of femoral traction is to limit blood loss into the thigh. For a constant surface area, the volume of a sphere is greater than the volume of a cylinder. Pulling (via traction) the thigh compartment back into its natural cylindric shape limits blood loss into the soft tissue. Enhanced victim comfort and decreased potential for neurovascular damage are important secondary benefits.

WHAT CRITERIA SHOULD BE USED TO EVALUATE A TRACTION SYSTEM?
Consider five key design principles when evaluating a femoral traction system:
1. Does the splint provide in-line traction, or does it incorrectly pull the victim's leg off to the side or needlessly plantar flex the victim's ankle?
2. Is the splint comfortable? Ask the victim how it feels.
3. Does the splint compromise neurologic or vascular function? Constantly check the victim's distal neurovascular function.
4. Is the splint durable, or will it break when subjected to backcountry stress? Try your traction design on an uninjured victim first.
5. Is the splint cumbersome? Many reasonable splint designs become so bulky and awkward that litter transport, technical rescue, or helicopter evacuation is impossible. For example, a full-length ski splint is not compatible with evacuation in certain small helicopters.

Box 13-3.

Femoral Traction Systems

Every femoral traction system has six components: ankle hitch, rigid support, traction mechanism, proximal anchor, method for securing, and padding. The ankle hitch and rigid support are outlined next. Box 13-4 lists traction mechanisms, proximal anchoring, method for securing, and padding.

ANKLE HITCH
Various techniques are used to anchor the distal extremity to the splint. Many work well, but some are difficult to recall in an emergency. Choose a technique that is easy to remember, and practice it.

Double-runner System
In this very straightforward technique, lay two short webbing loops ("runners") over and under the ankle (Fig. 13-12, *A*). Pass the long loop sides through the short loop on both sides and adjust (Fig. 13-12, *B*). This system is infinitely adjustable, enabling you to center the pull from any direction. Proper padding is essential, especially for a lengthy transport. Use the victim's boot to distribute the pressure over the foot and ankle, although this obscures visualization and palpation of the foot. You can leave the boot in place and cut out the toe section for observation.

Victim's Boot System
Use the victim's own boot as the hitch. Cut two holes into the side walls of the boot just above the midsole, in line with the ankle joint. Thread a piece of nylon webbing or a cravat through to complete the ankle hitch (Fig. 13-13). Because the boot is now functionally ruined, cut away the toe to allow direct neurovascular assessment.

Continued

Box 13-3.

Femoral Traction Systems—cont'd

ANKLE HITCH—cont'd
Buck's Traction
For extended transport, improvise Buck's traction using a closed-cell foam pad (Fig. 13-14). Wrap the pad around the lower leg, then loop a stirrup below the foot from medial calf to lateral calf. Fasten this assembly with a second cravat wrapped circumferentially around the calf over the closed-cell foam (duct tape or nylon webbing can be used instead of cravats). This system greatly increases the surface area over which the stirrup is applied and decreases the potential for neurovascular complications and dermal ischemia. It can also be used to manage a backcountry hip fracture. If Buck's traction is used for a hip injury, use a lesser amount of traction (5 pounds or less).

RIGID SUPPORT
This can be fabricated as a unilateral support, similar to the Sager traction splint or Kendrick traction device, or as a bilateral support, such as the Thomas half ring or Hare traction splint. Unilateral supports tend to be easier to apply than bilateral support.

Double–Ski Pole System
This is fashioned like a Thomas half ring, with the interlocked pole straps slipped under the proximal thigh to form the ischial support. Some mountain guides carry a prefabricated, drilled ski pole section or aluminum bar that can be used to stabilize the distal end of this system (Fig. 13-15).

Single–Ski Pole System
Use a single ski pole either between the legs, which is ideal for bilateral femoral fractures, or lateral to the

Box 13-3.

Femoral Traction Systems—cont'd

RIGID SUPPORT—cont'd
Single–Ski Pole System—cont'd
injured leg. The ultimate rigid support is an adjustable telescoping ski pole used laterally. You can elongate the pole to the appropriate length for each victim, making the splint very compact for litter work or helicopter evacuation (Fig. 13-16).

Tent Pole System
Fit conventional sectioned tent poles together to create the ideal length for rigid support. Because of their flexibility, make sure the tent poles are well secured to the leg to prevent them from flexing out of position. Place a blanket pin or bent tent stake (Fig. 13-17) in the end of the pole to provide an anchor for the traction system. Alternately, use a Prusik knot to secure the system to the end of the tent pole (Fig. 13-18).

Miscellaneous
You can use any suitable object, such as a canoe paddle, two ice axes taped together at the handles, or a straight tree limb, to fashion a rigid support. Although skis immediately come to mind as a suitable rigid component, they are often too cumbersome. Because of their length, skis may extend far beyond the victim's feet or require placement into the axilla, which is unnecessary and inhibits the victim's mobility (e.g., sitting up during transport). Premanufactured canvas pockets, available through the National Ski Patrol System, provide a ski tip and tail attachment grommet for use with the ski system.

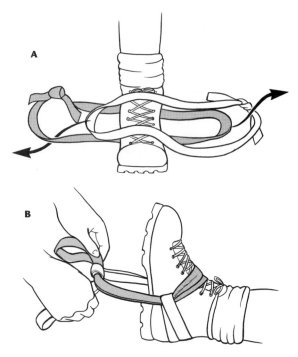

Fig. 13-12.   Double-runner ankle hitch.

wilderness use because of its minimal weight, low volume, and portability.

Distal Femur and Patella

Fracture of the distal end of the femur is frequently intraarticular and occurs with high-velocity loading when the knee is flexed. With axial loading of the femur, the patella becomes the driving wedge, and the femoral condyles are impacted.

Signs and Symptoms

1. Crepitus, significant instability (not seen with patellar fracture)

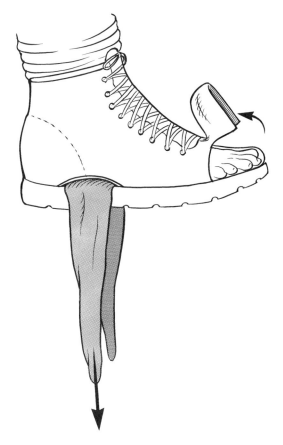

Fig. 13-13. Traction using cut boot and cravat.

2. Possible patellar fracture or splitting of the distal femoral condyles
3. With patellar fracture:
   a. Injury often obvious on deep palpation
   b. Injury often open because very little soft tissue overlies this sesamoid bone

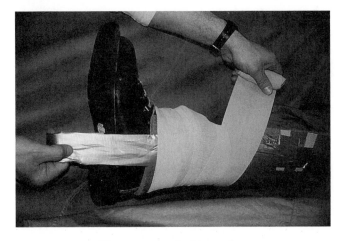

Fig. 13-14. Buck's traction.

Treatment
1. After initial examination of nerve and vessel function, realign the limb.
2. Apply a posterior splint to the realigned limb for transportation.
3. With an open wound in the region of the fracture or an abnormal nerve or vascular examination, arrange for immediate evacuation.

Tibia and Fibula

Tibial shaft fracture is associated with fibular shaft fracture in 90% of cases. These fractures result from high-impact trauma. The tibial plateau is the broad intraarticular surface of the upper tibia that articulates with the distal femur. This area can be fractured with a fall or jump from a height.

Signs and Symptoms
1. Pain, swelling, and deformity obvious on initial examination

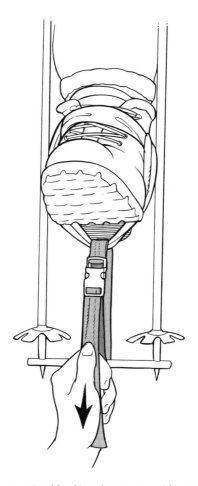

Fig. 13-15. Double–ski pole system with prefabricated cross-bar and webbing belt traction. Prefabricated, drilled ski section is used to attach ends of two ski poles. Traction is applied with a webbing belt and sliding buckle.

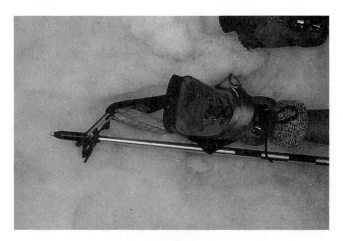

Fig. 13-16. Single–ski pole system. An adjustable telescoping ski pole is used as the rigid support. A stirrup is attached to a carabiner placed over end of pole. Traction is applied by elongating ski pole while another rescuer provides manual traction on victim's leg.

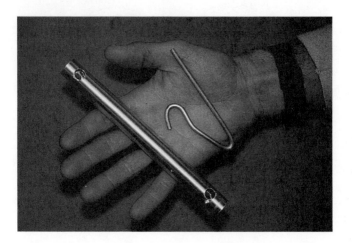

Fig. 13-17. Prefabricated, drilled tent pole section and bent stake, which serves as a distal traction anchor if a tent pole is used as the rigid support.

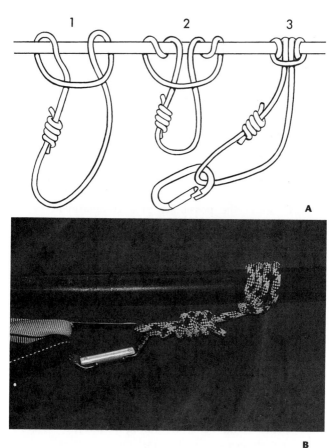

Fig. 13-18. **A,** Prusik knot made from a small-diameter cord is used as an adjustable distal traction anchor. **B,** Two Prusik wraps are shown. Three or four wraps provide additional friction and security. If Prusik knot slips, it can be easily taped in place.

2. With a tibial plateau fracture, hemarthrosis quickly noted, with significant swelling around the knee
3. Because of anatomic tethering of the popliteal artery by the fascia of the soleus complex, arterial injury possible, especially when associated with a knee dislocation

Treatment
1. When this injury is suspected, the entire limb must be inspected for distal sensory, motor, and circulatory function before realignment. Check distal pulses and capillary refill serially at 1-hour intervals.
2. Consider the possibility of a compartment syndrome.
3. Apply a posterior splint or U splint made from fiberglass or plaster.
4. Use a custom-made or improvised metal splint (e.g., SAM splint) that can be held in place with elastic bandages or tape. If SAM splints are used, at least two splints are needed for the medial and lateral component, and possibly a third for the posterior section.
5. Always pad the leg sufficiently before splinting.
6. Be aware that an air splint also provides adequate immobilization of the tibial-fibular fracture.
7. Make sure the ankle is held in neutral position.
8. Strap the injured leg to the noninjured leg to help reduce rotational forces during transport.
9. If materials are limited, fashion a crude splint by strapping the injured leg to the noninjured leg with a tree limb or walking stick placed between them for support.
10. Transport any victim with an unstable lower extremity fracture or dislocation with the limb elevated.
11. Take great care in serially examining the limb for the possibility of a compartment syndrome because this is the most common location for this problem.

Box 13-4.

Traction Mechanisms

Historically, the first traction mechanism that comes to mind is the Boy Scout–style "Spanish windlass." A windlass works, but it can be awkward to apply and is often not durable. The windlass can unwind if it is inadvertently jarred and can apply rotational forces to the leg.

The amount of traction required is primarily a function of victim comfort. A general rule is to use 10% of body weight or about 10 to 15 pounds for the average victim. After traction is applied, always recheck distal neurovascular function (circulation, sensation, movement). An improvised traction system invariably relaxes during transport and should be rechecked for proper tension.

CAM LOCK OR FASTEX SLIDER
This is a simple, effective system that uses straps that have Fastex-like sliders and are often used as waist belts or to strap items to packs. Alternatively, use a cam lock with nylon webbing. Attach the belt to the distal portion of the rigid support and then to the ankle hitch. Traction is easily applied by cinching the nylon webbing (Fig. 13-19).

TRUCKER'S HITCH
Fashion a windlass using small-diameter line (parachute cord) and a standard trucker's hitch for additional mechanical advantage (Fig 13-20). An adjustable tent pole allows traction to be applied by elongating the pole during manual traction.

PRUSIK KNOT
This is useful with almost any system (see Fig 13-18, A). Prusik knots provide traction from rigid supports

Continued

Box 13-4.
Traction Mechanisms—cont'd

PRUSIK KNOT—cont'd
with few tie-on points (e.g., a canoe paddle shaft or a tent pole). The Prusik knot can be used to apply the traction (by sliding the knot distally) or simply as an attachment point for one of the traction mechanisms already mentioned.

LITTER TRACTION
If no rigid support is available and a rigid litter (e.g., Stokes) is being used, apply traction from the rigid bar at the foot end of the litter. If this system is used, you must immobilize the victim on the litter with adequate countertraction, such as that using inguinal straps.

PROXIMAL ANCHOR
The simplest proximal anchor uses a single ischial strap, which can be made from a piece of climbing webbing or a prefabricated strap, belt, or cam lock (see Fig. 13-19). A cloth cravat can be used in a pinch. On the river a life jacket can be used (Fig. 13-21), and when climbing, a climbing harness is ideal. The preferred system is a proximal ischial strap, but a padded medial support (analogous to a Sager splint) can also be used. When using a medial traction system (Sager analog), generously pad the inguinal area. A folded SAM splint attached to the proximal end of the rigid support works well.

SECURING AND PADDING
All potential pressure points should be checked to ensure that they are adequately padded. An excellent padding system can be made by first covering the upper and lower parts of the leg with a folded length of

Box 13-4.

Traction Mechanisms—cont'd

SECURING AND PADDING—cont'd
Ensolite (Fig. 13-22). Folded Ensolite is preferred over the circumferential wrap because the folded system allows for visualization of the extremity if necessary. The victim will be more comfortable if femoral traction is applied with the knee in slight flexion (place padding beneath the knee during transport). The splint must be secured firmly to the leg. Almost any straplike object will work, but a 10- to 15-cm (4- to 6-inch) Ace bandage wrapped circumferentially will provide a comfortable and secure union. Finally, the ankles or feet should be strapped or tied together to give the system additional stability. Tying the ankles together also protects the injured leg from external rotation and jarring during transport.

Ankle

The intraarticular distal tibia, medial malleolus, distal fibula, or any combination of these may be involved in an ankle fracture, generally produced by large torsional forces around a fixed foot. With the distal tibia, axial loading from a fall or jump may also be involved.

Signs and Symptoms
Significant pain and swelling when the shoe is removed

Treatment
1. Palpate along the medial and lateral malleoli to confirm the clinical suspicion.

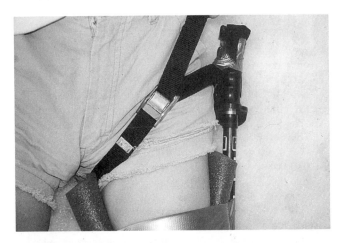

Fig. 13-19. Proximal anchor using cam-lock belt. Belt is applied as shown. Ski pole is used laterally as the rigid support. Duct tape is useful for securing components. Padding is helpful but not always necessary if victim is wearing pants.

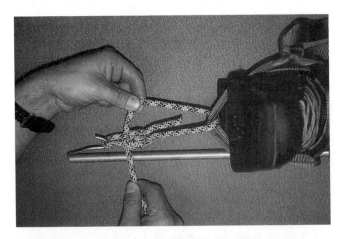

Fig. 13-20. Tent pole traction with trucker's hitch. A bent tent stake is placed into end of tent pole as the distal traction anchor. A simple trucker's hitch is used to provide traction.

2. After the shoe is removed to inspect the skin for open wounds, perform a neurocirculatory examination.
3. With a rotational deformity in the ankle, realign the ankle with gentle traction before applying a posterior splint with the ankle in neutral position.
4. Apply a U-shaped blanket roll or pillow splint.
5. During transport, make sure the limb is elevated above the level of the heart, with the victim supine on a backboard if possible.

Tarsals

Signs and Symptoms

1. Fracture of the calcaneus and talus during a fall or jump from a significant height when the victim lands on his or her feet
2. With calcaneal fracture, significant heel pain, deformity, and crepitus immediately evident after the boot is removed
3. With talar fracture, may be impossible to differentiate clinically from ankle fracture
   a. Occurs when the foot is forced into maximum dorsiflexion
   b. Tenderness and swelling distal to the malleoli
   c. Generally not associated with ankle fractures, but may be associated with dislocations of the subtalar joint, with which the deformity is more significant
4. With ankle fracture, tenderness and deformity at the level of the malleoli
5. Fractures of the other tarsal bones, while exceedingly rare, defined by localizing the tenderness to a specific site

Treatment

1. Apply a short-leg splint with extra padding for all these fractures.
2. Elevate the limb during transportation.
3. If a talar fracture is suspected, expedite evacuation of

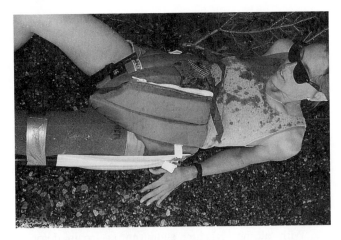

Fig. 13-21. Life jacket proximal anchor. An inverted life jacket worn like a diaper forms a well-padded proximal anchor. A kayak paddle is rigged to life jacket's side adjustment strap.

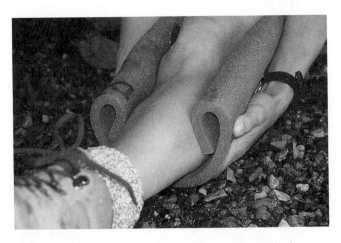

Fig. 13-22. Folding Ensolite padding often provides better visualization of extremity than does a circumferential wrap.

the victim because posttraumatic necrosis of the talar body is a common complication.

Metatarsals

Fracture at the base of a metatarsal often occurs in combination with a midfoot dislocation. Fractures frequently occur across the entire midfoot joint and are often associated with fractures at the bases of the second and fifth metatarsals. They usually occur with axial loading of the foot while it is in maximum plantar flexion.

Metatarsal shaft fractures occur with crush injuries and with falls or jumps from moderate heights. Midshaft metatarsal fracture also occurs as a stress, or so-called march, fracture. This injury is often the result of prolonged hiking or running.

Signs and Symptoms

1. With metatarsal base fracture
   a. Midfoot pain and swelling
   b. Once the shoe is removed, crepitus and tenderness at the base of the metatarsal
   c. Generally, overall alignment of the foot maintained, but instability is revealed with stressing the midfoot by stabilizing the heel and placing stress across the forefoot in the varus and valgus directions
2. With metatarsal shaft fracture
   a. Dull pain at the midshaft of a metatarsal (often the second or fifth) converted to more severe pain with associated crepitus by a jump from a log or rock
   b. Hallmarks: pain, localized tenderness

Treatment

1. For metatarsal base fracture, place the foot in a well-padded posterior splint and elevate it whenever possible.
2. Do not allow a victim with a suspected midfoot fracture/dislocation to ambulate under any circum-

stances because swelling will intensify and further injury to the midfoot may result.

3. For metatarsal shaft fracture, manage temporarily by having the victim wear a stiff-soled boot or orthotic insert. If fracture instability or extreme pain is present, apply a short-leg splint and allow no further weight bearing.

Phalanx

The great toe phalanx fracture is a significant problem functionally because of the necessary force placed on the great toe during the toe-off phase of weight bearing. A toe phalanx can be fractured by a crush injury or by having a heavy object drop onto the foot. This injury can be prevented by the use of a steel-toed or hard-toed boot.

Signs and Symptoms
1. Pain
2. Ecchymosis

Treatment
1. Manage any phalanx fracture by taping the toe to an adjacent uninjured toe with cotton placed in between.
2. Be aware that a stiff-soled boot minimizes the discomfort accompanying weight bearing.

LOWER EXTREMITY DISLOCATIONS
Hip

Posterior hip dislocation is produced by axial loading of the femur with the limb in relative adduction.

Signs and Symptoms
1. With posterior dislocation, severe pain around the hip
2. Affected limb apparently shortened and adducted, with any hip motion increasing the pain
3. Not clinically possible to determine presence of an associated acetabular fracture

4. With rare case of anterior dislocation, limb abducted and flexed; dislocation generally produced by wide abduction of the hip from a significant force

Treatment

1. Place the victim in a supine position, and perform a complete survey of all organ systems. Examine the distal limb carefully for associated fracture(s), and perform a careful sensory and motor examination.
2. When the victim is any distance from definitive care, attempt a closed reduction.
   a. Place the victim on a flat, hard surface.
   b. Provide analgesia with a narcotic, benzodiazepine, or both if available.
   c. Have an assistant stabilize the pelvis by placing both palms on the anterior iliac crests. Bend the victim's knee, and apply upward linear traction in line with the thigh (with an anterior dislocation) and with the hip flexed 30 degrees (with a posterior dislocation) (Fig. 13-23).
3. If this maneuver fails to reduce the hip, expedite evacuation because a direct relationship exists between the time to reduction and the incidence of osteonecrosis of the femoral head.

Knee

The tibia may be dislocated in any of four directions relative to the distal femur. The most common direction is anterior (tibia anterior to the femur). This injury represents a true emergency because of the high incidence of associated vascular injury, which occurs because of tethering of the popliteal vessels along the posterior border of the tibia by the soleus fascia.

Signs and Symptoms

1. Knee dislocation obvious because of the amount of deformity involved
2. Intimal flap tears, possibly producing delayed arterial thrombosis

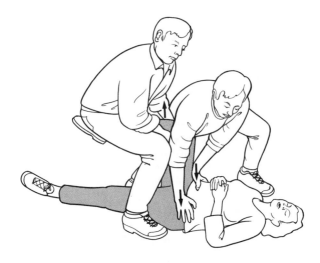

Fig. 13-23.   Reduction of dislocated hip.

Treatment
1. When this injury is suspected, perform a careful neurocirculatory screening examination. Be aware that intact distal pulses do not definitively rule out an arterial injury.
2. After the initial examination, apply linear traction to the lower limb to reduce the knee. This is generally successful regardless of the dislocation's direction.
3. For transport, apply a posterior splint to the limb and move the victim on a backboard.
4. Be vigilant to the possibility of an arterial lesion or emerging compartment syndrome. If this is suspected, arrange for emergency evacuation because of the risk of losing the limb.

Patellar Dislocation
Patellofemoral dislocation is seen frequently. Because of the increased femorotibial angle in a female, this injury is much more common in women. Generalized ligamen-

tous laxity may predispose to this problem. Dislocation of the kneecap may result from a twisting injury or asymmetric quadriceps contraction during a fall.

Signs and Symptoms
1. Pain
2. Malposition of patella

Treatment
1. Be aware that the patella lies lateral to the articular distal femur. Although neurovascular injury rarely occurs in association with this injury, conduct a screening examination.
2. Reduce the patella by simply straightening the knee, if possible.
3. If this is not successful, apply gentle pressure to the patella to push it back up onto the distal femoral articular groove.
4. Apply a knee splint with the joint in extension. Encourage the victim to avoid weight bearing, but if this is not possible, be aware that further damage is unlikely.
5. Keep the victim's knee in extension until definitive care can be obtained.
6. Note that a radiograph is ultimately required to rule out osteochondral fracture, which is frequently associated with an acute injury.

Ankle
Signs and Symptoms
1. Ankle dislocation almost always accompanied by fracture(s) of one or both malleoli
2. Swelling
3. Pain

Treatment
1. Align the ankle joint by grasping the victim's posterior heel, applying traction with the knee bent (to relax the gastrocnemius-soleus complex), and bringing the foot into alignment with the distal tibia.

2. After this maneuver, reexamine the foot, dress any wounds, and apply a posterior splint. Note that a U-shaped blanket roll or pillow splint can also be applied.
3. During transport, make sure the limb is kept elevated.
4. Be aware that this type of inversion injury is infrequently associated with fracture at the insertion of the peroneus brevis tendon. You may identify the presence of this injury with point tenderness at the base of the fifth metatarsal, but a radiograph is required for definitive diagnosis. Early management is the same as for a sprain.

Hindfoot

Signs and Symptoms
Calcaneus dislocated medially or laterally relative to the talus, the latter being slightly more common

Treatment
1. Attempt a reduction if it will be more than 3 hours until the victim can be transported to a definitive care center.
2. If no other injuries are apparent, give the victim a sedative during reduction.
3. Be aware that medial dislocation is reduced more easily than lateral dislocation, in which the posterior tibial tendon frequently becomes displaced onto the lateral neck of the talus, blocking the reduction. In either case, the maneuver is the same.
   a. Grasp the heel with the victim's knee flexed (relaxing the gastrocnemius-soleus complex), and apply linear traction to bring the heel over the ankle joint.
   b. Be aware that this maneuver is generally successful for medial dislocation, but lateral dislocation often requires open reduction.
4. After you attempt reduction, apply a posterior splint, U-shaped blanket roll, or pillow splint.

5. Make sure the limb is elevated.
6. Even if the reduction is successful, do not allow the victim to bear weight until definitive care is obtained.

Midfoot

Midfoot (Lisfranc's) dislocation is generally associated with one or more fractures at the base of the metatarsals, usually the second and fifth metatarsals. Midfoot dislocation occurs with axial loading of the foot in maximum plantar flexion.

Signs and Symptoms
1. Forefoot generally displaced laterally relative to the midfoot when the injury is initially unstable; more often the foot is normally aligned
2. Significant swelling with tenderness at the base of the second and fifth metatarsals
3. Instability and crepitus, with dorsoplantar-oriented force frequent

Treatment
1. After the neurocirculatory examination, stress the forefoot by stabilizing the heel and applying a varus- and valgus-directed force. If the forefoot is unstable and associated with significant swelling, pain, or crepitus, consider a midfoot dislocation to be present.
2. Apply a short-leg (posterior or U-shaped) splint.
3. Elevate the foot during transport.
4. Do not allow the victim to bear weight.

Metatarsophalangeal and Interphalangeal Joints

Metatarsophalangeal joint dislocation of a toe is relatively uncommon but can occur in the great toe with moderate axial force. An injury of this type at the great toe may be associated with a fracture of the metatarsal or phalanx; the dislocation is generally distal.

The lesser metatarsophalangeal joints are generally dislocated laterally or medially. The most common mechanism for this injury is striking unshod toes on immovable objects.

Signs and Symptoms
1. Open fracture
2. Pain
3. Swelling
4. Ecchymosis

Treatment
1. Because this may be an open fracture, perform a careful inspection of the foot.
2. Relocate the toe by applying linear traction with the victim supine and using the weight of the foot as countertraction.
3. Also, consider reduction of an interphalangeal joint by applying linear traction with gentle manipulation.
4. Once reduced, tape the injured toe to the adjacent toe for 1 to 3 weeks.
5. Have the victim wear a protective boot with a stiff sole and deep toe box.

CHAPTER 14

Wounds
(Laceration and Abrasion)

■ **LACERATION** ■

DEFINITIONS

A *laceration*, although the most obvious sign of trauma, is rarely life threatening. It represents an injury to the integument and may overlie an occult injury, such as a fracture, or may extend into the joint space.

GENERAL TREATMENT

The goals of wilderness wound management are to minimize infection, promote healing, and decrease the need for evacuation. Five specific steps should be followed: examination, anesthesia, cleaning and débridement, wound closure or packing, and bandaging. (See Box 14-1.)

Examination

1. For an extremity injury, evaluate the distal neurovascular function before administering local anesthesia.
   a. For wrist and hand lacerations, palpate the radial and ulnar pulses.
   b. Compare capillary refill, color, and temperature of each finger to the corresponding finger on the uninjured hand.
   c. Assess sensation of the radial and ulnar aspects of

Box 14-1.

First-aid Supplies Recommended for Wound and Abrasion Management

WOUND MANAGEMENT

10- to 15-ml irrigation syringe with an 18-gauge catheter tip

1 fl oz povidone-iodine solution USP 10% (Betadine)

Wound closure strips ¼ × 4 inches

Tincture of benzoin

Polysporin or double antibiotic ointment

Tweezers

Sterile surgical gloves

4 × 4-inch sterile dressings

Nonadherent sterile dressing (Aquaphor, Xeroform, Adaptic, Telfa)

Elastic conforming bandage

Assorted adhesive bandages

Tape

Surgical stapler, suture material, and suturing supplies

Cyanoacrylate glue ("superglue")

ABRASION MANAGEMENT

First-aid cleansing pads, 2% to 4% liquid lidocaine, viscous lidocaine jelly

Surgical scrub brush

Spenco 2nd Skin or other nonadherent dressing

Conforming stockinette bandage or nonwoven adhesive knit bandage

Aloe vera gel

Polysporin or double antibiotic ointment

Tape

each finger to sharp pain and two-point discrimination.

2. Explore the wound in good light conditions for tendon, muscle, or nerve injury; also look for foreign material. Test the motor function of each joint against resistance by isolating the joint and asking the victim to flex and extend the digit against resistance. A tendon that is 75% lacerated can still have function, but it should be decreased to resistance compared with the uninjured finger on the opposite hand.

Anesthesia

Topical Anesthesia

1. Mix equal parts of tetracaine 0.5%, adrenaline 1:2000, and cocaine 11.8% (TAC), and allow it to soak into a 2 × 2-inch sterile gauze pad. Place this directly around and in the wound for 7 to 10 minutes. The maximum dose of the solution is 2 to 5 ml for adults.

2. Do *not* use TAC on the ear, tip of the nose, or penis, and use it only with caution on highly permeable tissue, such as mucous membranes. Eliminating the cocaine, increasing the concentration of tetracaine to 1.87%, and decreasing the concentration of adrenaline to 1:15,000 may achieve an equivalent level of anesthesia.

Local Anesthesia

1. Infiltrate the wound with 1% lidocaine (Xylocaine) without epinephrine or 0.25% bupivacaine (Marcaine) using a 25-gauge needle and syringe.

2. The adult dose of lidocaine should not exceed 300 to 400 mg (30 to 40 ml). The maximum children's dose is 4 mg/kg body weight or 0.4 ml/kg of a 1% solution.

3. Buffering lidocaine reduces the pain of local anesthetic infiltration. To buffer, add 1 ml of sodium bi-

carbonate (1 mEq/ml solution) to 10 ml 1% lidocaine. Once buffered, the shelf life of the product is greatly reduced; discard the solution after 24 hours.

4. Alternative anesthetic strategies include the following:
   a. Diphenhydramine (Benadryl) has anesthetic properties similar to those of lidocaine. Dilute a 50-mg (1-ml) vial in a syringe with 4 ml normal saline (NS) solution to produce a 1% solution. Perform local infiltration as usual.
   b. Use NS solution alone as the injecting agent. This may provide just enough anesthesia to suture a small wound.
   c. Place ice directly over the wound to provide a short period of decreased pain sensation.

Cleaning and Débridement

1. Perform wound cleansing to remove as much bacteria, dirt, and damaged tissue as possible. The best method is to use a 10- to 15-ml syringe with an 18-gauge catheter attached to the end as a "squirt gun" to deliver a high-pressure stream.
2. Make sure the irrigating solution is clean and nontoxic to the tissues. Sterile NS solution, disinfected tap water, and 1% povidone-iodine solution (not "scrub") are all suitable for irrigation.
3. Use benzalkonium chloride to cleanse wounds inflicted by animals suspected of being rabid (see Chapter 30). The quantity of irrigation fluid should be at least 400 ml.

Irrigation Method

1. Draw the irrigation solution into a 10- to 15-ml syringe and attach an 18-gauge catheter tip.
2. Hold the syringe so the catheter tip is 2.5 to 5 cm (1 to 2 inches) above the wound and perpendicular to the skin surface. Push down forcefully on the plunger while prying open the edges of the wound

with your fingers, and squirt the solution into the wound (Fig. 14-1, *A*). Be careful to avoid being splashed by the irrigant after it hits the skin (put on a pair of sunglasses or goggles to protect your eyes from the spray).

3. Repeat this procedure until you have irrigated the wound with at least 200 ml of solution.
4. Remove any residual debris or devitalized tissue with a tweezers, scissors, knife, or any other sharp object. Even one or two particles of dirt left in a wound increase the likelihood of infection.
5. If the wound edges are macerated, crushed, or necrotic, perform sharp débridement.
6. Improvised wound irrigation requires only a puncturable container to hold water, such as a sandwich or garbage bag, and a safety pin or 18-gauge needle. Fill the bag with irrigation solution and puncture the bottom of the bag with the safety pin. Enlarge the hole if necessary by puncturing it a second time. Hold the bag just above the wound and squeeze the top firmly to begin irrigating (Fig. 14-1, *B*).

DEFINITIVE WOUND CARE

Lacerations that are not at high risk for infection can be safely closed in the backcountry. Time is a critical factor, however, and the longer closure is delayed, the more likely the wound is to become infected after it is closed. The "golden period" for closing most wounds is within 8 hours after the injury.

High-risk Wounds

High-risk wounds that should not be closed in the backcountry include animal or human bites to the hand, wrist, or foot, over a major joint, or through the cheek; any cat bite or scratch wound; deep puncture wounds; deep wounds on the hand or foot; wounds that contain a large amount of crushed or devitalized tissue; and wounds that are older than 8 hours.

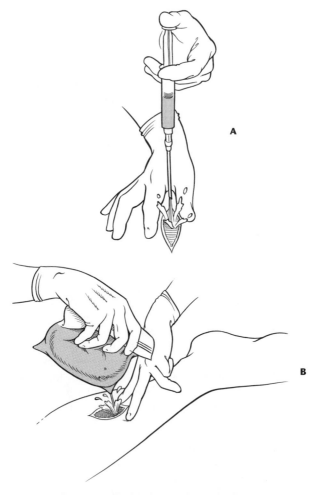

Fig. 14-1.   Wound irrigation. **A,** Syringe. **B,** Plastic bag.

Treatment

1. Pack the wound open with saline- or water-moistened gauze dressings, after irrigation and débridement.

2. Cover the packed wound with a conforming bandage, and splint the extremity in an elevated position.

3. Start the victim on an immediate course of antibiotic therapy. Options include amoxicillin-clavulanate 500 mg q6h, cephalexin 500 mg q6h, or penicillin 500 mg and dicloxacillin 500 mg q6h.

4. Change the packing at least once a day.

5. Close the wound with sutures or tape after 4 to 5 days if there is no sign of infection (delayed primary closure).

Low-Risk Wounds

Treatment

1. Wound taping is the preferred way to close a laceration in the backcountry. Use wound closure tape strips or butterfly bandages. Wound closure strips are stronger, longer, stickier, and more porous than butterfly bandages.

    a. Achieve hemostasis and dry the wound edges.

    b. Clip off hair near the wound with a scissors so that tape will adhere better. Hair farther from the wound edge can be shaved. Avoid shaving hair directly adjacent to the wound edge because shaving abrades the skin and increases the potential for infection.

    c. Apply a thin layer of tincture of benzoin evenly along both sides of the wound and allow it to dry (Fig. 14-2, *A*).

    d. Secure one half of the tape to one side of the wound. Oppose the other wound edge with a finger while using the free end of the tape as a handle to help pull the wound closed (Fig. 14-2, *B*). Avoid squeezing the wound edges tightly to-

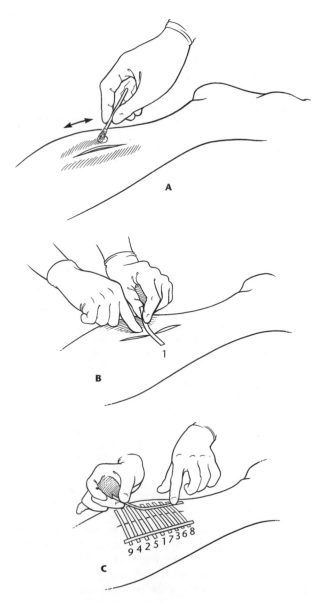

Fig. 14-2. Wound taping.

gether. They should just touch. Attach the other end of the tape to the skin.

   e. Allow the tape to overlap the wound edge by 2 to 3 cm (¾ to 1¼ inches) on each side, and space the strips 2 to 3 mm apart to allow drainage.

   f. Place cross-stays of tape perpendicular to and over the tape ends to prevent them from peeling off (Fig. 14-2, C).

   g. Note that wound closure strips can be improvised from duct tape or other self-adhering tape. Cut 1-cm (¼-inch) strips and then punch tiny holes along the length of the tape with a safety pin to allow drainage.

2. If no tape is available, glue strips of cloth or nylon from your clothes, pack, or tent to the skin with a "superglue."

   a. Place a drop of glue on the material and hold it on the skin until it dries.

   b. Use the other end of the strip to the pull the wound closed, and glue it to the skin on the other side of the wound.

   c. Avoid getting any glue into the wound. The glue is generally safe on intact skin but should not be used on the face.

   d. Expect the strips to fall off after about 3 days. The strips can be reapplied with fresh glue.

3. For a scalp laceration, assuming the victim has enough hair, close the wound by tying opposing strands of hair adjacent to the wound.

   a. Take a piece of heavy suture material or dental floss, and lay it on top of and parallel to the wound (Fig. 14-3, A).

   b. Twirl a few strands of hair on opposite sides of the wound and pull them together tightly, forcing the wound edges closed. Use the suture material to tie the opposing strands of hair together (Fig. 14-3, B).

4. Use sutures and staples for large gaping cuts, wounds that are under tension or that cross a joint, or

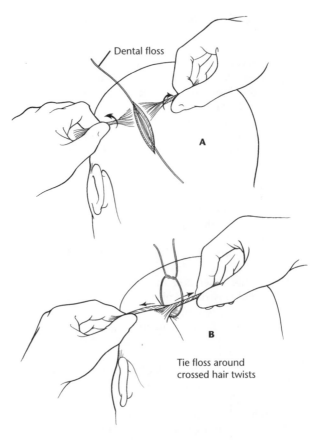

Dental floss

A

B

Tie floss around
crossed hair twists

Fig. 14-3. Scalp laceration closed using dental floss.

any other wounds that are difficult to keep closed
with tape.

a. Skin stapling is a relatively fast technique for closing wounds and is ideal for use in the wilderness,
   when evacuation to a medical facility is not
   readily available.

b. Staples are as strong as sutures, and more impor-

tantly, they produce less of an inflammatory response and have less chance of producing a wound infection.
  c. The cosmetic outcome is the same for both sutures and staples.
  d. Staples should not be used on the feet, hands, or face or if the laceration extends into tendons or muscles.
  e. Staples are left in place for the same length of time as sutures in similar anatomic sites.
  f. Staple removal requires a special device that is provided by each manufacturer.

Stapling Technique
1. Stapling devices have evolved significantly in the last several years. My choice for backcountry use is the 3M Precise Disposable Skin Stapler with 25 staples.
2. Squeeze the stapler partway until it clicks and you feel resistance. The two points of the staple should now be protruding out from the stapler (Fig. 14-4, *A*).
3. Grab one edge of the cut with one of the staples and use it as a hook to pull the wound closed. Use your index finger on the other hand to push the other wound edge in until the wound edges just meet (Fig. 14-4, *B*). Hold the stapler upright at a 90-degree angle to the wound, and make sure that the stapler is positioned evenly over the cut so that it does not overlap one wound edge more than the other. Gently and evenly squeeze the stapler with your thumb as shown to advance the staple into the tissue (Fig. 14-4, *C*).
4. Once the staple is seated, relax your thumb pressure fully on the stapler and back the stapler out to disengage it.

Wound Bandaging
1. The best dressing is one that does not stick to the wound. Many nonadherent dressings are available, including Aquaphor, Xeroform, Adaptic, and Telfa.
2. Apply an antiseptic ointment such as bacitracin or

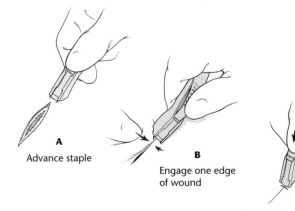

A
Advance staple

B
Engage one edge
of wound

C

Fig. 14-4. Wound stapling.

Polysporin to the surface of the wound before bandaging. Honey has certain antibacterial properties and can be combined if absolutely necessary with a gauze pad to create a nonadherent dressing.

■ ABRASION ■

DEFINITION
An *abrasion* is an area of scraped or denuded skin that is often embedded with dirt, gravel, and other debris, which can result in scarring or infection.

GENERAL TREATMENT (see Box 14-1)
1. Apply a topical anesthetic, such as 2% to 4% lidocaine or viscous lidocaine jelly, over the wound and let it sit for 5 to 10 minutes, or wipe the area with a lidocaine-containing cleansing pad.
2. Vigorously scrub the abrasion with a surgical brush or cleansing pad until all foreign material is removed.
3. Use a tweezers to pick out any embedded particles. Irrigate the abrasion with NS solution or water.

4. Apply a thin layer of topical antiseptic ointment, aloe vera gel, or, as a last resort, honey to the abrasion.

5. Cover with a nonadherent protective dressing and secure it in place with a bandage. Spenco 2nd Skin works well because it soothes and cools the wound while providing an ideal healing environment. The dressing can also be secured with a stockinette or nonwoven adhesive knit bandage and left in place for several days, as long as there is no sign of infection.

CHAPTER 15

Firearm and Arrow Injuries

FIREARM INJURY

Injuries caused by firearms differ in severity and type according to velocity of the bullet, whether fragmentation occurs, creation of a permanent cavity, presence of powder burns, and type of tissue struck.

General Treatment

1. Follow the basic principles of trauma care and resuscitation, including airway, breathing, circulation, control of bleeding, immobilization of the spine and fractured extremities, wound care, and stabilization of the victim for transport (see Chapter 7).
2. Remove the weapon from the vicinity where you are giving medical care. It may be wise to also remove the ammunition and open the firing chamber.
3. Perform endotracheal intubation as soon as possible if the victim has a neck wound and expanding hematoma. If endotracheal intubation is not possible and the airway becomes obstructed, perform a cricothyrotomy.
4. Provide immediate relief of a tension pneumothorax with a needle or tube thoracostomy, or occlusion of a sucking chest wound with petrolatum-impregnated gauze.

5. Control external bleeding by direct pressure and compression wraps.
6. Treat for shock and hypothermia.
7. Do *not* perform wide débridement of normal-appearing tissue.
8. Monitor the neurovascular status of an extremity wound; keep the extremity elevated to minimize swelling.
9. Be aware that the path of the bullet cannot be determined by connecting the entrance and exit wounds.
10. Note that removal of the bullet or bullet fragments is not necessary unless the bullet is intravascular, intraarticular, or in contact with nervous tissue.
11. Use forceps to remove from the skin any shotgun pellets that have minimal penetration.
12. For powder burns, remove as much of the powder residue as possible with a scrub brush because the powder will tattoo the skin if left in place.

ARROW INJURY
Arrowheads are designed to inflict injury by lacerating tissue and blood vessels, causing bleeding and shock.

General Treatment
1. Follow the same treatment principles of trauma care and resuscitation as for a firearm injury.
2. Irrigate the wound, remove any foreign material, and close lacerations primarily following the guidelines in Chapter 14.
3. Stabilize the victim for transport, leaving any embedded arrow in place during transport if possible. Cut the shaft of the arrow and leave about 10 cm (3 or 4 inches) protruding from the wound to make transport easier, if this can be accomplished with a minimum of arrow movement.
4. Fix the portion of the arrow that remains in the

wound with a stack of gauze pads or with cloth and tape.
5. Transfer the victim as quickly as possible to a medical care facility for removal of the arrow under controlled conditions.

CHAPTER 16

Fishhook Injury

Fishhooks have a barb or multiple barbs just proximal to the tip that are curved so that the more force that is applied to the hook, the deeper it penetrates. The barb does not allow the hook to be backed out.

GENERAL TREATMENT

1. Clean the skin surrounding the entry point with an antiseptic or with soap and water.
2. Remove the hook using one of the following techniques:
   a. Pass a string or shoelace through and around the bend of the hook. The hook can then be yanked from the skin while the shank of the hook is pressed against the skin surface to disengage the barb (Fig. 16-1).
   b. With a steady, firm motion, push the hook through the skin so that the barb completely appears. Cut off the barb or the shaft, and pull the remainder of the hook back out of the skin (Fig. 16-2).
3. Irrigate the wound with saline solution or water.
4. For a fishhook embedded in the eye, leave it in place and secure it with tape. Cover the eye with a metal patch or cup, and transport the victim to an ophthalmologist for definitive care.

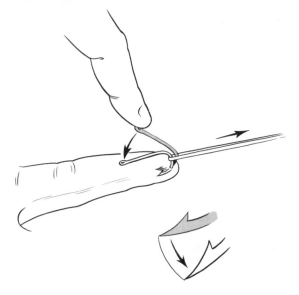

Fig. 16-1.   Fishhook removal.

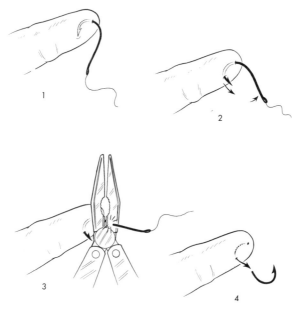

Fig. 16-2. Removal of a fishhook that has penetrated a fingertip.

CHAPTER 17

Sprains and Strains

DEFINITIONS

A sprain is the stretching or tearing of ligaments that attach one bone to another. Symptoms include tenderness at the site, swelling, ecchymosis, and pain with movement. Because these symptoms are also present with a fracture, it may be difficult to differentiate between the two.

A strain is an injury to a muscle or its tendon. Strains often result from overexertion or lifting and pulling a heavy object without using good body mechanics. Symptoms are initially the same as for sprains.

GENERAL TREATMENT

1. First-aid treatment for sprain and strain injuries is summarized by the acronym *RICES:* rest, ice, compression, elevation, and stabilization. Maintain RICES for the first 72 hours after any injury.

    a. *Rest.* Rest takes the stress off the injured joint and prevents further ligament and tendon damage.

    b. *Ice.* Ice reduces swelling and eases pain. For ice or cold therapy to be effective, apply ice early and for up to 20 minutes at least 3 or 4 times a day, followed by compression bandaging. If a compression wrap is not applied after ice therapy, the joint will swell as soon as the ice is removed.

c. *Compression.* A compression wrap prevents swelling and provides some support. Make the wrap by placing some padding (socks, gloves, pieces of Ensolite pad) over the sprained joint and then wrapping it with an elastic bandage. Wrap from distal to proximal. Make sure the wrap is comfortably tight. Monitor the extremity for numbness, tingling, or increased pain, which may indicate that the compression wrap is too tight and should be loosened.

    d. *Elevation.* Elevate the injured joint above the level of the heart as much as possible to reduce swelling.

    e. *Stabilization.* Tape or splint the injured part to prevent further injury.

2. Administer an NSAID, such as ibuprofen 600 to 800 mg q6-8h, to reduce pain and inflammation.

DISORDERS
Ankle Injuries
Ankle Sprain
Signs and symptoms

1. Ankle sprain: most commonly injured ligaments on the lateral aspect of the joint (anterior and posterior talofibular ligaments)
2. Ankle fracture: victim unable to bear weight or has bony tenderness to palpation at the posterior edge or tip of the lateral or medial malleolus
3. Foot fracture: victim unable to bear weight or has point bony tenderness to palpation at the base of the fifth metatarsal or navicular bone

Treatment

1. Follow RICES.
2. If the victim can walk, tape the ankle for support with an "open basket crossweave stirrup pattern" to prevent further injury (Fig. 17-1). An SAM splint can

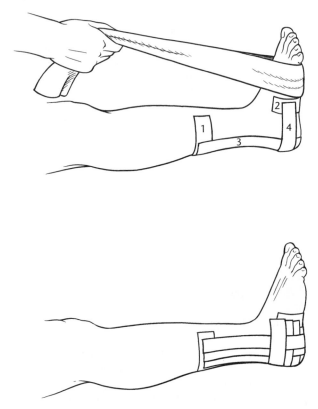

Fig. 17-1. Sprained ankle taped using an "open basket crossweave stirrup pattern."

also be wrapped around the foot and ankle, with the shoe in place, and secured with tape (Fig. 17-2).
3. To more securely tape an ankle:
   a. Apply an adhesive tape anchor strip halfway around the lower leg about 15 cm (6 inches) above the malleoli. Leave a 2.5- to 5-cm (1- to 2-inch) gap in front to allow for swelling.

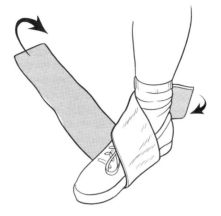

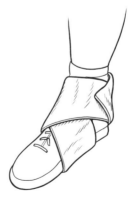

Fig. 17-2. SAM splint on ankle.

b. You can apply an additional anchor strip at the instep of the foot. Leave a 1- to 2-inch gap on the top of the foot.

c. Apply the first of five stirrup strips. Begin on the inside of the upper anchor, and wrap a piece of tape down the inside of the leg, over the inside medial malleolus, across the bottom of the foot, and up the outside part of the leg over the lateral malleolus, ending at the outer aspect of the upper anchor. Apply proper tension to prevent the ankle from inverting.

d. Apply the first of six to eight interconnecting horseshoe strips. Begin at the anchor on the inside of the foot, and wrap below the medial malleolus around the heel, below the lateral malleolus, and ending at the anchor on the outer part of the foot.

e. Repeat steps c and d. Remember to overlap the tape one half its width. These interlocking strips should provide excellent support for a walking person. At the end of these vertical and horizontal strips, a 1- to 2-inch gap on the top of the foot and ankle will allow for swelling.

f. On both sides, secure the tape ends with two vertical strips of tape running from the foot anchor to the calf anchor.

g. Beginning at the toes, wrap an elastic rolled bandage around the foot and ankle.

Ruptured Achilles Tendon
Signs and symptoms

1. An audible pop, with a feeling of being kicked in the calf
2. Inability to plantar-flex the foot
3. Swelling of the distal calf
4. Sometimes, a palpable defect in the tendon 2 to 6 cm (about 1 to 2½ inches) proximal to its insertion
5. No plantar flexion of the foot as the calf is squeezed (Thompson's test)

Treatment

1. If the tendon is strained and not completely torn or ruptured, follow RICES.
2. Have the victim gently stretch the tendon to keep it flexible, then gradually put weight on the foot, with walking as pain allows.
3. If the Achilles tendon is ruptured, walking will not be possible. Splint the ankle and evacuate the victim because surgery is needed to repair the torn tendon.

Knee Injuries

Overuse (Chronic) Knee Injury

Patellofemoral syndrome. This is the most common overuse syndrome and is also known as *chondromalacia patellae*.

Signs and symptoms

1. A dull aching pain under the patella or in the center of the knee that is aggravated by climbing or descending a hill or by sitting for a long period with the knee bent
2. Swollen knee
3. Crepitus, often heard when knee is flexed and extended

Treatment

1. Apply ice, and allow the victim to rest.
2. Administer an NSAID, such as ibuprofen 600 to 800 mg q8h.
3. Place a wide, supporting elastic band around the leg below the patella to help prevent pain during walking. This should not be overly tight.
4. Use two trekking or ski poles while hiking to help absorb impact and reduce pain.

Iliotibial band syndrome. This is an irritation of the connective tissue along the outside of the thigh.

Signs and symptoms

1. Stinging pain along the outside of the knee aggravated by running downhill or jumping
2. Pain reproduced by pressing on the outside of the upper knee

Treatment

1. Apply ice, and allow the victim to rest.
2. Administer an NSAID, such as ibuprofen 600 to 800 mg q8h.

Traumatic (Acute) Knee Injury

Ligament sprain. Twisting, rotating, or falling in an awkward position is more likely to produce a sprain injury to one of the major ligaments that support the knee than to create a fracture.

Signs and symptoms

1. An audible pop at the time of the injury and immediate pain that soon becomes a dull ache
2. For a severe sprain, instability of the knee while walking or turning
3. Severity based on percentage of ligament injured
   a. First-degree sprain: pain but no instability when the knee is stressed
   b. Second-degree sprain: pain and slight instability when the knee is stressed
   c. Third-degree sprain: significant instability but no pain when the knee is stressed, which denotes a completely torn ligament

Treatment

1. For first-degree sprain, use RICES. Walking can usually be resumed with little or no additional support.
2. For second-degree sprain, use RICES. Ensure that the victim wears a knee immobilizer while walking. This

device should be cylindrical and extend from the midthigh to the midcalf. Improvised materials that can be used include an Ensolite or Therm-a-Rest pad, life jacket, or internal-frame pack stays held in place with tape or bandannas. Cut a circular hole for the patella.

3. For third-degree sprain, use RICES. Do not allow the victim to walk without a knee immobilizer in place. If, after applying a knee immobilizer, the victim's knee still feels unstable and is prone to buckling with weight, evacuate the person without allowing walking.

Torn meniscus (cartilage). Menisci are crescent-shaped pieces of cartilage situated between the femur and tibia that act as shock absorbers for the knee. Partial or total tears of the meniscus often occur at the same time that ligaments are torn.

Signs and symptoms

1. Pain localized to the anterior joint space after activity (most common symptom)
2. Catching, clicking, or locking of the knee
3. Occasionally, joint painfully locked in a partially flexed position

Treatment

1. Apply ice, and allow the victim to rest.
2. Administer a NSAID, such as ibuprofen 600 to 800 mg q8h.
3. If the knee feels unstable, apply a complete immobilizer.
4. If the victim has a locked knee, attempt to unlock it by positioning the victim with the leg hanging over the edge of a table or flat surface with the knee in approximately 90 degrees of flexion. After a period of relaxation, apply longitudinal traction to the knee with internal and external rotation. Parenteral or oral

pain medication and a muscle relaxant may facilitate the reduction.

5. If the maneuver to unlock the knee is unsuccessful, perform arthrocentesis of the knee (*only under sterile conditions*). Instill 20 to 30 ml of 1% lidocaine. Generally, the victim will be able to relax the leg and straighten the knee joint after 10 to 15 minutes.

CHAPTER 18

Blisters and Hot Spots

DEFINITIONS
Hot spots are produced by friction. If the rubbing continues, a *blister* forms, characterized as a raised, fluid-filled bubble of skin.

DISORDERS
Hot Spots
Signs and Symptoms
Painful area of erythema

Treatment
1. Take a rectangular piece of moleskin or molefoam and cut an oval hole in the middle the size of the hot spot.
2. Center this over the affected area and secure it in place, making sure that the sticky surface is not on irritated skin (Fig. 18-1).
3. Reinforce the moleskin or molefoam with tape or a piece of nonwoven adhesive knit dressing.
4. If moleskin or molefoam is not available, place a piece of tape over the hot spot.

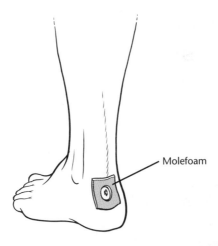

Fig. 18-1.   Hot spot treated with molefoam.

Blisters

Signs and Symptoms

1. Outer layer of skin that has separated from the more stable deeper layer
2. Fluid in the space between layers

Treatment

1. If the blister is small and still intact, do not puncture or drain it.
2. Place a piece of moleskin or molefoam, with a hole cut out slightly larger than the blister, over the site. Make sure it is thick enough to keep the shoe from rubbing against the blister. This may require several layers. Secure this with tape.
3. If the blister is large, but still intact, puncture it with a clean needle or safety pin at its base, and massage out the fluid.
4. Débride any necrotic skin with scissors.
5. Clean the area with an antiseptic towelette or with soap and water.

6. Apply antiseptic ointment or aloe vera gel, and cover with a nonadherent dressing.
    a. An excellent dressing for a blister is Spenco 2nd Skin. Made from an inert, breathable gel of 4% polyethylene oxide and 96% water, it absorbs anything oozing from the wound, helps prevent infection, relieves pain, and reduces further friction. It comes packaged between two sheets of cellophane.
    b. First, remove the cellophane from one side and apply the gooey side against the blister.
    c. Once it is adherent to the skin surface, remove the cellophane from the outside surface.
    d. Secure it in place with the adhesive knit bandage that comes with the product.
    e. Replace the entire dressing daily.
7. Place a piece of molefoam, with a hole cut out slightly larger than the blister, around the site. Secure this with tape or a piece of nonwoven adhesive knit dressing. Benzoin applied to the skin around the blister site will help hold the molefoam in place.
8. When supplies are limited, improvise by draining the fluid from the blister with a pin or knife and injecting a small amount of a superglue or benzoin into the evacuated space.
    a. Press the loose skin overlying the blister back in place, and cover the site with tape or a suitable dressing.
    b. Be aware that this can initially be quite painful, but it should allow the victim to continue hiking out of the wilderness.
9. You can improvise a blister dressing from a piece of gauze, antibacterial ointment, and water.
    a. Moisten the gauze with water.
    b. Squeeze out any excess water, then smear the ointment onto both sides of the gauze. Apply this to the blister.

PREVENTION

1. Make sure that shoes fit properly. A shoe that is too tight causes pressure sores; one that is too loose leads to friction blisters.
2. Wear a thin liner sock under a heavier one. Friction will then occur between the socks instead of between the boot or shoe and foot.
3. Dry feet regularly and use foot powder.
4. Apply moleskin to sensitive areas where blisters typically occur *before* hot spots develop.

CHAPTER 19

Life-threatening Emergencies
(Rescue Breathing/CPR/ Choking)

■ RESCUE BREATHING ■

ADULT

1. Check for breathing (see Fig. 7-2). If the victim is not lying on his or her back, gently roll him or her over, moving the entire body as a unit while maintaining spine precautions (see Fig. 7-1).
2. If no breathing is detected, open the airway with the head-tilt maneuver.
   a. Place the palm of one hand on the forehead and tilt the head back while the fingers of the other hand grasp and lift the chin.
   b. If a cervical spine injury is suspected, use the chin-lift or jaw-thrust technique to open the airway (see Figs. 7-3 and 7-4). Sweep two fingers through the victim's mouth to remove any foreign material or broken teeth.
3. If spontaneous breathing does not resume, pinch the victim's nostrils closed and place your mouth over the victim's mouth. Use a CPR Microshield or improvised barrier during mouth-to-mouth breathing to

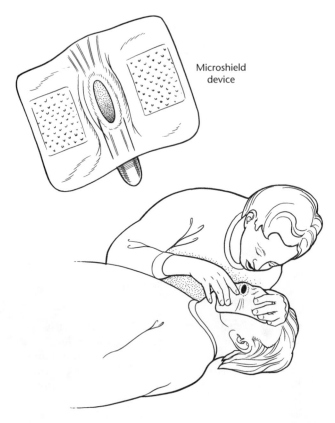

Microshield
device

Fig. 19-1. Rescue breathing using CPR Microshield device.

prevent physical contact with the victim's mouth (Fig. 19-1).
4. Blow air into the victim until you see the chest rise. Remove your mouth to allow the victim to exhale. Give two initial breaths.
5. Repeat this procedure, giving a vigorous breath every 5 seconds until the victim begins to breathe spontaneously, help arrives, or you are too exhausted to continue.

6. If air does not move in and out of the victim's mouth easily or chest movement is not detected, first try tilting the head farther back, or, if a cervical spine injury is suspected, repeat the jaw-thrust technique, pushing the victim's jaw further out. If breathing still does not occur, the airway may be obstructed by a foreign body (see p. 191).

7. During mouth-to-mouth breathing, the victim's stomach will often fill with air, eventually resulting in vomiting. If vomiting occurs, log-roll the victim in a manner that maintains cervical spine alignment, and clear the airway (see Fig. 9-1).

8. Check for a pulse by palpating the carotid artery in the victim's neck.
   a. If the victim is hypothermic, spend 1 full minute trying to detect a carotid pulse before assuming the person has no effective cardiac activity.
   b. If a pulse is present, continue rescue breathing.
   c. If no pulse is present, start chest compressions.

CHILD (OLDER THAN 1 YEAR)

1. Cover the child's mouth with your mouth.
2. Pinch the child's nose closed with the thumb and forefinger of the same hand that is placed on the forehead for the head tilt. Use your other hand to lift the chin.
3. Breathe two slow (lasting 1½ seconds) breaths into the child's mouth, with a 2-second pause between breaths. You should breathe in enough air to allow the child's chest to rise.
4. If the child does not start to breathe on his or her own, check for a pulse.
   a. If a pulse is present, continue rescue breathing with 20 breaths per minute.
   b. If no pulse is present, start chest compressions.

INFANT (YOUNGER THAN 1 YEAR)

1. Do not pinch the nose closed, but cover the infant's nose and mouth with your mouth. Apply the head-

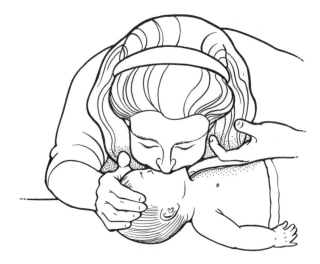

Fig. 19-2.   Rescue breathing—infant.

tilt maneuver, or use the jaw thrust if you suspect a cervical spine injury (Fig. 19-2).
2. Breathe two slow (lasting 1½ seconds) breaths (use only light puffs of air) into the infant's mouth, with a pause between breaths. You should breathe in enough air to allow the infant's chest to rise.
3. If the infant does not start to breathe on his own, check for a pulse.
   a. If a pulse is present, continue rescue breathing with 20 breaths per minute.
   b. If no pulse is present, start chest compressions.

■   CARDIOPULMONARY RESUSCITATION   ■

DEFINITION
CPR is the combination of rescue (mouth-to-mouth) breathing and chest compressions in a nonbreathing victim who has no pulse.

WHEN TO START CPR

1. Do not be afraid to initiate CPR, thinking you might be criticized for not continuing it indefinitely. People may blame themselves and each other for not doing extraordinary and heroic resuscitative measures. It is reasonable to give a victim the benefit of the doubt and start CPR, even if he or she has been without a heartbeat or breath for a prolonged time. It is difficult to know exactly how long a person found unconscious has actually been in cardiac arrest.

2. After assessing and initially managing the airway, take 10 seconds (60 seconds if the victim is hypothermic) to feel for a carotid pulse to determine if the heart is beating. If there is no pulse, begin chest compressions along with mouth-to-mouth breathing.

Chest Compressions

Adults

1. Place the victim on his or her back on a firm surface. Position the heel of one hand over the center of the victim's breastbone and the heel of your other hand over the bottom hand, interlocking the fingers (Fig. 19-3).

2. Be sure your shoulders line up directly over the victim's breastbone with elbows held straight.

3. Using a stiff-arm technique, compress the breastbone 4 to 5 cm (1½ to 2 inches) and then release. Using a smooth motion, the compression phase should equal the relaxation phase, with a rate of 80 to 100 compressions per minute (count out loud, "one-and-two-and-three-and . . ."). Do not remove your hands from the victim's chest between compressions (Fig. 19-4).

4. If you are working with a second rescuer, have the second rescuer give the victim a mouth-to-mouth breath with every fifth chest compression. If you are working alone, alternate 10 chest compressions with each two breaths. During CPR, check every few min-

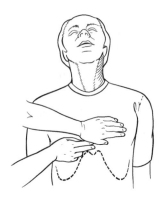
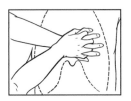

Fig. 19-3.   Hand position for chest compressions in CPR.

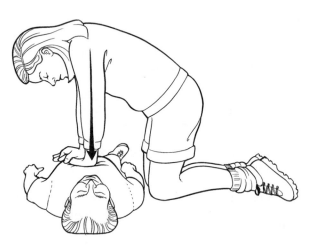

Fig. 19-4.   Chest compressions—adult.

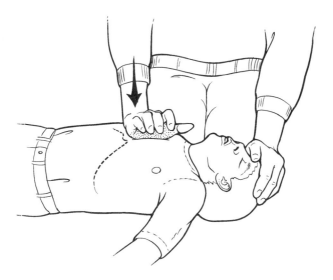

Fig. 19-5.   Chest compressions—child.

utes for return of a carotid pulse or spontaneous breathing.

Child (Older Than 1 Year)
1. Place the heel of your hand on the child's lower breastbone, with your fingers lifted off the chest (Fig. 19-5).
2. Compress the breastbone about one third to one half the thickness of the chest (2.5 to 4 cm [1 to 1½ inches]).
3. Compress the chest at a rate of approximately 100 per minute, stopping to give the child a breath every five compressions.
4. Continue the compression-to-breathing ratio of five to one. Use this same ratio whether one or two persons are doing the resuscitation. Stop to check for spontaneous breathing and a pulse after 1 minute, and then after every few minutes.

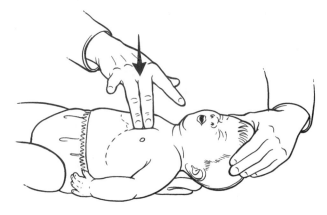

Fig. 19-6.   Chest compressions—infant.

Infant (Younger Than 1 Year)

1. Place your middle and ring finger on the lower part of the breastbone (Fig. 19-6).
2. Compress the breastbone about one third to one half the thickness of the chest (1.25 to 2.5 cm [½ to 1 inch]).
3. Compress the chest at a rate of approximately 100 per minute, stopping to give the infant a breath every five compressions.
4. Continue the compression-to-breathing ratio of five to one. Use this same ratio whether one or two persons are doing the resuscitation. Stop to check for spontaneous breathing and a pulse after 1 minute, and then after every few minutes.

WHEN TO STOP CPR

1. It has often been stated that, "Once started, CPR should never be terminated in the field." To adhere to this dictum is not only impractical, but it is potentially hazardous to rescuers.
2. It is well established that after 10 to 15 minutes of CPR, if a victim does not respond, he or she probably

never will. The rare exceptions have been victims who were profoundly hypothermic.

3. If CPR is not successful in resuscitating a victim after 15 to 30 minutes, and the victim is not profoundly hypothermic, then it is usually reasonable to discontinue CPR.

■ CHOKING/OBSTRUCTED AIRWAY ■

Choking is a life-threatening emergency that occurs when something obstructs the victim's airway so that he or she cannot breathe.

Signs and Symptoms

1. Suddenly agitated, clutching the throat, especially while eating
2. Inability to speak
3. Cyanosis

Treatment

1. For a choking adult or child, perform the Heimlich maneuver, as follows:
   a. Stand behind the victim and wrap your arms around the victim's waist.
   b. Make a fist with one of your hands and place it just above the victim's navel and below the rib cage, with the thumb side against the abdomen.
   c. Grasp your fist with the other hand and pull your hands forcefully toward you, into the victim's abdomen and slightly upward with a quick thrust.
   d. If unsuccessful, repeat the procedure to achieve a total of four or five thrusts (Fig. 19-7).
2. If the adult or child becomes unconscious, do the following:
   a. Lay the victim on his or her back and attempt rescue breathing (see p. 183).
   b. If rescue breathing is unsuccessful because of an airway obstruction, perform the Heimlich maneuver while kneeling down and straddling the vic-

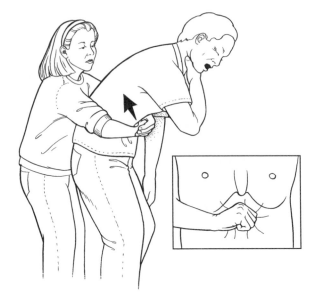

Fig. 19-7. Heimlich maneuver—standing.

   tim's thighs. Use the heel of the hand instead of a
   fist (Fig. 19-8).

  c. If still unsuccessful, sweep the mouth with one
    or two fingers to try to remove any foreign mate-
    rial.

  d. Continue to perform the Heimlich maneuver, and
    periodically attempt rescue breathing.

  e. If multiple attempts at clearing the airway and
    ventilating the victim are unsuccessful, perform a
    cricothyrotomy (see Fig. 7-6).

3. For a choking infant (younger than 1 year), do the
  following:

  a. If the infant is coughing and appears to be get-
    ting sufficient air, do not interfere with his or her
    attempts to cough the obstruction out of the air-
    way.

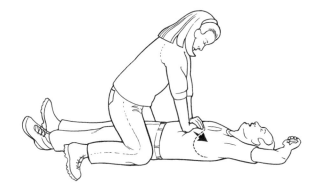

Fig. 19-8. Heimlich maneuver—supine.

b. If the infant cannot cough, cry, or get sufficient air, lay him or her face down, supported by and straddling your forearm, while resting your forearm on your thigh. Support the infant's head by grasping under the chin and holding onto the jaw. Make sure the infant's head is lower than the rest of the body.

c. Using the heel of your free hand, give up to five firm back blows between the infant's shoulder blades.

d. If the obstruction is not cleared, place your free hand on the infant's back, holding the back and head so they are sandwiched between both of your arms.

e. Carefully support the trunk and head while flipping the infant over to a supine position. Support the infant on your thigh, keeping the infant's head lower than the rest of the body. Give five quick, downward chest thrusts with two fingertips positioned over the infant's lower breastbone 1.24 cm (½ inch) below the nipples.

f. Look into the infant's mouth for a foreign object, and try to remove it.

g. If the infant becomes unconscious, try mouth-to-mouth rescue breathing. If you are unsuccessful at getting air into the infant's lungs, repeat steps a through e until you have removed the object or the child has started to breathe on his or her own.

CHAPTER 20

Allergic Reaction

■ **DEFINITION** ■

An allergic reaction can occur as a result of insect sting, food allergy, medication use, exposure to animals or plants, severe asthma, and other unknown reasons. An allergic reaction to insect sting is usually from the sting of a bee, wasp, hornet, or yellow jacket, or it can occur from the bite of a fire ant. The most severe form of an allergic reaction is anaphylactic shock, which can become life threatening within minutes. See specific chapters for information on stings, plant toxicities, or reactions to animals or animal products.

■ **DISORDERS** ■

ANAPHYLAXIS

Signs and Symptoms

1. Hives, diffuse epidermal erythema, soft tissue edema
2. Wheezing, cough, chest tightness, hoarseness, dyspnea
3. Dysphagia, nausea and vomiting, diarrhea, abdominal pain
4. Hypotension and tachycardia (shock), seizures
5. Edema involving the face, lips, tongue, pharynx, and larynx, producing an obstructed airway and respiratory arrest

6. The more immediate the reaction, the more severe the degree of anaphylaxis

Treatment
In the event of anaphylactic shock, there is no time to get the victim to medical facilities from the wilderness. The definitive treatment is epinephrine.

1. Obtain and maintain the airway, administering oxygen as needed.
2. Administer epinephrine.
   a. Begin with aqueous epinephrine 1:1000 subcutaneously in the deltoid region.
   b. The dose for an adult is 0.3 to 0.5 ml and for a child is 0.01 ml/kg, not to exceed a total dose of 0.3 ml. Repeat in 20 minutes if relief is partial.
   c. If the reaction is limited to pruritus and urticaria, with no wheezing or facial swelling, administer an antihistamine such as diphenhydramine (Benadryl) 50 to 75 mg q4-6h for an adult; for children, give 1 mg/kg. Reserve epinephrine for a worsened condition.
   d. Susceptible victims may use aerosolized epinephrine via a metered-dose inhaler (Primatene Mist, Medihaler-Epi) to counteract the effects of bronchoconstriction and laryngeal edema.
3. If the reaction is life threatening and the victim does not respond to subcutaneous or aerosolized epinephrine, administer epinephrine intravenously.
   a. For an IV infusion, the initial dose for an adult is 0.1 mg 1:1000 epinephrine (0.1 ml) diluted in 10 ml NS solution (final dilution 1:100,000). Repeat the dose at 5- to 10-minute intervals until the reaction has subsided.
   b. In an infant or child, the starting dose is 0.1 μg/kg/min up to a maximum of 1.5 μg/kg/min.
   c. Use epinephrine with caution in a person over age 45 because it can produce cardiac ischemia and arrhythmias.

d. Epinephrine is available in a spring-loaded injectable cartridge called the EpiPen (Meridian Medical Technologies, Inc.). This allows for self-administration of the medicine without dealing with a needle and syringe. The device contains 2 ml epinephrine in a disposable push-button spring-activated cartridge with a concealed needle. It delivers a single dose of 0.3 mg epinephrine injection, USP 1:1000 (0.3 ml) in a sterile solution intramuscularly. A child who weighs less than 30 kg (66 pounds) should receive EpiPen Jr., which delivers 0.15 mg epinephrine, USP 1:1000 (0.15 ml) in a sterile solution.

4. Treat bronchospasm and wheezing with albuterol, via a handheld, metered-dose inhaler with a spacer (adult dose is 4 to 8 puffs q15-20min prn).

5. Administer diphenhydramine 50 mg IV, IM, or PO. The dose for a child is 1 mg/kg.

6. Administer a corticosteroid. If IV access is available, administer 125 mg methylprednisolone (Solu-Medrol) or 15 mg dexamethasone (Decadron). If therapy is initiated orally, administer prednisone 60 to 100 mg for adults and 2 mg/kg for children.

7. For a hypotensive victim, place in Trendelenburg's position and inflate MAST suit if available.

8. Perform CPR if needed.

9. To decrease the absorption of antigen from an extremity, place the victim so that the extremity is in a dependent position, apply ice packs intermittently (10 minutes on, 10 minutes off) to produce local vasoconstriction, and loosely apply a constriction bandage to obstruct venous and lymphatic circulation. Release the bandage for 1 minute out of every 10 minutes, and completely remove it when the victim shows signs of improvement. Do not occlude the arterial circulation.

10. If a stinger remains after an insect sting, do not squeeze it because it may inject more venom into the victim. Gently flick it out if possible, or scrape it away.

11. Note that in severe cases, intubation may be needed. Be sure to visualize the vocal cords with a rigid laryngoscope because of the distortion caused by laryngeal edema. If an airway cannot be obtained immediately, perform a needle cricothyrotomy; for a child, perform a tracheostomy if oral intubation is not successful.

12. After treatment, be prepared to transport the victim immediately for medical evaluation because an anaphylactic reaction can recur once the effect of the epinephrine wears off.

CHAPTER 21

Diabetic Emergencies

DEFINITIONS AND CHARACTERISTICS

Insulin is a hormone that allows the body to use and store sugar. In diabetes, either the pancreas is unable to produce enough insulin to be physiologically useful (*type I, insulin-dependent diabetes*) or the insulin produced is ineffective (*type II, non–insulin-dependent diabetes*). Some diabetic patients need to take insulin injections to control their disease; others can control their blood sugar levels by diet and oral hypoglycemic medications. Anyone with diabetes should wear appropriate identification in case assistance is needed. Physiologic derangements seen with diabetes include high blood sugar levels, kidney failure, skin ulcers, bleeding into the vitreous of the eye, or other disorders associated with deterioration of the small blood vessels. If a diabetic person becomes confused, weak, or unconscious, he or she may be suffering from insulin-induced hypoglycemia or lapsing into a diabetic coma.

DISORDERS
Insulin-induced Hypoglycemia

If a diabetic patient takes too much insulin or, while taking an appropriate dose of insulin or a glucose-lowering agent, either fails to eat sufficient carbohydrate to match the insulin level or exercises at a greatly increased rate, a rapid drop in blood sugar level can occur.

Signs and Symptoms
1. Altered level of consciousness, possibly confusion, nervousness, belligerence, fainting, seizures, unconsciousness, or coma
2. Weakness, tremor, sweating, hunger, abdominal pain, ataxia, slurred speech, tachycardia
3. Minimal to absent prodrome, so that the victim becomes rapidly unarousable without warning

Treatment
1. If possible, obtain a blood glucose reading before beginning therapy. Dipstick readings are very helpful in permitting rapid, reasonably accurate blood glucose estimates. Check with the victim or others to see if glucagon has already been given because it will alter the blood glucose reading.
2. If the victim is still conscious and able to swallow, give him or her something containing sugar to drink or eat as soon as possible. This could be fruit juice, a banana, candy, or a nondiet soft drink. As soon as the victim feels better, have him or her eat a meal to avoid a recurrence.
3. If the victim is unconscious:
   a. Place tiny amounts of sugar granules, cake icing, or Glutose paste (one tube contains 25 g) under the victim's tongue, where it will be passively swallowed and absorbed.
   b. If available, administer 1 to 3 ampules of IV 50% dextrose in water while completing the ABCs (airway, breathing, circulation) of resuscitation. In a child under 8 years of age, give 25% dextrose in water in a dose of 2 to 4 ml/kg body weight or even 10% dextrose in water in a dose of 0.5 to 1 g/kg.
   c. As an alternative in a victim for whom you cannot quickly obtain IV access, give 1 to 2 mg of glucagon intramuscularly or subcutaneously. This dose may be repeated as needed.
   d. Be aware that families of insulin-dependent diabetic persons are often taught how to administer

intramuscular glucagon at home. In addition, an intranasal form is available. Check with the victim or others to see if glucagon has already been given because it will alter the blood glucose readings.

4. Provide supportive care, including airway management, aspiration and seizure precautions, administration of oxygen, and treatment for shock (see Chapter 8).

Diabetic Ketoacidosis

In diabetic ketoacidosis (DKA), blood sugar levels become dangerously high. The blood becomes acidotic as the by-products of metabolism (ketones) accumulate, dehydration occurs, and body chemistry falls out of balance.

Signs and Symptoms

1. History of recent polydipsia, polyuria, polyphagia, visual blurring, weakness, weight loss, nausea, vomiting, and abdominal pain
2. Early symptoms: polyuria, polydipsia, nausea and vomiting
3. Later symptoms: tachycardia, tachypnea with Kussmaul's breathing, hyperventilation, possibly fruity odor of ketones on the breath
4. Abdominal pain, especially in children
5. Skin dry with little sweating, hypotension or orthostatic blood pressure changes
6. Eventually, confusion, combativeness, or coma with signs of profound dehydration
7. Possibly an elevated temperature, resulting from the presence of sepsis

Treatment

1. If unsure whether the victim has hyperglycemia or hypoglycemia, assume it is hypoglycemia and administer sugar.
2. If the victim can drink, encourage him or her to consume large quantities of unsweetened fluids. Other-

wise, administer IV NS solution (2 L over 2 hours). Be aware that fluid resuscitation alone may help considerably in lowering hyperglycemia.

3. Provide supportive care, including airway management, administration of oxygen, and treatment for shock, while transporting the victim to a medical center.

4. If insulin is available, administer it as an IV infusion at a rate of 0.1 unit/kg/hr, or as appropriate for the measured blood sugar level.

Hyperglycemic Hyperosmolar Nonketotic Coma

Hyperglycemic hyperosmolar nonketotic coma (HHNC) represents a form of acute diabetic decompensation.

Signs and Symptoms

1. Prodrome significantly longer than that for diabetic ketoacidosis
2. Extreme dehydration, hyperosmolarity, volume depletion, altered level of consciousness
3. Fever, thirst, polyuria, oliguria
4. Orthostatic hypotension or frank hypotension, tachycardia, depressed sensorium, seizures, other changes in neurologic function

Treatment

1. Administer fluids rapidly. Give 2 to 3 L of NS solution over the first several hours.
2. Supplement the insulin levels using regular insulin 0.1 unit/kg/hr IV. Careful monitoring is required.
3. Correct electrolyte abnormalities, including sodium, potassium, phosphorus, and magnesium.
4. Correct the acidosis cautiously.
5. Transport to a medical facility.

Insulin Allergy

Signs and Symptoms

1. Local itching or pain
2. Delayed edema, urticaria, or anaphylaxis
3. Systemic reactions when the victim has discontinued insulin and then resumed therapy

Treatment

1. For mild reactions, administer diphenhydramine 50 mg q6h for adults and 1mg/kg for children.
2. For anaphylactic reactions, administer epinephrine (see Chapter 20).
3. Evacuate the victim immediately to a medical facility.

CHAPTER 22

Genitourinary Tract Disorders

Genitourinary (GU) tract disorders include urinary tract infections (UTIs), which can affect either the lower or the upper urinary tract; urinary stones; and scrotal pain.

■ DISORDERS ■

URINARY TRACT INFECTION

In women the primary cause of UTI is invasion of the urinary tract by bacteria that have ascended the urethra from the introitus. Most of these infections are caused by gram-negative aerobic bacteria, most often *Escherichia coli*. Infection of the urinary tract in a male is often associated with prostatic enlargement or infection.

Lower UTI (Uncomplicated UTI)

Signs and Symptoms
1. Bladder irritation (dysuria, frequency, urgency)
2. May lead to hematuria

Confirmation of the diagnosis by examination of the urine is typically impossible in the wilderness. Other GU processes that may mimic UTI include the following:

✢ Chills and fever, suggestive of upper UTI (pyelonephritis)

✢ Presence of risk factors in sexual history suggestive of chlamydial urethritis; more probable in sexually active women with multiple partners; chlamydial or gonococcal cervicitis often associated with cervical discharge

✢ Vaginal discharge, external irritation, or pain with intercourse suggestive of vaginal etiology, specifically vaginal infection

✢ Dysuria with flank pain, restlessness, and costovertebral angle (CVA) tenderness suggestive of urinary stone(s)

✢ In a male with dysuria, urethritis or prostatitis possible

Treatment

1. Perform a physical examination, including determination of temperature, abdominal examination, and assessment for CVA tenderness.

2. Perform a pelvic (bimanual) examination in a woman whose symptoms are associated with pelvic pain or vaginal bleeding. Although a formal pelvic examination using a speculum with the individual in a lithotomy position is virtually impossible in the wilderness, a simple bimanual examination can easily be performed to help identify an adnexal or uterine process (e.g., ectopic pregnancy, pelvic inflammatory disease [PID]).

3. Give antibiotic therapy (standard 3-day treatment) using one of the following:

   a. Trimethoprim/sulfamethoxazole (co-trimoxazole, Bactrim, Septra) one double-strength tablet bid for 3 days

   b. Ciprofloxacin (Cipro) 500 mg bid for 3 days

   c. Doxycycline 100 mg tid for 3 days (less effective)

4. If symptoms persist after standard therapy:
   a. Consider a resistant organism or pyelonephritis.
   b. In a male, consider a relapse caused by prostatitis. Extend treatment for 10 to 14 days or change to an extended-spectrum antibiotic (e.g., change from trimethoprim/sulfamethoxazole to ciprofloxacin).
5. In addition to the antibiotic therapy, provide for pain relief.
   a. When dysuria is a major component, give phenazopyridine (Pyridium) as a urinary anesthetic (200 mg tid for a maximum of 2 days).
   b. Warn the victim that the urine will turn orange.

Upper UTI (Pyelonephritis)

Pyelonephritis is an infection of the upper urinary tract (kidney) most often caused by ascending infection from the lower urinary tract.

Signs and Symptoms
1. Fever, chills, flank pain, dysuria, frequency, malaise, abdominal pain
2. May also present without fever, chills, or flank pain

Treatment
1. Administer an oral antibiotic if the victim is immunocompetent, without evidence of toxicity (fever, chills, or malaise), and can tolerate oral medication.
   a. Reasonable antibiotic choices include the same medications recommended for lower tract infection (see above) but require a full 10- to 14-day course.
   b. A quinolone antibiotic, such as ciprofloxacin 500 mg bid for 10 to 14 days, is an excellent first choice because of the low likelihood of bacterial resistance.
2. For a toxic victim, initiate therapy with a parenteral antibiotic, such as a third-generation cephalosporin (ceftriaxone [Rocephin] 1 g IM or IV q12h).

3. Treat nontoxic victims with a single parenteral dose, followed by 10 to 14 days of oral therapy.
4. When a high fever is present:
    a. Routinely administer acetaminophen or aspirin to make the victim more comfortable.
    b. If the fever persists, consider the possibility of a resistant organism, UTI, or an abscess.
5. Arrange for evacuation when protracted vomiting makes oral therapy impossible or when generalized toxicity (volume depletion, fever greater than 38.9° C [102° F], or marked CVA tenderness) is present. Additional risk factors include immunocompromise and extremes of age.
6. Instruct all victims to seek medical follow-up on return, even if symptoms resolve fully.

URINARY STONES

Signs and Symptoms

1. Pain, with location depending on stone's location, but typically felt in flank
    a. May radiate to groin as stone migrates distally
    b. Other causes for pain considered at this point: acute aortic dissection, back strain, herniated lumbar disk
2. Nausea and vomiting
3. Restlessness and inability to lie still
4. CVA tenderness
5. Absence of peritoneal signs; if these develop, indicates possible intraperitoneal process (e.g., appendicitis)
6. Absence of fever unless an associated UTI is present (which may develop in an obstructed ureter)
7. Gross hematuria possible, but microscopic hematuria more likely (urine dipstick test required for detection)

Treatment

1. Consider evacuation for severe nausea and vomiting (inadequate oral intake), fever (suggestive of an in-

fection proximal to the obstruction), or the presence of an intraperitoneal process.

2. Arrange for adequate hydration to help move the stone.

3. Although not usually practical in the wilderness, filtering the urine for stones is helpful for diagnosis.

4. Administer an antiinflammatory medication, such as ketorolac (Toradol) 30 mg IM or IV q6-8h, or an oral NSAID, such as ibuprofen 600 to 800 mg q6-8h, to reduce the pain of renal colic. You may also use these in addition to narcotic analgesia.

5. Administer a narcotic analgesic if needed.
   a. Use an oral narcotic combination drug, such as hydrocodone bitartrate 5 mg with acetaminophen 500 mg (Vicodin) 1 or 2 tablets q4-6h.
   b. For more severe pain, administer a parenteral narcotic, such as morphine sulfate 2 to 5 mg IV q5min, titrated for pain relief. Make sure that naloxone (Narcan) is available.

6. Administer an antiemetic drug if nausea and vomiting are factors.

7. Encourage the victim to seek medical follow-up even if symptoms resolve fully.

ACUTE SCROTAL PAIN

When palpation of the scrotum, including the testes, epididymis, and cord structures, reveals no abnormality or tenderness, consider referred pain as a possible consequence of renal, ureteral, or prostate disease.

Epididymitis

Epididymitis is an abrupt inflammation of the epididymis that spreads rapidly and can appear as generalized inflammation of the entire hemiscrotum (Fig. 22-1). The differential diagnosis includes torsion of the testicle, acute orchitis, or tumor of the testicle with hemorrhage or hydrocele. Most cases of epididymitis in young men are caused by *Chlamydia trachomatis*. At any age,

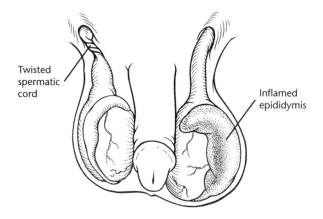

Fig. 22-1. Testicular disorders: twisted (torsed) spermatic cord and inflamed epididymis.

UTI caused by gram-negative rods can spread to the epididymis.

Signs and Symptoms
1. Acute scrotal pain in men over age 20 years (infectious epididymitis)
2. Testicular torsion in men under age 30 years (usually)
3. Gradual (over days) onset of pain
4. Dysuria or urethral discharge
5. Normal urinalysis in torsion, but pyuria in epididymitis (if urinalysis can be done, i.e., access to a urine dipstick)
6. Fever possible
7. Recent history of a UTI
8. Tenderness and swelling localized to one epididymis (usually at the superior pole)
9. Prehn's sign: relief of pain when elevating the testis (suggestive of epididymitis rather than torsion)

Treatment
1. Administer an antibiotic that covers *C. trachomatis.*
   a. Ofloxacin (Floxin) 300 mg bid for 14 days covers both gonorrheal and chlamydial organisms and is an excellent choice. Make sure the victim takes it on an empty stomach with a full glass of water.
   b. Doxycycline 100 mg or ciprofloxacin 500 mg bid can be given for 14 days, but these have inconsistent activity against *Neisseria gonorrhoeae.*
2. Allow the victim to rest supine with the scrotum elevated.
3. Give analgesic medication.
4. Arrange for the victim to wear men's supportive briefs or an athletic supporter to offer pain relief if the victim is expected to ambulate.
5. Be aware that relief after therapy usually occurs within 24 hours.
6. Inform the victim that induration and edema in the region of the epididymis may persist for 6 to 8 weeks.

Testicular Torsion

Signs and Symptoms
1. Only rarely in men over 30 years of age
2. May or may not occur during physical exertion
3. Nausea and vomiting
4. No preceding urethral discharge or fever
5. Testicle that rides high in the upper part of the scrotum
6. Relief of pain when the affected testicle is elevated (Prehn's sign), suggestive of epididymitis rather than torsion, but not reliable

Treatment
1. Be aware that testicular torsion of the spermatic cord requires surgical intervention. Therefore consider immediate evacuation if this diagnosis is suspected.

2. Attempt manual correction.
   a. Note that torsion most often occurs with the ante-rior portion of the testicle rotating from its lateral aspect to its medial aspect.
   b. To correct the torsion manually, attempt to turn the right testicle clockwise and the left testicle counterclockwise, when viewed from above.
   c. Be aware that extreme tenderness may make manual correction difficult.
   d. Relief of pain suggests that torsion has been cor-rected.
3. Advise the victim that evaluation by a urologist is in-dicated after successful detorsion.
4. Be aware that if the torsion is not corrected, loss of the affected testicle is likely.

Acute Bacterial Prostatitis

Signs and Symptoms
1. Abrupt onset, associated with systemic signs of in-fection
2. Fever, chills, perineal pain, low back pain, dysuria, frequency, and urgency
3. Hematuria possible
4. Tender, swollen ("boggy") prostate on palpation dur-ing rectal examination
5. Resultant acute urinary retention

Treatment
1. Initiate antibiotic treatment with either a quinolone, such as ciprofloxacin 500 mg bid for 14 days, ofloxa-cin 300 mg bid for 14 days, or norfloxacin (Noroxin) 400 mg bid for 14 days, or give trimethoprim/ sulfamethoxazole 1 double-strength tablet bid. Con-tinue therapy for a at least 2 weeks.
2. Arrange for "bed rest" if conditions permit.

MALE URETHRITIS

Male urethritis is typically sexually transmitted. It may be caused by *N. gonorrhoeae* (gonococcal urethritis) but more often is caused by *C. trachomatis* (the major cause of nongonococcal urethritis). *Ureaplasma urealyticum* and *Mycoplasma hominis* are thought to be responsible for most other cases.

Signs and Symptoms

1. Urethral discharge (mucopurulent with chlamydial and frankly purulent with gonococcal urethritis), dysuria, meatal pruritus
2. Flank or abdominal pain, fever, or hematuria not usually found; if present, suggests another etiology
3. Difficult to differentiate from a UTI in the field

Treatment

1. Treat suspected nongonococcal urethritis with doxycycline 100 mg bid for 7 to 14 days. Alternatively, administer azithromycin (Zithromax) 1 g as a single dose.
2. For suspected gonococcal urethritis, administer parenteral ceftriaxone 125 mg as a single dose plus doxycycline or azithromycin (as above), or ciprofloxacin 500 mg PO as a single dose plus doxycycline or azithromycin because of the likelihood of coexisting chlamydial infection. Note that oral ofloxacin 300 mg bid for 7 days covers both gonococcal and nongonococcal urethritis.
3. In the absence of a quinolone or doxycycline, substitute tetracycline 500 mg or erythromycin 500 mg qid for 7 days.
4. Notify any current sexual partners of the victim, and treat them with an appropriate regimen.

CHAPTER 23

Obstetric and Gynecologic Emergencies

Possible obstetric or gynecologic emergencies that could face rescuers in the wilderness include ectopic pregnancy, spontaneous abortion, ovulatory bleeding, dysfunctional uterine bleeding, vulvovaginal cellulitis and abscess, vaginitis, and PID.

■ DISORDERS ■

ECTOPIC PREGNANCY

Ectopic pregnancy is a medical emergency that requires prompt evacuation of the victim to a surgical facility. An episode of abnormal vaginal bleeding in the wilderness environment warrants early evaluation. Any history of salpingitis, PID, tubal surgery, use of fertility agents, use of intrauterine contraceptive device (IUD), or prior ectopic pregnancy should increase clinical suspicion. An ectopic pregnancy most often ruptures after 7 weeks' gestation (5 weeks from conception), although rupture can occur as early as 5 weeks' gestation (3 weeks from conception).

Signs and Symptoms

1. Late, missed, or prior menstrual period that was abnormal in some manner; however, a prior seemingly normal menstrual period also possible
2. History suggesting early pregnancy (e.g., breast tenderness and enlargement, morning nausea)
3. Rupture generally preceded by abnormal vaginal bleeding and abdominal pain
4. Normal or unstable vital signs
5. Dizziness or syncope if blood loss is substantial
6. Abdominal tenderness
7. After rupture, rebound tenderness and rigidity
8. On pelvic examination, adnexal tenderness or cervical motion tenderness in most but not all women
9. Adnexal mass (may not be palpable)
10. Uterine enlargement secondary to the effect of placental hormones

Treatment

1. Test the victim with a urinary beta-human chorionic gonadotropin (hCG) test (urine pregnancy test kit). (This should be included in remote expedition medical supplies.)
   a. If the test results are positive or there is clinical suspicion of ectopic pregnancy, arrange for early evacuation.
   b. If the test results are negative, the diagnosis cannot be excluded, but the likelihood of false-negative results is extremely rare (at the time an ectopic pregnancy becomes symptomatic).
   c. To ensure adequate performance of the test, only use a test with an internal positive reference.
2. Treat for shock (see Chapter 8).
3. Arrange for immediate evacuation.

SPONTANEOUS ABORTION

Spontaneous abortion, or "miscarriage," is defined as the natural termination of a pregnancy before the fetus is capable of extrauterine life (approximately 20 weeks' gestation).

Signs and Symptoms
All spontaneous abortions present with abnormal vaginal bleeding.

1. Threatened abortion
   a. No dilation of cervical os
   b. Common for woman to go on to complete the pregnancy
2. Inevitable abortion
   a. Increased bleeding and persistent pain
   b. Dilation of internal os
   c. No possibility of fetal survival
3. Incomplete abortion
   a. Increased bleeding and persistent pain
   b. Dilation of internal os
   c. No possibility of fetal survival
   d. Passing of some products of conception
4. Complete abortion
   a. Diagnosis is based on pathologic examination of all products of conception and cannot be made in the wilderness.
   b. Therefore a presumed complete abortion is handled as an incomplete abortion.

Treatment
1. Unless a pretrip ultrasound has verified an intrauterine pregnancy, immediately evacuate the victim to rule out ectopic pregnancy.
2. Keep the victim at "bed rest."
3. Direct all field treatment to volume replacement.

MITTELSCHMERZ (OVULATORY BLEEDING)
Signs and Symptoms
1. Sudden onset of right or left lower quadrant abdominal pain, occurring at mid-cycle (e.g., between days 12 and 16) in a woman of reproductive age

2. Presentation **not** associated with marked gastrointestinal, genitourinary, or systemic symptoms
3. Symptoms usually lasting less than 8 hours
4. Vaginal bleeding or spotting usually **not** associated; may indicate ectopic pregnancy
5. Mild referred pain; rebound tenderness; when right-sided tenderness noted, difficult to exclude appendicitis
6. Pelvic (bimanual) examination needed to exclude PID (often less adnexal tenderness than with PID)

Treatment
1. Evaluate the possibility of more serious problems (ectopic pregnancy, appendicitis).
2. Perform an examination immediately if symptoms worsen.
3. Keep the victim at "bed rest" for 12 to 24 hours.
4. Administer a mild nonnarcotic analgesic (e.g., acetaminophen) for pain relief.
5. Obtain a urinary beta-hCG reading if a test kit is available.

DYSFUNCTIONAL UTERINE BLEEDING

Dysfunctional uterine bleeding refers to unexpected menstrual bleeding in the absence of an anatomic cause. It may result from various hormonal imbalances. In women taking oral contraceptive pills, bleeding most frequently results from a deficiency of estrogen relative to progesterone at the level of the endometrium. In women not taking these pills, dysfunctional uterine bleeding may be caused by either a deficiency or an excess of estrogen.

Signs and Symptoms
Unexpected menstrual bleeding

Treatment
1. Perform a urine pregnancy test to reach the diagnosis, ruling out the possibility of a complication of pregnancy.

2. Only consider treatment if the woman has had normal menstrual periods, denies abdominal pain, and has a normal pelvic examination (i.e., no adnexal mass or tenderness).
3. Supply estrogen or progestin, depending on the cause (estrogen deficiency or excess).
   a. Bleeding typically comes under control within 12 to 36 hours.
   b. High doses of oral contraceptive pills of the combination monophasic type are usually effective, such as Lo/Ovral (norgestrel 0.3 mg and ethinyl estradiol 30 μg).
   c. The usual dose for this purpose is 3 pills/day for 7 days.
   d. Side effects, such as headache, fluid retention, and depression, sometimes occur.
   e. After administration of the oral contraceptive pills (i.e., after 7 days), expect the bleeding to recur.
4. If abdominal or pelvic pain develops or bleeding persists, arrange for immediate evacuation of the victim.
5. Note that any victim with dysfunctional uterine bleeding in the field should seek follow-up as soon as practical.

VULVOVAGINAL CELLULITIS AND ABSCESS

This usually results from polymicrobial infection of a Bartholin gland. Causative organisms include *Neisseria gonorrhoeae* and *Chlamydia trachomatis*.

Signs and Symptoms
1. Severe localized vulvar pain and tenderness just lateral to the posterior vaginal introitus
2. Unilateral vulvar erythema and edema
3. Tender, fluctuant mass palpable lateral to the posterior introitus

Treatment
1. Perform incision and drainage if adequate equipment is available.

a. Make the incision over the mucosal (medial) side of the point of maximal fluctuation.
   b. Insert a hemostat through the mucosal incision and spread the tips in the deeper tissue to ensure entrance into the actual abscess cavity.
   c. Irrigate the cavity with a syringe technique (see Chapter 14).
   d. Apply gauze packing to maintain drainage for 24 to 48 hours.
2. Administer antibiotic coverage if there is evidence of surrounding cellulitis.
   a. A reasonable choice is cephalexin (Keflex) 500 mg 3 times a day for 7 to 10 days.
   b. No antibiotic is required after routine incision and drainage.
3. If the availability of water and conditions permit, arrange for the victim to have a sitz bath daily.
4. Change the dressing once or twice a day until the wound is healing well without drainage.
5. Be aware that recurrence is common with simple incision and drainage. Instruct the victim to seek follow-up treatment on return.

VAGINITIS
Bacterial Vaginosis (*Gardnerella Vaginitis*)
Signs and Symptoms
1. Gray or yellow, foul-smelling discharge
2. Minimal itching and vulvar irritation

Treatment
1. Administer metronidazole (Flagyl) 1 g bid for 48 hours, then 500 mg bid for 7 days.
2. For a pregnant or allergic victim, consider ampicillin 500 mg qid for 7 days (less effective method).

Candida **Vulvovaginitis**

Signs and Symptoms

1. Thick, white vaginal discharge
2. Vulvar itching or burning
3. Dysuria
4. Dyspareunia

Treatment

1. Apply an imidazole (clotrimazole, miconazole, buto-conazole, or terconazole) cream.
2. The dosage options for clotrimazole are:
   - ❖ 100 mg vaginally for 7 days
   - ❖ 200 mg vaginally for 3 days
   - ❖ 500 mg vaginally in a single dose
3. Note that creams can also be used externally for vulvar irritation.
4. Use oral fluconazole (Diflucan) 150 mg as an effective alternative that has a considerable weight and volume advantage.
   a. Administer 150 mg as a single oral dose.
   b. If symptoms do not resolve completely, you may need to re-treat the victim.

Trichomonas **Vaginitis**

Signs and Symptoms

1. Dry or yellowish-gray discharge
2. Minimal odor
3. Severe pruritus
4. Dysuria (common)

Treatment

1. Administer a 2-g single oral dose (or 1 g PO bid, to lessen gastrointestinal side effects) of metronidazole for both the victim and her sexual partner.
2. Alternatively, administer 500 mg bid for 7 days.

PELVIC INFLAMMATORY DISEASE

PID is a syndrome caused by pathogens ascending from the lower genital tract, usually the cervix, resulting in infection of the fallopian tubes and adjacent structures. Risk factors include the presence of other sexually transmitted diseases, previous episode of PID, multiple sexual partners, and IUD use. PID is typically a polymicrobial process.

Signs and Symptoms
1. Clinical diagnosis often difficult, with symptoms including fever, chills, malaise, anorexia, nausea, vomiting, dyspareunia, vaginal discharge, and unilateral or bilateral (more common) abdominal pain
2. Mild to severe lower abdominal pain
3. Physical examination showing tachycardia, fever, yellowish endocervical discharge, bilateral lower abdominal tenderness, adnexal tenderness and/or mass (unilateral or bilateral), and cervical motion tenderness

Treatment
1. Attempt to differentiate PID from other serious diseases such as appendicitis, septic abortion, or pyelonephritis.
2. Perform a urinary beta-hCG pregnancy test (if available) to rule out ectopic pregnancy.
3. At the first opportunity, examine male sexual contacts and test them for *N. gonorrhoeae* and *C. trachomatis*.
4. For severe PID, give intravenous or intramuscular antibiotics.
   a. Ceftriaxone (Rocephin) 250 mg IM one dose, followed by doxycycline 100 mg PO bid for 10 to 14 days.
   b. In the absence of this regimen, administer ofloxacin (Floxin) 400 mg PO bid plus metronidazole (Flagyl) 500 mg PO bid for 14 days.
5. Evacuate the victim if any of the following is present:
   a. Pregnancy
   b. Adnexal mass (to rule out abscess)

    c. Peritoneal signs
    d. Toxic appearance (e.g., temperature greater than 39° C [102.2° F]) with severe malaise
    e. Severe nausea and vomiting
    f. Presence of an IUD

CHAPTER 24

Wilderness Eye Emergencies

THE WILDERNESS EYE KIT

The wilderness kit for treating eye disorders and injuries should include ophthalmic antibiotic solutions, topical anesthetic agents, mydriatic-cycloplegic solutions, topical steroids, topical vasoconstrictors and decongestants, fluorescein strips or drops, artificial tears, cotton-tipped applicators, prednisone 20-mg tablets, a headlamp or flashlight, and a small magnifying lens (see Appendix H).

OCULAR PROCEDURES
Eye Patching

1. Use a pressure patch to hold the eyelid closed and thereby facilitate healing of a corneal defect and protect the injured eye from bright light.
   a. A pressure patch is indicated in many common eye emergencies and whenever the surface of the cornea has been injured, especially with a large corneal defect.
   b. Small corneal defects may heal rapidly without patching.
   c. After patching, the victim often experiences less pain and tearing.
2. Do not use patching when the corneal epithelial de-

fect is secondary to an active infection (e.g., conjunctivitis, corneal ulcer).
3. Never apply a pressure patch to an eye after a penetrating injury. After eye penetration or trauma, tape a protective cup (e.g., padded drinking cup) over the eye or fashion a cloth "donut" from a cravat or other cloth to avoid placing pressure or inflicting any further trauma during evacuation.

Equipment
1. Two gauze eye patches (gauze 2 × 2-inch or commercial patches)
2. 1-inch (2.5 cm) tape
3. Antibiotic ointment
4. Mydriatic-cycloplegic

Procedure
1. Before patching a corneal abrasion, apply both a drop or two of a mydriatic-cycloplegic and a thin ribbon of antibiotic-antiseptic ointment.
   a. The cycloplegic will relax the ciliary muscle spasm that accompanies corneal abrasion.
   b. Check the victim for a narrow anterior chamber before instilling the drop (see Estimation of Anterior Chamber Depth), although this is usually not realistic in the field.
2. Use antibiotic ointment for prophylaxis, although corneal abrasions rarely become infected.
3. For the patch to be effective, you must put it on just tightly enough to keep the eyelid shut, but do not put undue pressure on the eye.
4. Use two patches.
   a. Double the first patch by folding vertically, and place it over the closed lid. If a second patch is not available, this patch can be held in place with a single piece of tape.
   b. Put the unfolded second patch over the first folded patch.
5. Prepare the skin near the eye with tincture of benzoin

to help the tape adhere. Be careful to keep the benzoin out of the eye.

6. Place the tape diagonally from the center of the forehead to the cheekbone. Make sure the tape completely covers the patch to minimize slippage but does not extend onto the angle of the mandible.

7. Remove the patch every 24 hours so that the eye can be reexamined and the patch changed. Using a clean patch every 24 hours helps to prevent infection.

8. Instruct the victim with an eye patch to rest the uninjured eye. Discourage reading because rapid involuntary movement of the patched eye occurs.

Upper Eyelid Eversion

1. Place the end of a cotton-tipped applicator horizontally above the tarsal plate while you pull the eyelashes and the lid margin down and out (Fig. 24-1, *A*).

2. Flip the lid up to evert it. Hold the everted lid in position by pressing the lashes against the superior orbital rim (Fig. 24-1, *B*).

Fluorescein Examination

1. Use fluorescein staining to evaluate all red or painful eyes.

2. Wet the fluorescein strip with a drop of saline (artificial tears) or a drop of the topical anesthetic being used.

3. When examining an eye with a possible infectious process, always use a separate fluorescein strip for each eye to avoid cross-contamination.

4. Next, apply the wetted strip to the inside of the victim's lower lid.

5. Ask the victim to blink, which will spread the fluorescein over the surface of the eye. Areas of corneal disruption stain a brilliant green.

6. Use a small, blue filter placed over a penlight, which works well in the dark.

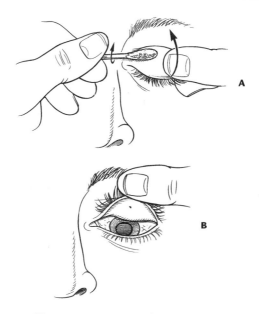

Fig. 24-1.   Upper eyelid eversion.

a. Outside during the day, simple sunlight causes any significant corneal lesion to fluoresce.
b. Fluorescein permanently stains soft contact lenses, so instruct victims to remove these lenses before the fluorescein examination and leave them out for several hours after the examination.

Examination of Pupils

Examine the pupils for size, equality, shape, and reaction to light.

a. An irregularly shaped pupil may indicate pupillary sphincter injury or spasm caused by intraocular inflammation.
b. A pointed "teardrop pupil" suggests an ocular

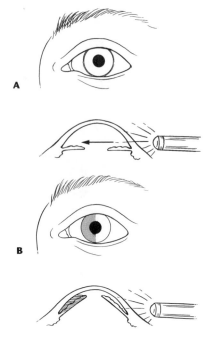

Fig. 24-2.   Estimating depth of anterior chamber.

penetration injury. Approximately 10% of the population has anisocoria (unequal pupils).

c. When evaluating a red or painful eye, a significant difference in pupillary size provides a helpful clue to diagnose iritis (constricted) or glaucoma (dilated).

Estimation of Anterior Chamber Depth

Shine a small flashlight obliquely from the temporal side of the eye (Fig. 24-2, *A*).

a. If the nasal iris is well illuminated, it suggests a normal anterior chamber.

b. If the nasal iris lies in shadow, it suggests a shallow anterior chamber (narrow angle) (Fig. 24-2, *B*).

c. This may be a difficult test to interpret. It is helpful to compare one eye with the other or the victim's eye with that of another person.

Extraocular Muscle Testing

Have the victim follow a flashlight or finger through the extremes of gaze in six directions.

a. Grossly limited extraocular motion with bulging of the eye from the orbit suggests acute orbital inflammation or retro-orbital hemorrhage.

b. If the eye appears sunken within the orbit, and the victim exhibits limited upward gaze, suspect a blowout fracture of the orbital floor.

Visual Fields Testing

1. Ask the victim to cover one eye completely and look directly at your nose from a distance of about 1 m (3 feet).

2. Place your fingers outside the victim's field of peripheral vision and slowly move them centrally.

3. Ask the victim to inform you when he or she can see your fingers. The victim's fields are generally normal when they correspond with those of the examiner.

■ **DISORDERS** ■

SUDDEN LOSS OF VISION IN WHITE "QUIET" EYE

Acute and significant visual loss is an ophthalmologic emergency. The common causes of acute visual loss include the following:

1. Retinal detachment
2. Central retinal artery occlusion

3. Anterior ischemic optic neuropathy
4. Optic neuritis
5. Central retinal vein occlusion
6. Vitreous hemorrhage
7. Arteritic anterior ischemic optic neuropathy

Each of these conditions requires immediate evacuation and definitive follow-up. However, giant cell or temporal arteritis (a type of arteritic anterior ischemic optic neuropathy) requires immediate field treatment to avoid bilateral loss of vision.

Giant Cell (Temporal) Arteritis

Signs and Symptoms
1. Rare under age 50 years
2. Associated with temporal headache
3. Jaw claudication
4. Low-grade fever
5. History of associated weight loss
6. History of polymyalgia rheumatica
7. Transient visual obscurations
8. Usually affects one eye first, then the second eye within hours to days

Treatment
1. Because this disease can cause significant visual loss in the absence of effective treatment, initiate care immediately with a high-dose steroid (prednisone 80 to 100 mg qd for 4 to 6 weeks).
2. Evacuate the victim so that a high-dose IV steroid can be administered.
3. When treated, symptoms often improve within 1 to 3 days. However, steroids are typically continued for many weeks.

THE RED EYE
Acute-Angle-Closure Glaucoma

Acute-angle-closure glaucoma results from a sudden rise in intraocular pressure (IOP) and is characterized by a red painful eye and decreased vision. Victims at risk include elderly persons and farsighted individuals.

Signs and Symptoms

1. A red eye, often with the pupil mid-dilated and a steamy (edematous) cornea
2. The affected eye (palpated through the eyelid) often feeling appreciably harder than the unaffected eye (palpate through the lid **gently and with extreme caution.**)
3. May be intermittent
4. Symptoms beginning in low light
5. Acute onset of severe pain and blurred vision with red eye
6. Possible nausea, vomiting, and generalized head pain

Treatment

1. Instill timolol 0.5% (Timoptic) 1 gtt bid.
2. Instill pilocarpine 2% (Pilocar) 1 gtt q15min × 4, then qid.
3. Administer acetazolamide (Diamox) 250 mg PO qid.
4. Arrange for immediate evacuation for emergency ocular surgery (laser iridotomy).

Corneal Abrasion

Signs and Symptoms

1. Conjunctival redness
2. Intense pain localized to the cornea after an injurious event
3. Identification of a corneal lesion sometimes made using visible light but often enhanced by fluorescein staining
   a. During daytime, use of a cobalt-blue filter not necessary because fluorescein fluoresces from incident ultraviolet (UV) radiation associated with sunlight
   b. Credit-card-size "Fresnel" magnifying lens possibly helpful

Treatment
1. Apply a topical antibiotic solution. A solution is preferable to an ointment when the victim is expected to remain active. If the victim is sleeping or if the eye is patched, an ointment has greater longevity.
2. If the abrasion is extensive (>30% of the corneal surface) or painful, add a mydriatic-cycloplegic agent to the regimen.
3. Instruct the victim to avoid activity requiring frequent active eye movement.
4. If the eye is not patched, apply cool compresses over the eye after the topical antibiotic to soothe the area.
5. Be aware that many small (<3 mm) abrasions resolve as quickly with or without corneal (eye) patching.
   a. Base the decision to patch the eye on abrasion size and patient comfort (many victims with severe corneal defects feel more comfortable after patching).
   b. If the decision is made to patch, apply the patch with enough pressure to prohibit the eyelids from opening and closing but without putting undue pressure on the cornea.
6. Give an oral analgesic or antiinflammatory drug to provide symptomatic relief
7. Be aware that a corneal abrasion typically resolves within 24 to 48 hours, although a large abrasion may take longer. Evacuate promptly any victim with a corneal lesion that does not resolve within 4 days or that is progressing (enlarging or becoming more painful).

Corneal Erosion

This occurs when a small portion of corneal epithelium is torn as the eyelid opens, usually in a person with a prior history of corneal abrasion. The cause of recurrent corneal erosion is failure of complete bonding of the healing corneal epithelium to its basement membrane.

Signs and Symptoms

1. Acute ocular pain, photophobia, and tearing, often occurring at the time of awakening, just after the eyes are first opened
2. Typically, bright fluorescein staining of the erosion but with the erosion sometimes healing before the examination, revealing a normal cornea; erosion often recurring the next morning

Treatment

1. Apply antibiotic ointment to the eye (above lower eyelid) before patching.
2. Apply the cycloplegic one time only.
3. Patch the affected eye for 12 hours, then remove the patch to inspect the eye. If total resolution has not occurred, replace the patch for another 12 hours.
4. Use hypertonic ophthalmic saline solution (Muro-128) after the patch is removed, 1 to 2 gtt q3-4h. Recurrence rate is high unless hypertonic saline solution is used.
5. If hypertonic ophthalmic saline solution is not available, instill artificial tears 4 to 8 times per day.
6. If the corneal epithelium is loose and not healing, consider gentle débridement, following the topical anesthetic, with a sterile applicator to remove cautiously the loose epithelium.
7. If the victim with corneal erosion does not respond to treatment, encourage evacuation.

Contact Lens–Related Corneal Abrasion

A lens-related corneal abrasion is at high risk for transformation into a corneal ulcer.

Signs and Symptoms

Same as for other corneal abrasions

Treatment

1. **Do not patch.**
2. Apply an antibiotic solution. Ciprofloxacin (Ciloxan)

ophthalmic solution 0.3% is preferable, 1 to 2 gtt
q2-4h for 5 to 7 days.

Corneal Ulcer

This usually occurs after an injury or in a soft contact
lens wearer. Soft contact lenses allow pathogens to adhere to the corneal surface, creating deposits of organisms that can then go on to invade the stroma. This is
especially true if the soft lens is worn continuously.

Signs and Symptoms
1. Red painful eye
2. Photophobia
3. Discharge
4. Decreased visual acuity in the affected eye
5. A white or gray spot (white cell infiltrate) on the cornea that is visible without fluorescein

Treatment
1. Instill ciprofloxacin (Ciloxan) 0.3% ophthalmic solution 1 gtt q15min for 6 hours, then 1 gtt q30min, continued during the evacuation. If ciprofloxacin is not
   available, use another ocular antibiotic. These may
   have reduced efficacy.
2. Apply a cycloplegic agent.
3. **Do not patch the eye.**
4. **Do not wear contact lenses.**
5. Administer an analgesic as needed.
6. Be aware that immediate ophthalmologic consulta-
   tion is required for appropriate culturing and antimicrobial treatment. Do not withhold antibiotics pend-
   ing evacuation.

Corneal Foreign Body

Signs and Symptoms
1. Pain, irritation, tearing, redness, and a sensation of
   "something in the eye"
2. Sometimes visualized with the naked eye, often enhanced with fluorescein staining (highlighting any
   corneal damage)

Treatment

1. Note that a foreign body can often be removed by simple irrigation with a copious amount of the cleanest water available (disinfected drinking water).
2. If simple irrigation is unsuccessful, use a moistened cotton swab to **gently** brush away the foreign body. The corneal epithelium can be easily damaged by forceful or repetitive use of this technique.
3. After removal of the foreign body, instill topical antibiotic drops. You may apply a corneal pressure patch if there is an epithelial defect.
4. Apply a cool compress to ease discomfort.
5. Inform the victim that the foreign body sensation will return after the anesthetic wears off.
6. Be aware that if the foreign body is metallic, a rust ring may develop. This is not dangerous and can be removed later by an ophthalmologist.
7. If the foreign body cannot be easily removed or if symptoms (pain, irritation, redness) persist for more than a day after removal, initiate evacuation.

CONJUNCTIVITIS

The specific determination of the cause for conjunctivitis can be difficult in the field. Fortunately, most cases are self-limited or are bacterial and respond to an antibiotic. Visual acuity should always be checked, even though conjunctivitis typically does not cause a change. Any deterioration is cause for concern and potential evacuation.

Acute Bacterial Conjunctivitis (Pinkeye)

Signs and Symptoms

1. Irritation and tearing
2. Eyelids that stick together during sleep
3. Hyperemia of the conjunctivae
4. Purulent discharge

Treatment

1. Apply topical antibiotic solution 1 to 2 gtt q2-6h for at least 5 to 7 days.

2. If the infection progresses (increasing symptoms) despite an antibiotic, arrange for evacuation.
3. If corneal opacification is noted (e.g., corneal ulcer, more common in a soft contact lens wearer), arrange for evacuation.
4. **Do not patch the eye.**

Viral Conjunctivitis (Acute Follicular Conjunctivitis)

Signs and Symptoms
1. Tearing (with scant or no purulent discharge)
2. Redness of the conjunctivae
3. Tender preauricular lymph nodes
4. Redness and edema of the eyelids

Treatment
1. Consider instilling a topical antibiotic (because specific diagnosis is difficult in the field), 1 to 2 gtt q2-6h for at least 5 to 7 days.
2. Apply cool compresses for symptomatic relief. Be careful not to cross-contaminate the noninvolved eye.
3. Apply a vasoconstricting topical eye solution.
4. Be aware that viral conjunctivitis may last 2 weeks.
5. Evacuate the victim if the condition is not resolving or if any corneal opacification is noted.
6. **Do not patch the eye.**

Chemical Conjunctivitis and Chemical Injury to the Cornea

Chemical conjunctivitis may be caused by any irritant (e.g., sunscreen, insect repellent, stove fuel) accidentally introduced into the eye. More serious burns affecting the cornea may be caused by caustic substances. Alkali and acid burns are true emergencies.

Signs and Symptoms
Immediate pain, tearing, and irritation

Treatment
1. Irrigate the eye with a copious amount of the cleanest water available **as soon as possible.** In most cases, 1 L of irrigation water is sufficient. However, for an alkali burn, use 3 L.
2. Cool compresses may provide relief. Be careful not to cross-contaminate the noninvolved eye.
3. Use an antibiotic ophthalmic ointment for prophylaxis.
4. Apply a light pressure patch.
5. If the injury was from an acid or alkali, serious permanent damage may occur. Irrigate the eye(s) and transport the victim rapidly to definitive care.
6. Evacuate any victim with a corneal burn associated with corneal opacification or significant defect on fluorescein staining.

Inclusion (Chlamydial) Conjunctivitis

Chlamydial conjunctivitis is a sexually transmitted disease seen most often in young adults.

Signs and Symptoms
1. Similar to those for acute bacterial conjunctivitis
2. Swollen eyelids
3. Many small follicles (raised pale bumps) in the palpebral conjunctivae (especially of the lower lid)

Treatment
1. Administer doxycycline 100 mg bid PO for 21 days.
2. Apply cool compresses to provide relief. Be careful not to cross-contaminate the noninvolved eye.
3. Inclusion conjunctivitis may be difficult to differentiate from other, more common forms of bacterial conjunctivitis, but consider it when conjunctivitis does not resolve after 4 to 5 days of using a conventional topical antibiotic.

Allergic Conjunctivitis

Signs and Symptoms
1. Itching and tearing (without purulent discharge)
2. At times, swelling and redness of the conjunctivae

Treatment
1. Instill vasoconstrictive drops qid for 1 to 2 days.
2. Apply cool compresses.
3. If desired, add an oral antihistamine to relieve itching.

Herpes Simplex Viral Keratitis

Ocular herpes can result from sexually transmitted herpes simplex virus (HSV). However, it is usually caused by HSV-1, the virus responsible for cold sores. Bilateral involvement is seen in about 12% of cases.

Signs and Symptoms
1. Symptoms mimicking those of corneal abrasion
   a. Eye diffusely reddened
   b. Pain, photophobia, tearing, foreign body sensation
2. In early herpetic infection, only small punctate lesions or a single vesicle of the cornea seen
3. Over time, typical dendritic (branching) pattern of corneal involvement becoming apparent on fluorescein staining

Treatment
1. Instill a topical antiviral agent (trifluridine [Viroptic] 1% ophthalmic solution) q2h while the victim is awake until the corneal epithelium has healed. Then instill this agent qid for 1 week.
2. Evacuate the victim.

BLEPHARITIS

Signs and Symptoms
1. Itching and burning of the eyelids, often with crusting around the eyes on awakening

2. Red eyelid margins that are crusty and thickened
3. Possibly injected conjunctivae

Treatment
1. Gently scrub the eyelid margins with baby shampoo bid using a washcloth or cotton-tipped applicator.
2. Apply warm compresses for 15 to 20 minutes tid to qid.
3. Instill artificial tears, for associated mild ocular irritation or dry eyes, 4 to 8 times a day.
4. If symptoms are severe, apply antibiotic ointment qid to the eyelid margin for 1 week, then qhs for 1 more week.

IRITIS

Iritis may result from a specific etiology (e.g., infection, trauma, overexposure to ultraviolet light) or may occur independently.

Signs and Symptoms
1. Moderate to severe pain that does not respond to topical anesthesia
2. Photophobia
3. Blurred vision
4. Pupil of the involved eye constricted and less reactive
5. Redness surrounding the cornea; ciliary vessels running through the sclera beneath the conjunctivae becoming injected, causing a purplish area of injection around the cornea ("ciliary injection")

Treatment
1. Address any specific etiology.
2. Administer prednisolone (Pred-Forte) 1 gtt qh for 1 to 3 days.
3. Evacuate the victim if the condition persists or progresses. The iritis associated with UV photokeratitis or corneal abrasion is usually self-limited.

UV PHOTOKERATITIS (SNOWBLINDNESS)

UV-induced photokeratitis represents corneal damage. Intense exposure to UV light may cause a corneal burn in 1 hour, although symptoms may not become apparent for 6 to 12 hours.

Signs and Symptoms

1. Pain, although there is typically a 6- to 12-hour symptom-free interval just after exposure
2. Severe gritty sensation in the eyes
3. Photophobia
4. Tearing
5. Marked conjunctival erythema and chemosis
6. Eyelid edema
7. Ciliary injection with iritis
8. Usually bilateral
9. On fluorescein staining, a horizontal bandlike uptake that corresponds with the shielding effect of the squinting eyelids

Treatment

1. Spontaneous healing generally occurs in 24 hours. However, take steps to minimize pain and disability.
2. Remove contact lenses.
3. Instill a single dose of a topical anesthetic to help control pain during the examination. **Do not use the anesthetic more than once** because prolonged use can impair corneal reepithelialization.
4. Apply an antibiotic solution. If a pressure patch is used, apply the topical antibiotic ointment before patching.
5. Administer an antiinflammatory drug, such as ibuprofen, to control symptoms.
6. Administer a systemic narcotic analgesic, if necessary.
7. Apply cold compresses to provide some relief.
8. If needed, instill a mydriatic-cycloplegic agent to reduce pain greatly by reducing ciliary spasm.

9. Note that topical steroids are not recommended because of the potential for delayed epithelial healing.
10. Patch the affected eye for 12 hours, then remove the patch to inspect the eye. If total resolution has not occurred, replace the patch for another 12 hours.

Prevention
1. Wear sunglasses that block more than 90% of UVB.
2. Add side shields to sunglasses to prevent reflected UV light from striking the cornea.
3. Always carry spare sunglasses.
4. Create a makeshift shield by cutting narrow horizontal slits in a piece of cardboard, foam padding, or duct tape and securing this over the eyes.

EFFECTS OF HIGH ALTITUDE ON PATIENTS AFTER RADIAL KERATOTOMY
Radial keratotomy (RK) is a common corneal surgical procedure that corrects for myopia (nearsightedness). Recent reports have documented hyperopic shifts in refractive error in RK patients going to very high altitudes. This means that patients with prior RK are at risk for loss of visual acuity at very high altitudes. Patients whose eyes have been undercorrected seem to have fewer problems than those with complete correction.

EPISCLERITIS
Signs and Symptoms
1. Localized inflammation and dilation of the episcleral vessels
2. Little discomfort or discharge
3. Often in only one sector of the eye
4. Results from irritants or is idiopathic
5. Often a history of prior similar episodes

Treatment
1. If irritation exists, instill 0.3% pheniramine maleate plus 0.025% naphazoline ophthalmic solution (Naphcon-A) up to qid.

2. Ensure that this condition is evaluated on the victim's return.

SUBCONJUNCTIVAL HEMORRHAGE

This condition is usually caused by local trauma, coughing, or straining.

Signs and Symptoms
1. Usually asymptomatic
2. Blood seen underneath the conjunctivae, often localized to one sector of the eye
3. After trauma, critical to consider the presence of a conjunctival lesion or a ruptured globe

Treatment
1. In general, no treatment is required.
2. Administer artificial teardrops qid to relieve mild ocular irritation.
3. Subconjunctival hemorrhage usually resolves spontaneously in 1 to 2 weeks.
4. If the condition does not resolve or recurs, seek ophthalmologic care.

HYPHEMA

Hyphema usually results from a blunt injury to the eye, resulting in hemorrhage into the anterior chamber.

Signs and Symptoms
1. Meniscus or layering of blood along the lower anterior chamber (in front of the iris) after the victim has been upright for 5 to 10 minutes
2. Decreased vision and eye pain
3. Lethargy and vomiting possible as a result of acutely increased IOP

Treatment
1. Allow the victim to rest in an upright (e.g., sitting) position.

2. Do not instill any ocular medicine or perform any manipulation.
3. Arrange for immediate evacuation.

DACRYOCYSTITIS (INFLAMMATION OF THE LACRIMAL SAC)

Signs and Symptoms

1. Pain, redness, and swelling over the lacrimal sac (innermost aspect of lower eyelid)
2. Mucoid or purulent discharge expressed from the nasolacrimal punctum when pressure is applied

Treatment

1. Administer cephalexin (Keflex) 500 mg tid to qid for 10 days or ciprofloxacin (Cipro) 750 mg bid for 7 to 10 days.
2. Be aware that topical antibiotics are minimally effective.
3. Apply warm compresses.
4. Administer pain medication as needed.
5. Because chronic dacryocystitis often requires surgical correction, seek follow-up on return.

RUPTURED GLOBE

Signs and Symptoms

1. Reduced vision; gross visual acuity assessed by testing the victim for the following abilities (in order of decreasing visual acuity):
   ✤ To read print
   ✤ To count fingers
   ✤ To detect hand motion
   ✤ To localize a light source
   ✤ To perceive light
2. Pupil appearing distorted and teardrop shaped, pointing toward the rupture
3. Conjunctival hemorrhage with dark specks of uveal tissue underneath
4. Limited extraocular mobility

Treatment
1. **Do not press on the eye.**
2. Elevate the victim's head to decrease IOP.
3. Cover the eye with a cup or improvised shield to avoid any pressure on the globe.
4. Avoid any activities that may cause the victim to blink excessively or to strain (including further ocular examination).
5. Administer a systemic antibiotic such as ciprofloxacin (Cipro) 750 mg PO bid or a third-generation cephalosporin (ceftriaxone [Rocephin]) 1 g IV ql2h if available.

PRESEPTAL CELLULITIS
Signs and Symptoms
1. Tenderness and redness of the eyelid often associated with fever
2. Unlike orbital cellulitis, no pain with eye movement or restriction of extraocular movement
3. Inability to open the eye because of marked eyelid edema
4. Appearance resembling and easily confused with an allergic eyelid reaction or insect bite
5. With an allergic or inflammatory process, usually itching without tenderness

Treatment
1. Administer ciprofloxacin (Cipro) 750 PO bid for 7 to 10 days.
2. Alternatively, administer cephalexin (Keflex) 500 mg tid to qid for 7 to 10 days.
3. Apply warm compresses to the inflamed region qid.
4. For a severe lesion with a fluctuant mass (abscess), perform incision and drainage if necessary.
5. *Consider* evacuation for any victim with the following conditions:
   a. Toxic appearance
   b. Child under 5 years of age

c. No improvement or any worsening after 2 to 3 days of oral antibiotics

    d. Requires instrumentation

ORBITAL CELLULITIS

Pathogens that cause orbital cellulitis include *Staphylococcus* and *Streptococcus* species, *Haemophilus influenzae* (common in children), *Bacteroides,* and various gram-negative rods (especially after trauma).

Signs and Symptoms

1. Red eye, blurred vision, diplopia, headache, fever, eyelid edema
2. Erythema, warmth, and tenderness over the affected area
3. Conjunctival chemosis and injection
4. Restricted ocular motility and pain developing on attempted ocular motion
5. Possible coexisting meningitis

Treatment

1. Evacuate the victim immediately.
2. Administer ceftriaxone (Rocephin) 1 to 2 g IV q12h.
3. Although oral antibiotics are considered suboptimal for this condition, a reasonable regimen initiated during transport might include any of the following:
    a. Ciprofloxacin 750 mg (Cipro) PO bid (first choice)
    b. If available, a second- or third-generation oral cephalosporin (e.g., cefpodoxime [Vantin] 400 mg bid)
    c. Cephalexin (Keflex) 500 mg qid

INFECTION OF THE EYELID
Hordeolum

Hordeolum is a common infection in a gland of the eyelid. A small hordeolum that forms an external pustule and points toward the skin is called a *stye.*

Signs and Symptoms
1. Localized pain, swelling, and redness of the eyelid, often associated with a purulent discharge
2. Infection pointing to either the skin or to the conjunctival side of the lid

Treatment
1. Apply warm compresses for 15 to 20 minutes several times per day.
2. Gently scrub the eyelid with soap and water several times per day.
3. Apply a topical antibiotic q4-6h for 7 to 10 days, such as gentamicin (Garamycin) 3 mg/ml ophthalmic solution.
4. If cellulitis is present, administer a systemic antibiotic for 7 to 10 days.
5. Rarely, perform incision and drainage if there is no response to treatment.

Chalazion
Signs and Symptoms
1. Noninflamed, nontender mass in the upper or lower lid
2. May follow a hordeolum
3. Usually points toward the conjunctival side of the lid

Treatment
1. Apply warm compresses.
2. Note that incision and curettage are often necessary if the condition persists (this should be done by an ophthalmologist).

CHAPTER 25

Dental Emergencies

The most common dental emergencies are the result of inflammation, infection, or trauma.

■ DISORDERS ■

TOOTHACHE (PULPITIS)
The common toothache is caused by inflammation of the dental pulp and is often associated with dental caries.

Signs and Symptoms
1. Pain, which may be severe, intermittent, and difficult to localize
2. Pain that is often made worse by hot or cold foods or liquids
3. Carious lesion in the painful tooth; rarely sensitive to percussion or palpation

Treatment
1. If the offending carious lesion can be localized, first apply a piece of cotton soaked with eugenol (oil of cloves).
2. Place a temporary filling material, such as Cavit or zinc oxide–eugenol (ZOE) cement (Intermediate Restorative Material [IRM]), into the lesion to protect the nerve. Softened candle wax can also be used.
3. If the episodes of pain last longer, indicating a mod-

erate pulpitis, fill the lesion as above, and give the victim a nonnarcotic analgesic.
4. For severe pulpitis, with continuous and severe pain, administer a local anesthetic, then evacuate the victim. You can achieve a nerve block with bupivacaine 2% with 1:200,000 epinephrine (Marcaine) that lasts for about 8 hours and does not produce central nervous system depression. Even large doses of narcotics may not provide pain relief and might compromise the victim's ability to participate in evacuation.
5. In extraordinary circumstances, locate the offending tooth, expose the pulp, remove the inflamed tissue with a barbed broach, and cover the lesion with temporary filling material.

INFECTIONS
Apical Abscess and Cellulitis
Signs and Symptoms
1. Dental pain associated with swelling and fluctuation in the gum line at the base of the tooth; swelling much more common on the facial side than on the lingual side
2. Pain caused by percussion of the offending tooth
3. No sensitivity to hot or cold in the affected tooth

Treatment
1. Incision and drainage is the treatment of choice (Fig. 25-1).
   a. Infiltrate the area with a local anesthetic. Adequate anesthesia may also be obtained by applying cold (ice or snow) to the area to be incised.
   b. Make an incision at the point of maximum fluctuation down to bone in one swift movement.
   c. Spread the incision with a hemostat or knife handle.
   d. Place a T-shaped drain into the wound. Drain material can be improvised from a piece of surgical glove or gauze dressing.

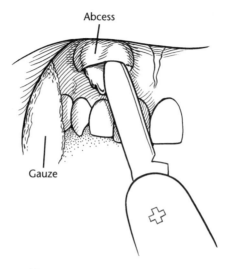

Fig. 25-1. Apical dental abscess.

2. Administer warm saline rinses every q2h.
3. If incision and drainage cannot be performed, administer an oral antibiotic (penicillin 500 mg or erythromycin 500 mg every q6h).
4. Make every effort to locate a dentist because this condition can lead to a systemic infection and often requires extraction of the tooth or root canal therapy.

Pericoronitis

Pericoronitis is an infection of the gingival flap around a partially erupted tooth. The most common site is the mandibular third molar.

Signs and Symptoms
1. May mimic streptococcal pharyngitis or tonsillitis
2. Pain at the site of infection
3. Trismus

Treatment
1. Initiate field treatment, which consists of curettage of the area around the tooth and under the flap. In the absence of proper dental instruments, use a small, curved hemostat.
2. Irrigate the space under the flap with disinfected water or sterile normal saline solution using a syringe and catheter.
3. Begin hot saline rinses q2h, and administer an oral antibiotic (penicillin 500 mg or erythromycin 500 mg q6h).

Deep Fascial Space Infection
Apical infection occasionally spreads beyond the local area to the canine, buccal, and masticator spaces and to the floor of the mouth.

Signs and Symptoms
1. Hallmark—trismus
2. Fever and sepsis
3. Swelling minimal because of the overlying muscle mass
4. Submandibular space infection (Ludwig's angina) that produces elevation of the tongue and brawny, painful edema of the submandibular area
5. Continued swelling that restricts neck motion and produces dysphonia, odynophagia, and drooling; possible progression to acute airway obstruction and asphyxia
6. Mediastinitis and cavernous sinus venous thrombosis

Treatment
1. Be aware that airway management with early intubation or cricothyroidotomy may be necessary.
2. Administer an IV antibiotic (penicillin 2 million units) or oral antibiotic (penicillin 1000 mg) if IV therapy is not available.

3. Evacuate the victim immediately to the nearest medical facility.

TRAUMA
Uncomplicated Crown Fracture
Signs and Symptoms
1. Fractured tooth, but no pulp tissue visible
2. Possible sensitivity to cold or heat

Treatment
1. Smooth any sharp edges with a fingernail file or cover with wax.
2. If thermal sensitivity is severe, apply ZOE (IRM), Cavit, or softened candle wax to the fractured crown.

Uncomplicated Crown-Root Fracture
Signs and Symptoms
Similar to uncomplicated crown fracture, except that the fracture is nearly vertical, leaving a small, chisel-shaped fragment attached only by the palatal gingiva

Treatment
1. Treatment is the same as for an uncomplicated crown fracture.
2. Remove the mobile fragment to make the victim more comfortable.

Complicated Crown Fracture
Signs and Symptoms
1. Tooth fractured
2. Pulp exposed

Treatment
1. Stop the bleeding by placing a moistened tea bag into the socket or next to the bleeding gum.
2. Cap the exposed area with IRM, Cavit, or softened candle wax.

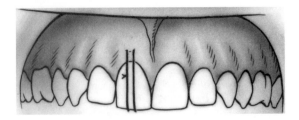

Fig. 25-2. Suture used to stabilize a loosened or avulsed tooth.

Complicated Crown-Root Fracture

Signs and Symptoms
Obliquely fractured tooth, resulting in pulp exposure and a mobile fragment attached to the palatal gingiva

Treatment
1. Remove the mobile fragment.
2. Cap the exposed area with IRM or Cavit.

Root Fracture

Signs and Symptoms
Slight to severe malposition of the crown

Treatment
1. Reposition the tooth as precisely as possible and splint the tooth by suturing it to the gum (Fig. 25-2).
2. If the coronal fragment cannot be stabilized and you are days away from a medical facility, remove the mobile fragment. **Do not attempt to extract the apical fragment.**

Extrusion

Signs and Symptoms
Tooth that is partially displaced from its socket and extremely mobile

Treatment

1. Reposition the tooth with gentle, steady pressure, allowing time to displace the blood that has collected into the apical region of the socket.
2. Observe the victim's occlusion as a guide to proper reduction. If the victim bites and contacts only the injured tooth, further positioning is necessary.
3. Splint the tooth for 2 to 3 weeks, if possible.

Lateral Luxation

Signs and Symptoms

1. Tooth displaced but not mobile because the apex is locked into its new position in the alveolar bone
2. High, metallic tone on percussion

Treatment

1. Use one finger to guide the apex gently down and back, while another finger repositions the crown (Fig. 25-3). The tooth may snap back into place and be stable or may require splinting.
2. Use a suture to splint the tooth in place (see Fig. 25-2).

Total Avulsion

If a tooth is totally avulsed from the bone, it may be salvageable if replaced within 30 to 60 minutes.

Signs and Symptoms

1. Tooth no longer attached to the bone
2. Bleeding in the socket site

Treatment

1. Clean the debris off the tooth by rinsing gently (**do not scrub**) with either saline solution or milk. Handle the tooth only by the crown.
2. Remove any clotted blood from the socket with gentle irrigation and suction.
3. Gently replace the tooth in the socket with slow, steady pressure.

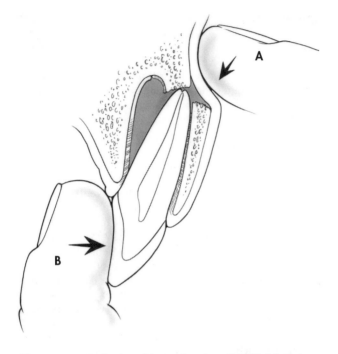

Fig. 25-3. Reduction of lateral luxation. *(Modified from Andreasen JO, Andreasen FM: Essentials of traumatic injuries to the teeth, Copenhagen, 1990, Munksgaard.)*

4. Splint or suture the tooth in place.
5. If the tooth cannot be replaced immediately, store it in balanced Hank's solution, tissue culture medium, physiologic saline solution, white milk, or saliva, in that order of preference.
6. Relieve bleeding by placing a moistened tea bag into the socket that is bleeding.

CHAPTER 26

Snake and Reptile Bites

DEFINITIONS AND CHARACTERISTICS

Two main families of venomous snakes indigenous to the United States are Crotalidae (pit vipers) and Elapidae (coral snakes). Most snakebites are caused by the pit vipers, so called because of a depression, or pit, in the maxillary bone. Rattlesnakes (Plates 5 and 6), the cottonmouth (water moccasin) snake (Plate 7), and the copperhead snake (Plate 8) are members of the pit viper family. The major snakes of medical importance outside of North America are the cobras, mambas, kraits, coral snakes, Australian elapids, sea snakes, vipers, rattlesnakes, asps, and colubrids (rear-fanged snakes).

Identifying characteristics of pit vipers include the following (Fig. 26-1):

1. Depression, or pit, in the maxillary bone, located midway between and below the level of the eye and the nostril on each side of the head
2. Vertical elliptic pupils ("cat's eye")
3. Triangular head that is distinct from the remainder of the body
4. Single row of subcaudal scutes, or scales
5. May have rattles on the tails
6. One or two fangs on each side of the head

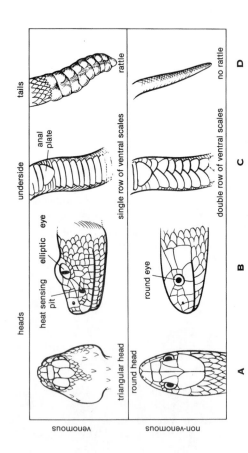

Fig. 26-1. Identification of venomous pit vipers. **A,** Triangular head. **B,** Elliptic eye; heat-sensing facial pits on sides of head near nostrils. **C,** Single row of ventral scales leading up to anal plate. **D,** Rattles on tail (baby rattlesnakes have only "buttons" but are still quite venomous).

Two members of the coral snake family, Elapidae, occur in the United States: the western coral snake *(Micruroides euryxanthus),* found in Arizona and New Mexico, and the eastern coral snake *(Micrurus fulvius)* (Plate 9), distributed from coastal North Carolina through the Gulf states to western Texas. The elapids differ from pit vipers in having very short fangs, round pupils, and subcaudal scales in a double row. Because many nonpoisonous mimics occur in coral snake territory, the rule of thumb for identifying a venomous species is red bands bordered by yellow or white indicate a venomous animal, whereas red bands bordered by black indicate a nonvenomous animal. *This rule applies to all coral snakes native to the United States but **does not apply** to species found south of Mexico City and in other foreign countries.*

DISORDERS
Pit Viper Envenomation

Not all bites result in significant, or any, envenomation. Observe the victim closely for signs and symptoms.

Signs and Symptoms

1. Common: local burning pain immediately after the bite, weakness, nausea and vomiting, paresthesias, pain, fang marks, swelling (usually within 5 minutes)
2. Less common: ecchymoses, fasciculations, hypotension, bullae, necrosis
3. Without treatment
   a. May have rapidly progressing edema that can involve an entire extremity within 1 hour if envenomation is severe (Table 26-1)
   b. Usually spreads more slowly, over 6 to 12 hours
   c. Edema that is soft, pitting, and limited to subcutaneous tissues
4. Hemorrhagic blebs and bullae developing at the site of the bite within 6 to 36 hours; may progress proximally along the involved extremity

Table 26-1.

Grades of Envenomation	
ENVENOMATION	**CHARACTERISTICS**
None	Fang marks, but no local or systemic reactions
Minimal	Fang marks, local swelling and pain, but no systemic reactions
Moderate	Fang marks and swelling progressing beyond the site of the bite; systemic signs and symptoms, such as nausea, vomiting, paresthesias, or hypotension
Severe	Fang marks present with marked swelling of the extremity, subcutaneous ecchymosis, severe symptoms, including manifestations of coagulopathy

5. Paresthesias of the scalp, face, and lips, along with periorbital muscle fasciculations
   a. Indicate that a significant envenomation has occurred
   b. May be complaints of a rubbery or metallic taste in the mouth
   c. General symptoms: weakness, sweating, nausea, faintness
6. Hemorrhage manifested as skin petechiae, epistaxis, hematemesis, melena, hemoptysis, and blindness; pulmonary edema possible
7. *With some Mojave Desert rattlesnakes, bites produce neuromuscular blockade, leading to respiratory paralysis, in the absence of a significant local tissue reaction.* Paralysis initially appears as cranial nerve deficits (hoarseness, difficulty swallowing, ptosis) and progresses to involve the diaphragm.

Treatment

1. Direct treatment at reducing venom effects, minimizing tissue damage, and preventing complicated sequelae.
2. Provide prehospital management.
   a. Avoid panic. Instruct the victim to back out of the snake's striking range, which is approximately the length of the snake.
   b. If the snake has been killed, transport it with the victim for identification purposes. However, it is not necessary to identify the snake to treat the bite appropriately. If the snake is killed, do not handle it directly; arrange to transport it in a closed container. Collect the snake using a stick that is longer than the snake. Decapitated head reactions persist for 20 to 60 minutes, and even the severed head of a snake can envenom a person.
   c. Immobilize the bitten extremity by splinting as if for a fracture.
   d. Obtain medical assistance. Arrange for the victim to be transported to the nearest medical facility, with minimal exertion.
   e. Encourage the victim to drink liquids to maintain adequate hydration.
3. Implement other first-aid measures.
   a. The *pressure immobilization technique* (Fig. 26-2) has been used successfully to manage certain elapid snakebites and funnel-web spider bites in Australia and marine envenomations. The efficacy of the technique depends on collapsing small, superficial lymphatic and venous vessels to retard venom uptake and distribution. Possible disadvantages include increased local tissue damage in crotalid bites because of the necrotizing effect of the venom if it remains localized to certain sites over time. Therefore it is not recommended for routine use, but it should be considered when the deleterious local effects must be weighed against a life-

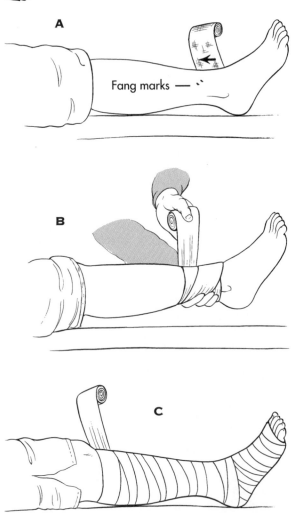

Fig. 26-2. Australian compression and immobilization technique. This technique has proved effective in management of elapid and sea snake envenomations. Its efficacy in viperid (true viper) bites has yet to be evaluated clinically.

D

E

F

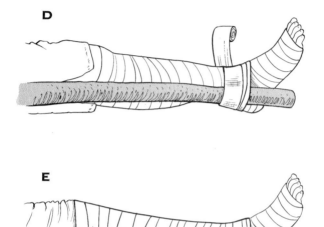

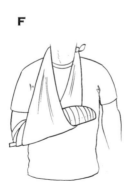

Fig. 26-2, cont'd   For legend see facing page.

threatening situation that follows the systemic distribution of venom.

   (1) To apply the pressure immobilization technique for venom sequestration, if the bite location permits, place a cloth or gauze pad (approximate dimensions 6 to 8 cm [2½ to 3 inches] × 6 to 8 cm × 2 cm [1 inch] thick) directly over the area and hold it firmly in place with a circumferential bandage 15 to 18 cm (6 to 8 inches) wide applied at lymphatic-venous occlusive pressure. If the cloth or gauze pad is not available, a rolled bandage may be used alone. Take care not to occlude the arterial circulation, as determined by the detection of arterial pulsations and proper capillary refill.

   (2) Splint the limb, and do not release the bandage until after the victim has been brought to proper medical attention and you are prepared to provide systemic support, or after 24 hours. Take care to check frequently that swelling beneath the bandage has not compromised the arterial circulation.

b. The classic recommendation to apply a tourniquet is controversial. An arterial-occlusive tourniquet represents a decision to sacrifice a limb to minimize systemic symptoms and save a life. A lympho-occlusive constriction band applied proximal to the bite may be beneficial, but take care to allow arterial inflow to the affected limb.

c. The classic recommendation to incise and suck the wound also is controversial. With regard to suction, a negative-pressure device called The Extractor (Sawyer Products) may remove a clinically significant amount of venom if it is applied over the bite site within 3 minutes of the bite and left in place for 30 minutes.

d. Electroshock therapy can be dangerous to victims and has no proven value in managing bites by pit vipers.

e. Cryotherapy is not recommended because freezing or vasoconstricting already compromised tissues may contribute to necrosis.

f. Use of antivenin in the field is unwise. Backpacking the extensive equipment and drugs necessary to administer IV antivenin is cumbersome, and severe anaphylaxis must be anticipated.

g. Administer a broad-spectrum antibiotic, such as dicloxacillin or cephalexin 250 to 500 mg PO qid for 7 to 10 days.

h. Immobilize the bitten extremity in a position of function within a well-padded splint.

Coral Snake Envenomation

The coral snake clinical envenomation syndrome is attributed to the eastern coral snake. The bite of the western coral snake is generally of lesser severity; no fatal bite has been reported from this species.

Signs and Symptoms

1. Little or no pain and no local edema or necrosis; venom primarily neurotoxic
2. Within 90 minutes of envenomation, weak or numb feeling in bitten extremity
3. Several hours later, systemic symptoms appearing, including tremors, drowsiness or euphoria, and marked salivation
4. After 5 to 10 hours, slurred speech and diplopia, heralding the onset of cranial nerve palsies
   a. Bulbar paralysis: manifested as dysphagia and dyspnea
   b. Total flaccid paralysis possible
5. Symptoms possibly delayed as long as 13 hours after the bite
6. Paresthesias and muscle fasciculations common at the site of the bite
7. Flaccid paralysis, respiratory failure
8. Nausea and vomiting, weakness, dizziness, difficulty breathing

9. Less common: local edema, diplopia, dyspnea, diaphoresis, myalgia, confusion; death extremely rare

Treatment
1. Follow the recommendations for field management of a pit viper bite (see above). Note that the pressure immobilization technique may be efficacious and poses less of a theoretic hazard because coral snake venom does not produce local tissue necrosis.
2. Note that because it is difficult to ascertain early whether envenomation by a coral snake has occurred, treatment and observation are mandatory. Early treatment with antivenin is advised in any suspected bite with envenomation because signs and symptoms can be delayed for up to 13 hours. Therefore transport the bitten victim to a medical facility where definitive antivenin therapy can be undertaken.
3. Be aware that management of envenomation by the western coral snake is purely supportive because no antiserum is commercially available.

Envenomation by Non–North American Snakes
Signs and Symptoms
1. For elapids (cobras, mambas, kraits, Australian venomous snakes, coral snakes):
   a. Local—findings absent or minimal; significant pain with some species, regional lymphadenopathy and necrosis with some species, edema with some species
   b. Systemic—neurotoxicity (cranial nerve dysfunction, ptosis, dysphonia, blurred vision, altered mental status, peripheral weakness and paralysis, respiratory failure) with delayed (up to 10 hours) onset possible, hypersalivation, diaphoresis, cardiovascular failure, coagulopathy, myonecrosis, renal failure
   c. Eye exposure to venom from any of the spitting

cobras or ringhals—immediate burning pain and tearing, which may lead to corneal ulceration, uveitis, and permanent blindness

2. For sea snakes:
   a. Local—trivial; fang marks difficult to identify
   b. Systemic—neurotoxicity (cranial nerve dysfunction, peripheral weakness and paralysis, respiratory failure), hypersalivation, dysphagia, dysarthria, trismus, muscle spasm, myotoxicity with resulting muscle pain and tenderness, myoglobinemia, myoglobinuria, hyperkalemia

3. For vipers and pit vipers:
   a. Local—pain, soft tissue swelling, regional lymphadenopathy, ecchymosis, bloody exudate from fang marks, hemorrhagic bullae; early absence of findings does not rule out significant envenomation; local necrosis possibly significant
   b. Systemic—essentially any organ system potentially involved; cardiovascular toxicity (hypotension, pulmonary edema), neurotoxicity (cranial nerve dysfunction, peripheral weakness) with some species, hemorrhagic diathesis, renal failure, altered taste sensation, headache, diarrhea, vomiting, fever, abdominal pain, hypotension

4. For burrowing asps:
   a. Local—single fang puncture mark common, severe pain, some swelling, lymphadenopathy, occasional local necrosis
   b. Systemic—nausea, vomiting, diaphoresis, fever, respiratory distress, cardiac arrhythmias

5. For colubrids:
   a. Local—mild to moderate local swelling, pain, ecchymosis, bloody exudate from fang marks
   b. Systemic—nausea, vomiting, coagulopathy, renal dysfunction, headache

Treatment

1. Initiate same field treatment as for North American pit viper envenomation, with the notation to use the

pressure immobilization technique for bites of elapids, sea snakes, burrowing asps, colubrids, and any
unknown snake when the bite does not produce significant local pain.
2. For viper and pit viper bites or when the bite does
produce significant local pain, apply a proximal constriction band and local suction. In either case, splint
the extremity at heart level.
3. Arrange to transport the victim as quickly as possible
to the nearest appropriate medical facility where antivenin therapy can be initiated.

Venomous Lizard Bites

The Gila monster and Mexican beaded lizard are
found in North America. Both possess venom glands
and grooved teeth. Human envenomation most often
occurs when the lizard retains its grasp and chews on
the victim.

Signs and Symptoms
1. Usually simple puncture wounds, although teeth
   may break off or be shed during the bite and remain
   in the wound
2. Pain, often severe and burning, at the wound site
   within 5 minutes
   a. Pain radiating up the extremity
   b. Intense pain lasting 3 to 5 hours and then subsid-
      ing after 8 hours
3. Edema at the wound site, usually within 15 minutes,
   that progresses slowly in variable degrees up the extremity
4. Cyanosis or blue discoloration around the wound
5. Weakness, fainting, diaphoresis
6. Tenderness at the wound site for 3 to 4 weeks after
   the bite, but usually little tissue necrosis
7. Hypotension rare; no coagulation defects noted

Treatment

A Gila monster may hang on tenaciously during a bite, and mechanical means may be required to loosen the grip of the jaws.

1. Cleanse the wound thoroughly with a soap and water scrub or with a dilution of povidone-iodine.
2. Infiltrate the puncture wounds with 1% lidocaine using a 25-gauge needle.
3. Then probe the wounds to detect the presence of shed or broken teeth, helping to prevent future infection from a foreign body.
4. Administer an analgesic appropriate for the degree of pain.

CHAPTER 27

Bites and Stings From Arthropods

The principal disorders involving the bites or stings of arthropods are spider bites; bee, wasp, and ant stings; caterpillar spine irritation; interactions with sucking bugs, beetles, flies and other winged insects, lice, fleas, mites, and ticks; and stings from scorpions.

■ DISORDERS ■

SPIDER BITES
Brown Spiders

Necrotic arachnidism, or "loxoscelism," is caused by spiders of the genus *Loxosceles* and other spiders that deposit a venom characterized by its local dermonecrotic activity. The "fiddleback" spider (Plate 10) carries the characteristic violin-shaped marking on the dorsum of its cephalothorax. The clinical spectrum of loxoscelism ranges from mild and transient skin irritation to severe local necrosis accompanied by hematologic and renal pathologic conditions.

Signs and Symptoms
1. Most common presentation is an isolated cutaneous lesion
2. Local symptoms beginning the moment of the bite,

with a sharp stinging sensation, although some victims report no awareness of having been bitten
3. Stinging subsiding over 6 to 8 hours, then replaced by aching and pruritus
4. Site becoming edematous, with an erythematous halo surrounding an irregularly shaped violaceous center of incipient necrosis (Plate 11)
5. Often erythematous margin spreading irregularly, in a gravitationally influenced pattern that leaves the original center near the top of the lesion
6. In more severe cases, serous or hemorrhagic bullae arising at the center within 24 to 72 hours, with an underlying eschar
7. Systemic reactions: hemoglobinuria within 24 hours of envenomation; fever, chills, maculopapular rash, weakness, leukocytosis, arthralgias, nausea, and vomiting within 24 hours of the bite

Treatment
1. Apply cold compresses intermittently for the first 4 days after the bite. **Do not apply heat.**
2. If the wound appears infected, apply a topical antiseptic (mupirocin, bacitracin) under a sterile dressing. Administer an oral antibiotic, such as cephalexin, dicloxacillin, or erythromycin.

Widow Spiders
Female spiders of the genus *Latrodectus* (Plate 12) carry the characteristic hourglass marking on the ventral abdomen.

Signs and Symptoms
1. Initial bite sometimes sharply painful, but often nearly painless, with only a tiny papule or punctum visible; surrounding skin slightly reddened and sometimes indurated; in many cases, no further progression of symptoms occurs
2. Neuromuscular symptoms: can become dramatic within 30 to 60 minutes as involuntary spasm and ri-

gidity affect the large muscle groups of the abdomen, limbs, and lower back
3. Predominantly abdominal presentation resembling an acute abdomen
4. Priapism, fasciculations, weakness, ptosis, thready pulse, fever, salivation, diaphoresis, vomiting, bronchorrhea, pulmonary edema, rhabdomyolysis, hypertension
5. Characteristic pattern of facial swelling, known as *Latrodectus* facies, possible hours after the bite

Treatment
1. Be aware that the natural course of an envenomation is to resolve completely after a few days, although pain may last for a week or more.
2. Apply a cold pack (ice pack) to the bite site.
3. For muscle spasm, administer diazepam or another benzodiazepine.
4. Administer pain medication.
5. Monitor the victim for hypertension.
   a. Administer a centrally acting or vasodilating antihypertensive if the victim develops urgent hypertension and such a drug is available.
   b. Be alert for a seizure associated with rapid acceleration of hypertension.

Funnel-Web Spiders
Funnel-web spiders are large, aggressive spiders that deliver a potent neurotoxin.

Signs and Symptoms
1. Intense pain at the bite site
2. Phase I
   a. Begins minutes after venom injection, with local piloerection and muscle fasciculation; becomes generalized over the next 10 to 20 minutes
   b. Severe hypertension, tachycardia, hyperthermia, and coma developing next
   c. Diaphoresis, salivation, lacrimation, diarrhea,

sporadic apnea, and grotesque muscle writhing after the previous symptoms
3. Phase II
   a. Begins 1 to 2 hours after envenomation, as phase I symptoms begin to subside
   b. May be a return of consciousness and the appearance of recovery
   c. In severe cases, gradually worsening hypotension, with periods of apnea and the onset of pulmonary edema

Treatment
1. In the field, apply the pressure immobilization technique for venom sequestration at the bite site (see Chapter 26).
2. Give specific antivenin, which is developed in rabbits and is the mainstay of treatment.
3. Be aware that general management, in addition to antivenin administration, is based on symptoms and is supportive.
   a. Give oxygen and IV fluid support.
   b. Use atropine 0.6 to 1.0 mg to lessen salivation and bronchorrhea.
   c. Administer a beta-adrenergic blocking agent to control severe hypertension and tachycardia.

Banana Spiders
The *Phoneutria* spiders of South America are large nocturnal creatures noted for their aggressive behavior and painful bites.

Signs and Symptoms
1. Severe local pain that radiates up the extremity into the trunk, followed within 10 to 20 minutes by tachycardia, hypertension, hypothermia, profuse diaphoresis, salivation, vertigo, visual disturbances, nausea and vomiting, and priapism
2. If death occurs in 2 to 6 hours, usually a result of respiratory paralysis

Treatment
1. Treat mild envenomation symptomatically by infiltrating the bite site with a local anesthetic or by applying peripheral vasodilating warmth.
2. Be aware that narcotics may potentiate the venom's respiratory depressant effect and should *not* be used.
3. For severe envenomation, administer polyvalent antivenin (Sero Antiaracidico Polivalente, Instituto Butantan).

Wolf Spiders
Wolf spiders are diurnal predators that are usually a mottled dark gray or brown.

Signs and Symptoms
1. Local pain, swelling, and erythema
2. Rarely, necrosis

Treatment
1. Apply a cold (ice) pack to the bite site.
2. Administer oral pain medication or infiltrate the area with an anesthetic agent.

Tarantulas
Tarantulas are large, slow spiders capable of inflicting a painful bite when threatened. Several varieties possess urticating hairs, which they flick by the thousands through the air into an attacker's skin and eyes.

Signs and Symptoms
1. Intense inflammation where hairs land, which may remain pruritic for weeks
2. Aching or stinging pain at the bite site

Treatment
1. Be aware that therapy is supportive and based on symptoms.
2. Elevate the bitten extremity and immobilize it to reduce pain.

3. Administer pain medication.
4. Note that topical or systemic corticosteroids and oral antihistamines can be used for urticating hair exposure.

Hobo Spiders

The hobo spider, also called the Northwestern brown spider *(Tegenaria agrestis),* can cause a necrotic bite similar to that induced by the brown recluse spider.

Signs and Symptoms
1. Local redness, vesiculation, and necrosis
2. Systemic effects: headache, visual disturbances, hallucinations, weakness, lethargy

Treatment
1. Apply cold compresses intermittently for the first 4 days after the bite. **Do not apply heat.**
2. If the wound appears infected, apply a topical antiseptic (mupirocin, bacitracin) under a sterile dressing. Administer an oral antibiotic, such as cephalexin, dicloxacillin, or erythromycin.

Running Spiders and Sac Spiders

Running and sac spiders are often nondescript spiders with yellow, brown, green, or olive coloration.

Signs and Symptoms
1. Vary with species
2. May include dyspnea, varying degrees of weakness, local redness, pain and edema, headache, fever, nausea, and necrosis

Treatment
1. Be aware that this lesion usually heals without problems provided secondary infection does not develop.
2. Apply cool compresses, elevate the involved area, immobilize the victim, and give analgesics as needed.

BEES, WASPS, AND ANTS

By far the most important venomous insects are members of the order Hymenoptera, including bees, wasps, and ants (Fig. 27-1).

Signs and Symptoms

1. Instantaneous pain, followed by a wheal-and-flare reaction, with variable edema
2. With fire ants, vesicles that subsequently become sterile pustules from insects grasping the skin with their mouthparts and inflicting multiple stings (Plate 13)
3. With multiple bee, wasp, yellowjacket, or hornet stings, vomiting, diarrhea, generalized edema, dyspnea, hypotension, and collapse
4. Large local reactions relatively common, spreading more than 15 cm (6 inches) beyond the sting and persisting longer than 24 hours
5. Allergic sting reactions
   a. Occur in areas remote from the sting and typically include pruritus, hives, difficulty breathing, and nausea
   b. When become life threatening, marked respiratory distress, hypotension, loss of consciousness, and arrhythmias
   c. Most fatalities within 1 hour of sting

Treatment

1. Be aware that the treatment of anaphylactic reaction follows conventional guidelines, as follows:
   a. Maintain the airway and administer oxygen.
   b. Obtain IV access. Administer lactated Ringer's or NS solution to support the blood pressure at a level of 90 mm Hg systolic.
   c. Administer epinephrine. Begin with aqueous epinephrine 1:1000 subcutaneously (SC) in the deltoid region. The dose for adults is 0.3 to 0.5 ml, and for children 0.01 ml/kg body weight. An alternative is to inject the contents of an EpiPen or

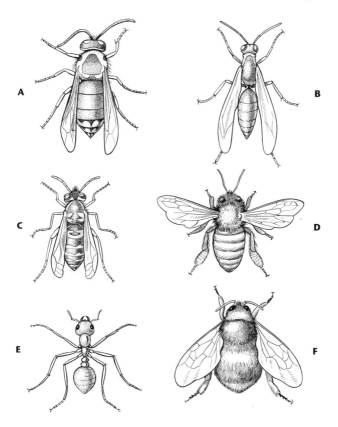

Fig. 27-1.   Representative venomous Hymenoptera: **A,** Hornet *(Vespula maculata);* **B,** wasp *(Chlorion ichneumerea);* **C,** yellowjacket *(Vespula maculiforma);* **D,** honey bee *(Apis mellifera);* **E,** fire ant *(Solenopsis invicta);* **F,** bumblebee *(Bombus species).*

EpiPen Jr IM into the lateral thigh region. Repeat in 20 minutes if relief is partial. If the reaction is limited to pruritus and urticaria, there is no wheezing or facial swelling, and the victim is older than 45 years, administer an antihistamine and reserve epinephrine for a worsened condition.

d. If the reaction is life threatening and there is no response to SC epinephrine, administer epinephrine IV. Give an adult a 0.1-mg bolus of 1:1000 aqueous epinephrine (0.1 ml) diluted in 10 ml NS solution (final dilution 1:100,000) infused over 10 minutes. Prepare a mixture for continuous infusion by adding 1 mg 1:1000 aqueous epinephrine (1 ml) to 250 ml NS solution, thus creating a concentration of 4 μg/ml. This infusion should be started at 1 μg/min (15 minidrops/min) and increased to 4 to 5 μg/min if the clinical response is inadequate. In infants and children, the starting dose is 0.1 μg/kg/min up to a maximum of 1.5 μg/kg/min, with the awareness that infusion rates in excess of 0.5 μg/kg/min may be associated with cardiac ischemia and arrhythmias.

e. Relieve bronchospasm. Administer micronized albuterol or metaproterenol by handheld metered-dose inhaler.

f. Administer antihistamines. Manage mild reactions with diphenhydramine 50 to 75 mg IV, IM, or PO. The dose for children is 1 mg/kg. Nonsedating antihistamines, such as fexofenadine 60 mg or cimetidine 300 mg, are adjuncts.

g. Administer corticosteroids. If the reaction is severe or prolonged or if the victim is regularly medicated with corticosteroids, administer hydrocortisone 200 mg, methylprednisolone 50 mg, or dexamethasone 15 mg IV with a 10-day oral taper to follow. The parenteral dose of hydrocortisone for children is 2.5 mg/kg. If the therapy is initiated orally, administer prednisone 60 to 100 mg for adults and 1 mg/kg for children.

2. For mild hymenopteran stings, apply ice packs to provide relief.

3. Be aware that a honeybee or yellowjacket may leave a stinger in the wound. Scrape or brush this off with

a sharp edge; do not remove the stinger with a forceps because it may squeeze the attached venom sac and worsen the envenomation.

4. Note that a home remedy, such as a paste of unseasoned meat tenderizer or baking soda, is of variable usefulness, although some report the former to be effective. Topical anesthetics in "sting sticks" have limited usefulness.

5. Because infection is common, apply antimicrobial ointment, such as mupirocin, to cover the wound. Breaking fire ant blisters is not recommended.

6. Be aware that envenomation from multiple hymenopteran stings may require more aggressive therapy, including IV calcium gluconate (5 to 10 ml of 10% solution) in conjunction with a parenteral antihistamine and corticosteroid to relieve pain, swelling, and nausea and vomiting. A corticosteroid, such as methylprednisolone 24 mg the first day, then tapered over 5 days, often hastens resolution of a large local reaction to a bee or wasp sting.

7. Manage delayed serum sickness in response to multiple hymenopteran stings with a corticosteroid, such as prednisone 60 to 100 mg for adults and 1mg/kg for children, tapered over 2 weeks.

CATERPILLARS

Injury usually follows contact with caterpillars and is less frequent with the cocoon or adult stage. The largest outbreaks have been associated with spines detached from live or dead caterpillars and cocoons.

Signs and Symptoms

1. With caterpillars that have hollow spines and venom glands, instant nettling pain, followed by redness and swelling, after direct contact with the live insect
   a. Ordinarily, no systemic manifestations; symptoms subsiding within 24 hours
   b. Possibly intense pain with central radiation, ac-

companied by nausea and vomiting, headache, fever, and lymphadenopathy
  c. Rarely, coagulopathy
2. With attached or detached spines from certain caterpillars or moths, itching and erythematous, papular, or urticarial rash within a few hours to 2 days after contact
  a. Rash persisting for up to 1 week
  b. Lesions rarely bullous
  c. Conjunctivitis, upper respiratory tract irritation, rare asthmalike symptoms with or without dermatitis

Treatment
1. Apply adhesive tape, a commercial facial peel, or a thin layer of rubber cement to remove spines.
2. Administer an oral antihistamine and/or NSAIDs. If the dermatitis is severe and persistent, consider administering a corticosteroid, such as prednisone 60 to 100 mg for adults and 1 mg/kg for children, tapered over 10 days.

SUCKING BUGS
"Sucking bugs" have sucking mouthparts, generally in the form of a beak. Included are the assassin bugs, kissing bugs (see Fig. 27-3), and flying bedbugs. Many of these bugs bite at night on exposed parts of the body. The bites themselves may be painless.

Signs and Symptoms
1. On initial exposure, usually no reaction.
2. With repeated bites, reddish itching papules that may persist for up to 1 week; bites often grouped in a cluster or line and may be accompanied by giant urticarial wheals, lymphadenopathy, hemorrhagic bullae, and fever
3. Systemic anaphylaxis possible
4. Possible pain at the sting site
  a. Local swelling that last several hours

b. With bedbugs, usually a pruritic wheal with central hemorrhagic punctum, followed by a reddish papule that persists for days

Treatment
Be aware that treatment is supportive and not particularly effective.

BEETLES
Several families of beetles, such as the blister and rove beetles, produce toxic secretions that may be deposited on the skin.

Signs and Symptoms
1. With the blister beetle, contact painless and seldom remembered by the victim; blisters induced by cantharidin toxin and appear 2 to 5 hours after contact, generally as single or multiple areas, usually 5 to 50 mm in diameter and thin walled; unless broken or rubbed, not usually painful
2. With the rove beetle, vesicant substance is an alkaloid; if the beetle is crushed or rubbed on the skin, redness occurs after several hours, followed by a crop of small blisters that persist for 2 to 3 days; conjunctivitis occurs if the secretion is rubbed into the eyes

Treatment
1. Treat beetle vesication as a superficial chemical burn.
2. Note that topical preparations containing corticosteroids and antihistamines are not particularly effective.

TWO-WINGED FLIES, BITING MIDGES, AND MOSQUITOES (Fig. 27-2)
Signs and Symptoms
1. Immediate pruritic wheals followed after 12 to 24 hours by red, swollen, and itchy lesions; can have blistering or necrosis

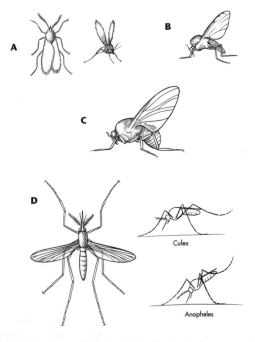

Fig. 27-2. Blood-feeding biting flies (not drawn to scale): **A,** Sand fly; **B,** biting midge; **C,** blackfly; **D,** mosquito.

2. Rarely, immune response leading to asthma, bullous eruptions, fever, lymphadenopathy, or hepatomegaly

Treatment
1. Immediately after the bite, apply a cold (ice) pack.
2. Apply a topical antipruritic lotion or cream.
3. If the reaction is severe or prolonged, consider the administration of a corticosteroid, such as prednisone 60 to 100 mg for adults and 1 mg/kg for children, tapered over 7 to 14 days.

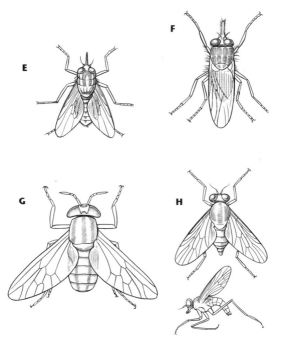

Fig. 27-2, cont'd **E,** stable fly; **F,** tsetse fly; **G,** tabanid fly; **H,** snipe fly.

CUTANEOUS MYIASIS

Parasitism by fly larvae occurs when an insect, such as the human botfly, deposits an egg on human skin. The egg hatches immediately, and the larva enters the skin through the bite of the carrier or through some other small break in the skin. The larvae grow to 15 to 20 mm under the skin.

Signs and Symptoms

1. As the larvae grow under the skin, initial pruritic papule becomes a furuncle with a characteristic cen-

tral opening from which serosanguineous fluid exudes.
2. Pain often accompanies movement of the older larvae, but lesion is not particularly tender to palpation.
3. Tip of the larva may protrude from the central opening, or bubbles produced by its respiration may be seen.
4. Lymphadenopathy, fever, and secondary infection are rare.

Treatment
1. Sometimes, exert simple pressure to extrude the organism, particularly if it is small.
2. Be aware that occlusion of the breathing hole with heavy oil, nail polish, or animal fat (e.g., bacon) may cause the larva to emerge sufficiently for it to be grasped and withdrawn.
3. Alternatively, inject about 2 ml of local anesthetic into the base of the lesion, thus extruding the larva by fluid pressure.
4. If you attempt surgical excision under local anesthesia, take care not to break or rupture the larva because this might result in an inflammatory reaction that leads to infection.

LICE
Lice are very active, but nits (eggs) are easily identified as whitish ovals, about 0.5 mm long, attached firmly to one side of the hair.

Signs and Symptoms
1. Small red macule in response to secretions released by the louse during biting and feeding
2. Characteristic body louse bite: a central hemorrhagic punctum in many of the macules
3. Excoriations, crusts, eczematization in a parallel pattern from scratching, particularly on the shoulders, trunk, and buttocks (favorite sites for bites)

4. Severe pruritus and inflammation caused by sensitization after repeated exposure to bites; victim possibly infested for weeks before pruritus becomes marked
5. Occipital and posterior cervical adenopathy associated with head lice

Treatment

1. Treat head lice with 1% gamma benzene hexachloride (lindane) shampoo. Apply it to the wet hair, lather, and leave it in place for 4 minutes before rinsing it out. Repeat the treatment 7 to 10 days later as a precaution in case some nits were not killed by the first application.
2. Treat body lice with the same medication, but be aware that parasites and nits are not usually found on the skin. These must be eradicated from the clothing. Take a good bath and launder all clothing.
3. Treat pubic lice with 1% gamma benzene hexachloride lotion or shampoo as for head lice. Rub crotamiton lotion into the affected area daily for several weeks to destroy hatching ova and prevent a persistent infection. Manage eyelash infection by careful application of physostigmine ophthalmic ointment, using a cotton-tipped applicator.

FLEAS (Fig. 27-3)

Signs and Symptoms

1. Small central hemorrhagic punctum surrounded by erythema and urticaria; bullae or even ulceration after bite in highly sensitive individuals
2. Intensely pruritic, with scratching often resulting in crusting and the development of impetigo
3. Tungiasis caused by burrowing flea (jigger, chigo, sand flea), usually on the feet, buttocks, or perineum of a person who wears no shoes or frequently squats

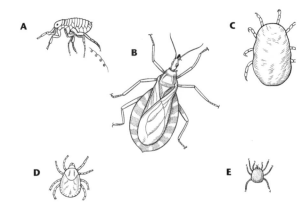

Fig. 27-3. Various blood-feeding arthropods (not drawn to scale): **A,** Flea; **B,** kissing bug; **C,** soft tick; **D,** hard tick; **E,** chigger mite.

    a. Firm itchy nodule with posterior end of the flea visible as a dark plug or spot in the center of the nodule

    b. Numerous papules aggregating into plaques with a honeycomb appearance

    c. Secondary infection around each flea inevitable, resulting in ulceration and suppuration

Treatment

1. Relieve pruritus by applying calamine lotion with phenol.
2. Administer a systemic antihistamine to help control itching.
3. Clean excoriations and apply a topical antiseptic ointment, such as mupirocin.
4. With a burrowing flea infestation (tungiasis), remove the burrowing flea or a pustule will rupture, leaving an ulcer.

MITES

The human scabies mite is *Sarcoptes scabiei* var. *hominis.* The adult female burrows into the epidermis.

Signs and Symptoms
1. Hallmark of scabies: severe nocturnal pruritus
   a. Itching also provoked by any warming of the body
   b. Elapsed time of 4 to 6 weeks between infestation and onset of severe pruritus
2. Cutaneous manifestations: an epidermal burrow (a linear or serpentine track, rarely longer than 5 to 10 mm) with a predilection for the interdigital spaces, palms, flexor surfaces of the wrists, elbows, feet and ankles, belt line, anterior axillary folds, lower buttocks, and penis and scrotum

Treatment
1. Be aware that in most cases a single overnight application of 1% gamma benzene hexachloride cream or lotion is curative, although symptoms may persist for over a month until the mite and mite products are shed with the epidermis. Apply the chemical even beneath the fingernails.
2. Note that alternative scabicides may be desirable for use in infants and pregnant women.
   a. For infants over age 2 months, permethrin cream 5% is approved for use, as is sulfur in petrolatum (5% to 10%).
   b. Another alternative is crotamiton cream 10% or lotion applied for 2 consecutive nights.

TICKS (see Fig. 27-3)
Local Reaction to Tick Bites
Signs and Symptoms
1. Vary from small pruritic nodule to extensive area of ulceration, erythema, and induration
2. Possibly accompanied by fever, chills, and malaise

Treatment
1. If tick mouthparts or the head remain embedded in the wound, remove them surgically using a needle or the sharp tip of a knife or scalpel.
2. Manage wound infection with an antibiotic.

Tick Paralysis

Tick paralysis (Plate 14) occurs most frequently during the spring and summer when ticks are feeding. Girls are more often affected than boys because the ticks can hide more easily in girls' longer scalp hair.

Signs and Symptoms
1. From 5 to 6 days after the adult female tick attaches: restlessness, irritability, paresthesias in the hands and feet
2. Over the ensuing 24 to 48 hours: ascending, symmetric, and flaccid paralysis with loss of deep tendon reflexes; weakness usually greater in the lower extremities
3. Within 1 to 2 days: severe generalized weakness possible, accompanied by bulbar and respiratory paralysis
   a. Cerebellar dysfunction with incoordination and ataxia possible
   b. Facial paralysis an isolated finding in persons with ticks embedded behind the ear

Treatment
1. Note that the diagnosis is established when the paralysis resolves after tick removal. In North America, most victims show improvement within hours of tick removal, with a return to normal in several days.
2. Be aware that, aside from tick removal, treatment is supportive.

Lyme Disease

Lyme disease, caused by *Borrelia burgdorferi,* is transmitted most often by the deer tick *Ixodes scapularis* and the western black-legged tick *I. pacificus.*

Signs and Symptoms

1. Stage I
   a. Average 7 days (range 3 to 32 days) after inoculation, victim develops an expanding, annular, and erythematous skin lesion (erythema migrans) (Plate 15).
   b. Initially, central red macule or papule, but as lesion expands, partial central clearing usually seen, while outer borders remain bright red.
   c. Borders usually flat but may be raised.
   d. Center of some early lesions intensely red and indurated, vesicular, or necrotic; sometimes area develops multiple red rings within the outside margin, or the central area turns blue before clearing.
   e. Lesion diameter 15 cm (6 inches) (range 3 to 68 cm [1 to 27 inches]) and may be anywhere on the body, although most common sites are thigh, groin, and axilla.
   f. Lesion warm to the touch and usually described as burning, but occasionally as itching or painful.
   g. Rash fading after an average of 28 days (range 1 to 14 weeks) without treatment; with antibiotics, lesion resolves after several days.
   h. Constitutional symptoms accompany erythema migrans, but usually mild and consisting of regional lymphadenopathy, fever, and malaise.
   i. Annular erythematous lesions occur hours after bite, representative of hypersensitivity reaction and not to be confused with erythema migrans.
2. Stage II
   a. During hematogenous spread of microorganisms (a few days to weeks after bite), multiple annular skin lesions in 20% to 50% of victims

        (1) Generally smaller, migrate less, and lack indurated centers

        (2) Located anywhere except palms and soles

        (3) No blistering or mucosal involvement

  b. Other skin manifestations: malar rash; rarely, urticaria

  c. Most common constitutional symptoms: malaise and fatigue, which may be severe and are usually constant throughout the duration of the illness

  d. Fever, typically low grade and intermittent, common

  e. Tender regional lymphadenopathy along distribution of erythema migrans or posterior cervical chains

  f. Generalized lymphadenopathy and splenomegaly

  g. Symptoms of meningeal irritation in some victims, including severe intermittent headaches, stiff neck with extreme forward flexion, and lack of Kernig's or Brudzinski's signs

  h. Mild encephalopathy with somnolence, insomnia, memory disturbances, emotional lability, dizziness, poor balance, and clumsiness

  i. Dysesthesias of the scalp

  j. Musculoskeletal complaints, including arthralgias; migratory pain in tendons, bursae, and bones; and generalized stiffness or severe cramping pain, particularly in the calves, thighs, and back

  k. Symptoms of hepatitis and generalized abdominal pain

  l. Conjunctivitis in 10% to 15% of victims

  m. Neurologic manifestations an average of 4 weeks after the onset of erythema migrans, including meningoencephalitis, with headache as a major symptom; facial nerve palsy (in 50% of victims with Lyme disease meningitis, but may be isolated finding); radiculoneuritis (The triad of meningitis, cranial neuritis, and radiculoneuritis suggests Lyme disease in the differential diagnosis.)

n. Cardiac abnormalities in 4% to 10% of victims, including atrioventricular block that can progress to complete heart block

o. Arthritis in about 60% of untreated persons with erythema migrans
  (1) Develops in a few weeks to 2 years (median 4 weeks) after onset of illness
  (2) Typical pattern of brief recurrent episodes of asymmetric, oligoarticular swelling and pain in large joints, separated by longer periods of complete remission
  (3) Knee most frequently involved, followed by the shoulder, elbow, temporomandibular joint, ankle, wrist, hip, and small joints of the hands and feet

Treatment

If the diagnosis of Lyme disease is made by clinical or serologic determination, initiate antibiotic therapy.

1. For stage I disease, give amoxicillin 1 g PO tid for 4 weeks; an alternative is doxycycline 200 mg PO bid for 3 days, then 100 mg PO bid for a total of 4 weeks. Another alternative not yet approved by the U.S. Food and Drug Administration is azithromycin 200 mg PO bid for 3 weeks.

2. Treat any manifestations of stage II disease with ceftriaxone 1 g IV q12-24h for 2 to 4 weeks.

Relapsing Fever

Relapsing fever is an acute borrelial disease characterized by recurrent paroxysms of fever separated by afebrile periods.

Signs and Symptoms

1. Abrupt onset of fever lasting about 3 days, afebrile period of variable duration (average 6 to 7 days), and relapse with return of fever and other clinical manifestations
   a. Fever usually high, greater than 39° C (102.2° F)
   b. Initial febrile period averaging 3 days but possibly lasting 1 to 17 days
   c. Febrile period terminating with rapid defervescence (the crisis), accompanied by drenching sweats and intense thirst
2. Pruritic eschar at the site of the tick bite possible but usually absent by the onset of clinical symptoms
3. Incubation period of about 7 days, then fever, frequently accompanied by shaking chills, severe headache, myalgias, arthralgias, muscular weakness, lethargy, upper abdominal pain, nausea, and vomiting
4. Splenomegaly, hepatomegaly, altered sensorium, peripheral neuropathy, pupillary abnormalities, pathologic deep tendon reflexes
5. Rash, ranging from a macular eruption to petechiae and erythema multiforme, developing in about 25% of victims

Treatment

1. Be aware that tetracaine and erythromycin are both effective. A 5- to 10-day course (500 mg PO qid) of either drug is recommended.
2. Note that a Jarisch-Herxheimer reaction is common after the first dose of antibiotics. It is often severe and may be fatal.
   a. The reaction begins with a rise in body temperature and exacerbation of existing signs and symptoms. Vasodilation and a fall in blood pressure follow.
   b. Pretreat any victims who will be receiving the initial dose of an antibiotic to treat relapsing fever with an IV infusion of isotonic saline solution in

anticipation of the Jarisch-Herxheimer reaction.
  c. Note that a lower initial dose of antibiotic may reduce the frequency of this reaction.

Rocky Mountain Spotted Fever

Rocky Mountain spotted fever (RMSF) is caused by *Rickettsia rickettsii*. Most cases in the United States occur between the months of April and September, when the vector ticks are active.

Signs and Symptoms

1. Ranges from mild, subclinical illness to fulminant disease with vascular collapse and death within 3 to 6 days of onset
2. Incubation period 2 to 14 days, with severe disease associated with the shorter incubation period
3. Typically, a sudden onset of fever, chills, headache, and myalgias; fever is usually high, greater than 39 C° (102.2° F)
4. Most characteristic feature: rash, which develops 2 to 5 days after the onset of illness
    a. Typically develops first on the wrists, hands, ankles, and feet, spreading rapidly in centripetal fashion to cover most of the body, including the palms, soles, and face
    b. Lesions initially pink macules, 2 to 5 mm in diameter, that readily blanch with pressure
    c. After 2 to 3 days: lesions fixed, darker red, papular, and finally petechial
    d. Hemorrhagic lesions coalescing to form large areas of ecchymoses
    e. *Unfortunately, rash often absent on initial presentation, making diagnosis more difficult; in 10% to 15% of victims, no rash ever noted ("spotless fever")*
5. Other signs and symptoms: abdominal pain, vomiting, diarrhea, confusion, conjunctivitis, peripheral edema
6. Seizures possible during acute phase of illness, but rarely persist

7. Lethargy and confusion common, possibly progressing to stupor or coma
8. Cough, chest pain, dyspnea, or coryza also noted

Treatment

1. Initiate antibiotic therapy at the earliest suspicion for RMSF. Unfortunately, the classic triad of rash, fever, and tick bite is rarely present.
2. Give either tetracycline or chloramphenicol, both of which are very effective, although neither drug is rickettsicidal. These antibiotics inhibit the rickettsiae until an adequate immune response by the victim eradicates the infection.
   a. Give tetracycline 25 to 50 mg/kg/day PO in four divided doses (2 g/day for adults).
   b. Give chloramphenicol 50 mg/kg/day PO for adults and 75 mg/kg/day for children.
3. Continue treatment until the victim is afebrile for 48 hours, or for a minimum of 5 to 7 days. Be aware that relapses are common but may be treated with the same drug when they occur.

Ehrlichiosis

Ehrlichiae are tick-borne rickettsial organisms that cause disease in humans and animals throughout the world. Human ehrlichiosis has a broad clinical spectrum, ranging from a subclinical infection to a mild viral-like illness to a life-threatening disease.

Signs and Symptoms

1. After an average incubation period of 7 days (range 1 to 21 days): high fever, headache, chills or rigors, malaise, myalgia, anorexia
2. Rash, which may be maculopapular or petechial, in 20% to 40% of victims about 8 days after onset of illness
3. Severe complications: more likely in older persons and include cough, pneumonitis, dyspnea, respiratory failure, encephalopathy, and renal failure

Treatment

Give tetracycline 500 mg PO qid or doxycycline 200 mg PO bid for 5 to 10 days.

Colorado Tick Fever

Colorado tick fever is caused by a small ribonucleic acid (RNA) virus that is transmitted by ticks to humans. The incubation period is 3 to 6 days (range 0 to 14 days).

Signs and Symptoms
1. Usually begins with an abrupt onset of fever
   a. Most characteristic feature of illness (seen in 50% of victims): biphasic, or "saddleback," fever pattern
   b. From 2 to 3 days of fever, followed by 1 or 2 days of remission, then an additional 2 to 3 days of fever
   c. During fever, also have severe headache, myalgias, lethargy
2. Photophobia, ocular pain, anorexia, nausea, vomiting, abdominal pain
3. Macular or maculopapular rash in 5% to 12% of victims
4. Usually mild, but severe complications possible, especially in children under age 10 years; include meningoencephalitis or hemorrhagic diathesis
5. Three weeks or longer required for full recovery, with most common persistent symptoms malaise and weakness

Treatment

Be aware that treatment is supportive and based on symptoms.

Babesiosis

Babesia organisms are intraerythrocytic protozoan parasites. The vector tick may be the same as that which carries the infectious agent of Lyme disease. The presence of an intact spleen appears to play an important role in resistance to *Babesia* organisms.

Signs and Symptoms

1. Acute babesiosis: gradual onset of malaise, anorexia, and fatigue followed within several days to a week by fever, sweats, and myalgias
2. Less common symptoms: headache, nausea, vomiting, depression, shaking chills, splenomegaly, jaundice, hepatomegaly
3. No rash associated with disease
4. Hemolytic anemia more pronounced in splenectomized victims

Treatment

1. Note that limited or no efficacy has been shown with antimalarial agent therapy.
2. Give a combination of quinine 650 mg PO and clindamycin 600 mg PO q6h to adult victims with serious disease. Currently, treatment is only recommended for the seriously ill victim.

Prevention of Tick-Borne Diseases and Tick Removal

Close and regular inspection of all parts of the body should be performed when traveling in tick-infested areas. Protective clothing (long pants cinched at the ankles or tucked into boots and socks) should be worn when in tick-infested areas. Spraying clothes with an insect repellent may provide an additional barrier against ticks (Box 27-1). Adult ixodid ticks are generally on the body for 1 or 2 hours before attaching.

Procedure

1. Grasp the attached tick as close as possible to the skin surface with blunt curved forceps, tweezers, or fingers protected with tissue. Note that medium-tipped angled forceps are best because sharp forceps can puncture an engorged tick and straight

Box 27-1.

Insect Repellents

✤ Wear proper clothing to prevent the insect from obtaining access to the skin. Light-colored clothing makes it easier to spot ticks and is less attractive to biting flies.

✤ Use screens over windows, screened enclosures, or bed nets with fine mesh.

✤ Avoid unnecessary use of lights. Camp in a site that is high, dry, open, and uncluttered.

✤ Apply a repellent containing *N,N*-diethyl-3-methylbenzamide, commonly known as DEET (from its former chemical name). Bathing, excessive sweating, wiping, or other abrasive action that depletes the supply of available repellent on skin may justify reapplication. Avoid prolonged use of high concentrations (in excess of 35%) of DEET, particularly with small children.

✤ Use premethrin-impregnated fabric (Fig. 27-4). Note that the insecticidal action can noticeably reduce the density of the biting population in the immediate area. After contact, pests drop or fly away from the treated clothing, but they are not necessarily killed.

ones make the angle of approach to grasp the tick more difficult.

2. Pull the tick out counter to the direction that the mouthparts entered the skin; be sure to use steady pressure and take care not to crush or squeeze the tick's body because expressed fluid may contain infective agents.

3. After the tick is removed, disinfect the bite site.

4. Be aware that traditional methods of tick removal, such as applying fingernail polish, using isopropyl

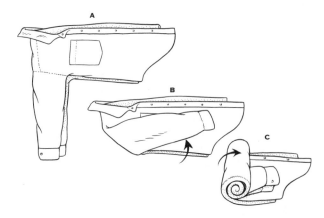

Fig. 27-4. Technique for impregnating clothing or mosquito netting with premethrin solution. **A** to **C,** Lay jacket flat
and fold it shoulder to shoulder. Fold sleeves to inside, roll
tightly, and tie middle with string. For mosquito net, roll tightly
and tie.

    alcohol, or applying a hot extinguished match, do not
effect tick detachment and may induce the tick to
salivate or regurgitate into the wound.

SCORPIONS
Centruroides exilicauda, the bark scorpion (Plate 16) of
Arizona, is usually less than 5 cm (2 inches) long, yellow
to brown, and possibly striped. It carries the identifying
subaculear tooth beneath its stinger.

Signs and Symptoms
1. Begin immediately after envenomation and progress
   to maximum severity in 5 hours
2. Infants: extreme illness possible 15 to 30 minutes after a sting
3. Improvement without administration of antivenin
   within 9 to 30 hours
4. Paresthesias and pain persisting for days to 2 weeks
5. Grade I: local pain and paresthesias at the site of en-

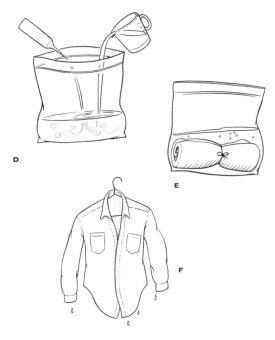

Fig. 27-4, cont'd **D,** Pour 2 ounces permethrin into plastic bag. Add 1 quart water. Mix. Solution will turn milky white. **E,** Place garment or mosquito netting in bag. Shut or tie tightly. Let sit for 10 minutes. **F,** Hang garment or netting for 2 to 3 hours to dry. Fabric can also be laid on clean surface to dry. *(Modified from Rose S: International travel health guide, Northampton, Mass, 1993, Travel Medicine.)*

venomation, which can be elicited by tapping on the sting site

6. Grade II: pain and paresthesias remote from the sting bite, along with local findings
7. Grade III: either cranial nerve or somatic skeletal neuromuscular dysfunction
   a. Cranial nerve dysfunction: blurred vision, wandering eye movements (involuntary, conjugate,

slow, roving), hypersalivation, difficulty swallow-ing, tongue fasciculation, upper airway obstruc-tion, slurred speech
   b. Somatic skeletal neuromuscular dysfunction: jerk-ing of the upper extremities, restlessness, arching of the back, and severe involuntary shaking and jerking that may be mistaken for a seizure (true seizures caused by other scorpion species)
8. Grade IV: both cranial nerve and somatic skeletal neuromuscular dysfunction
9. Hypertension, nausea, vomiting, hyperthermia, tachycardia, and respiratory distress also possible

Treatment
1. Control local pain with ice packs, which may be ap-plied for 30 minutes each hour. Give oral analgesics as necessary.
2. Observe the victim of a grade I or II envenomation for progression to more severe symptoms.
3. Avoid the use of narcotics, barbiturates, benzodiaz-epines, or other potent analgesics to control symp-toms of agitation or motor hyperactivity because these agents may lead to apnea and loss of protective airway reflexes.
4. Manage hyperthermia from uncontrolled muscular activity with cooling (see Chapter 4).
5. Be aware that antivenin administration is controver-sial. Some recommend it for reversal of grade III en-venomation with respiratory distress or grade IV en-venomation. Administration carries the risk of anaphylaxis because the antivenin is derived from goat serum. Generally, it should be administered in a hospital critical care setting.

CHAPTER 28

Plant-Induced Dermatitis

Plants can induce reactions that reflect sensitivity, including urticaria or hives, and chemical irritation. Plants that typically produce these reactions include poison oak, poison ivy, and poison sumac.

■ DISORDERS ■

SENSITIVITY TO POISON OAK, IVY, AND SUMAC

Sensitivity to poison ivy (Fig. 28-1), poison oak (see Fig. 28-1; Plate 17), and poison sumac represents the single most common cause of allergic skin reactions in the United States. The plant genus responsible is *Toxicodendron* (formerly *Rhus*) and includes all three of these plants. Each species has a distinct geographic range (Box 28-1).

About 50% of the U.S. adult population are clinically sensitive to poison ivy, oak, and sumac. Another 35% have negative skin test reactions but react to high concentrations of urushiol, the antigen in all three plants (Box 28-2). These people typically do not manifest poison oak or ivy dermatitis until they have experienced sufficient sensitization, after which they may develop severe dermatitis. A smaller group (15% of the popula-

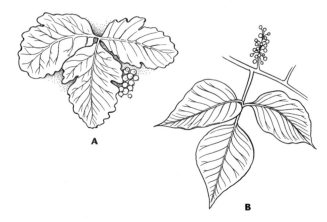

Fig. 28-1. **A,** Poison oak. **B,** Poison ivy.

tion) does not react to higher concentrations of urushiol
and cannot be sensitized. This group is considered to be
naturally tolerant, but it is unclear whether the tolerance results from early antigenic exposure or a genetic
predisposition.

Signs and Symptoms
1. Itching
2. Within hours to days: erythematous, edematous, vesicular, or bullous eruption; papular and granuloma-
   tous eruptions also possible.
3. Eruptions revealing "scratch marks"
   a. Correspond to where the plant touched the skin
   b. Sharply demarcated margins also possible, corre-
      sponding to where the person's clothing covered
      the skin
4. In extreme cases, fever and malaise

Treatment
1. Follow these guidelines for limited, mild eruption
   (area of involvement well localized and does not include the face, hands, or genitalia).

Box 28-1.

Identification and Geographic Range of Poison Oak, Ivy, and Sumac*

✤ The plants have an odd number of leaflets (usually three) that vary in color depending on the season. With poison oak and ivy, three leaflets arise from a single point on the stem. With poison sumac, leaves are paired across the stem, with a single terminal leaf.

✤ The plants grow best along streams and lakes and thrive in hot sunny weather.

✤ The plants do not survive well in deserts or mountains.

✤ The plants can be found in every state of the continental United States.

✤ Along the Pacific Coast, poison oak can grow at elevations of up to 1500 m (5000 feet).

✤ Poison ivy is found throughout the East, Midwest, and South.

✤ Poison sumac inhabits swampy areas in the East and South.

✤ No species of *Toxicodendron* grows wild in Alaska or Hawaii.

*The plants have different configurations in different regions, but these guidelines generally apply.

a. Apply a potent (class 1) topical steroid in a gel, cream, or ointment to speed resolution. Many preparations are available, such as betamethasone 0.05% gel (Diprolene), clobetasol 0.05% gel (Temovate), and halobetasol 0.05% ointment (Ultravate).

b. Limit the use of any high-potency topical steroid to 2 weeks, and avoid the face and groin area.

c. Do not use high-potency topical steroids on the skin of infants to prevent unintended dermal striae and atrophy.

Box 28-2.

Facts About Urushiol

- ✤ Urushiol differs among poison ivy, oak, and sumac only slightly in structure and biologic cross-reactivity. A person who is sensitive to poison ivy can be expected to react to poison oak and poison sumac.
- ✤ Contrary to popular belief, blister fluid **does not** contain antigen and does not transmit the rash to other sites.
- ✤ Urushiol resin can be carried by smoke if the plant is burned.
- ✤ The amount of urushiol in poison ivy, poison oak, and poison sumac is about equal year-round, even during the winter, when the plants have shed their leaves. As the leaves turn red and dry up in the fall, urushiol returns to the stem and roots. Thus, when the dead leaves fall to the ground, they are virtually devoid of urushiol. However, the remaining plant continues to pose a hazard.
- ✤ Once contaminated with urushiol, the average person has only about 10 minutes in which to wash it off with soap and water to prevent dermatitis. Organic solvents used as washes (e.g., Technu Poison Oak-N-Ivy Cleanser) may reduce the incidence and severity of dermatitis, even when used up to 48 hours after exposure. Highly sensitive individuals may experience a reaction within minutes of contact.

    d. For pruritus, use a topical nonsensitizing anesthetic such as pramoxine (Prax, PrameGel), Aveeno anti-itch lotion, or Sasna.

    e. For weepy (exudative) lesions, apply soaks of Burow's solution (aluminum acetate, Domeboro) or soak the victim in a tepid bath with 1 cup of Aveeno colloidal oatmeal or 2 cups of linnet starch per tub. Note that calamine lotion may also offer relief.

    f. To prevent secondary superficial bacterial soft tissue infections, insist on cleanliness. If a secondary superficial bacterial infection occurs and becomes severe, treat with an antiseptic, such as topical mupirocin (Bactroban) tid for 3 to 5 days and/or an oral antibiotic, such as cephalexin (Keflex) 250 to 500 mg tid for 7 days.

    g. For modest ancillary value, administer an antihistamine, aspirin, or an NSAID.

2. For severe involvement (generalized or involvement of the face, hands, or genitalia), observe the following guidelines.

    a. Administer prednisone 60 to 120 mg initial dose, tapered over 14 to 28 days. Alternately, administer triamcinolone (Aristocort) 40 mg IM.

    b. Be aware that relative contraindications to systemic corticosteroids include active infection, diabetes, hypertension, recent vascular accident, endocrinopathy, or a family history of glaucoma.

    c. Note that steroid regimens prescribed for less than 10 days often result in recurrence of the dermatitis. A sudden flare-up after drug therapy is less responsive to additional steroids.

    d. As the dermatitis heals, the pruritus can resurge. Left untreated, this can lead to a patch of chronic neurodermatitis. Use a topical steroid cream or ointment judiciously to alleviate symptoms (e.g., triamcinolone acetonide 0.025%, desonide 0.025%, hydrocortisone 1%).

CONTACT URTICARIA (HIVES)

Signs and Symptoms

1. Redness, itching, and swelling that develop as discrete wheals or widespread edema 1 to 2 hours after exposure to the offending plant
2. Anaphylaxis if the hypersensitive individual has also ingested some of the plant

Treatment

1. Treat anaphylaxis when present (see Chapter 20).
2. For a severe case, administer epinephrine 0.2 to 0.4 ml of a 1:1000 aqueous solution subcutaneously.
3. Administer diphenhydramine (Benadryl) 50 to 100 mg (adult dose) IM to limit wheal formation.
4. Give diphenhydramine 50 mg q6-8h PO or hydroxyzine 25 to 50 mg tid PO to help control itching.
5. Check the victim's clothing and gear for parts of the plant.

CHEMICAL IRRITATION

Exposure to certain plants can lead to chemical irritation caused by hundreds of naturally occurring chemical substances.

Signs and Symptoms

1. Many forms possible, but most mild and self-limited, although severe local reactions possible
2. Local swelling and redness, large blisters, exudative and serosanguineous crust
3. Wheals; itching; occasionally, intense local pain

Treatment

1. Be aware that treatment of primary irritant dermatitis is often unsatisfactory.
2. Remove the victim from further exposure to the plant irritant.
3. Cleanse the area gently with soap and water. Note that medicated soaks and compresses, such as Bu-

row's aluminum acetate (Domeboro), diluted 1:20 and applied bid or tid to the affected area, can speed resolution.

4. If medicated soaks are not available, use cool soaks to soothe the victim.

5. Note that antihistamines usually have little effect and corticosteroids are of no use in controlling primary irritation.

6. Reassure the victim that the dermatitis usually heals in less than 5 days if no complications develop and if tissue damage is minimal.

CHAPTER 29

Mushroom Toxicity

The four major types of mushroom toxins are: gastrointestinal toxins, disulfiram-like toxins, neurotoxins, and protoplasmic toxins.

■ DISORDERS ■

DISORDERS CAUSED BY GASTROINTESTINAL TOXINS (Table 29-1)

Signs and Symptoms

1. Nausea, vomiting, intestinal cramping, and diarrhea within 1 to 2 hours of ingestion
2. Stools usually watery and occasionally bloody with fecal leukocytes
3. Spontaneous remission of symptoms in 6 to 12 hours

Treatment

1. Initiate supportive treatment, including IV or oral fluid and electrolyte replacement.
2. For a severe case, administer an antiemetic, such as prochlorperazine (Compazine), 2.5 to 10 mg IV or a 25-mg suppository.
3. Treat diarrhea with loperamide (Imodium 4 mg initially, followed by 2 mg after each loose stool, up to 8 mg a day).

Table 29-1.

Gastrointesinal Disorders—Causative Mushrooms and Identification

NAME	DESCRIPTION
Chlorophyllum molybdites (green-spored parasol) (Plate 18)	This summer mushroom has a large whitish cap (often 10 to 40 cm [4 to 16 inches] in diameter) that is initially smooth and becomes convex with maturity. Tan or brown warts may be present. The gills are free from the stalk, initially white to yellow and becoming green with maturity. The stalk is 5 to 25 cm (2 to 10 inches) long, smooth, and white. The ring is generally brown on the underside.
Omphalotus illudens (jack-o'-lantern) (Plate 19)	This bright-orange to yellow mushroom has sharp-edged gills. It often grows in clusters at the base of stumps or on buried roots of deciduous trees. The cap is 4 to 16 cm (1½ to 6½ inches) in diameter on a stalk that is 4 to 20 cm (1½ to 8 inches) long. Gills are olive to orange, with white to yellow spores.
Amanita flavorubescens and *Amanita brunnescens*	Both have broad caps (3 to 15 cm [1¼ to 6 inches] in diameter) with loosely attached warts. The caps are yellowish to brown. The stalks are 3 to 18 cm (1¼ to 7 inches) long, enlarging toward the base with a superior ring.

DISORDERS CAUSED BY DISULFIRAM-LIKE TOXINS (Table 29-2)

Signs and Symptoms

1. If a person ingests these mushrooms and subsequently ingests alcohol, symptoms similar to those of an alcohol-disulfiram (Antabuse) reaction
   a. Severe headache, flushing, and tachycardia within 15 to 30 minutes of alcohol ingestion
   b. Hyperventilation, shortness of breath, palpitations
2. Sensitivity to alcohol ingestion 2 to 6 hours after ingestion and lasting for up to 72 hours

Treatment

1. Initiate supportive treatment.
2. Note that symptoms resolve spontaneously within 3 to 6 hours.
3. Be aware that activated charcoal is not beneficial.

Table 29-2.

Disulfiram-like Disorders—Causative Mushroom and Identification	
NAME	**DESCRIPTION**
Coprinus atramentarius (inky cap) (Plate 20)	This mushroom has a 2- to 8-cm (1- to 3-inch) cylindric cap on a 4- to 5-cm (1½- to 2-inch) thin stalk. The cap is white, occasionally orange or yellow at the top, with a surface that is characteristically shaggy. The mature cap often develops cracks at its margins, which turn up. The cap blackens as it matures and then liquefies.

DISORDERS CAUSED BY NEUROLOGIC TOXINS (MUSCARINE) (Table 29-3)

Signs and Symptoms

1. Symptoms developing within 15 to 30 minutes of ingesting muscarine-containing mushrooms
2. Salivation, urination, lacrimation, diarrhea, diaphoresis, abdominal pain, gastrointestinal upset, vomiting
3. Bradycardia and bronchospasm
4. Constricted pupils

Table 29-3.

Muscarine Disorders—Causative Mushrooms and Identification	
NAME	DESCRIPTION
Amanita muscaria (Plate 21)	This mushroom has a cap 5 to 30 cm (2 to 12 inches) in diameter that is scarlet red with white warts. The stalk is white, often hollow, and grows 15 to 20 cm (6 to 8 inches) long, tapering upward. It has a prominent cup and volva and numerous rings. Gills are free and white.
Inocybe patouillardii (Plate 22)	The Inocybe family contains small brown mushrooms with conical caps up to 6 cm (2½ inches) in diameter. Stalks are 2 to 10 cm (¾ to 4 inches) long, covered with fine brown to white hairs. Gills are brown and notched.
Clitocybe dealbata	Clitocybe mushrooms are whitish tan to gray, with 15- to 33-mm (¾- to 1½-inch) caps on hairless stalks 1 to 5 cm (½ to 2 inches) long. Gills run down the stalk.

5. Copious bronchial secretions that may cause respiratory failure, requiring mechanical ventilation

Treatment

1. Treatment consists of supportive care with oxygen, suctioning, and IV fluid replacement if available.
2. Administer atropine 0.01 mg/kg IV or IM for children and 1 mg for adults to manage profound secretions or bradycardia. Repeat the dose prn until secretions are manageable.
3. Note that symptoms resolve spontaneously within 6 to 24 hours.

ISOXAZOLE REACTIONS (Table 29-4)

Signs and Symptoms

1. Begin within 30 minutes of ingestion and last 2 hours
2. With mild ingestion (10 mg), dizziness and ataxia

Table 29-4.

Isoxazole Reactions—Causative Mushrooms and Identification	
NAME	DESCRIPTION
Amanita muscaria	See Table 29-3
Amanita pantherina (Plate 23)	This mushroom is 5 to 15 cm (2 to 6 inches) long with a cap 5 to 15 cm in diameter. The cap is white to pink early and becomes reddish-brown or brown with maturity. The stalk has a distinct ring, with a volva or cup at the bottom. When the flesh is cut or injured, it develops a pinkish tinge. Gills are free and produce white spores.

3. With ingestion of 15 mg or more:
   a. Pronounced ataxia, visual disturbances
   b. Delirium or manic behavior
   c. Visual hallucinations, seizures, muscle twitching, hyperactivity

Treatment
1. Note that treatment is primarily supportive.
2. Provide appropriate sedation with IV phenobarbital (30 mg qh) or diazepam (5 mg q15-20min prn in an adult or 0.1 to 0.3 mg/kg in a child) if necessary, but use it with caution in the wilderness.
3. Be aware that atropine may worsen the central nervous system symptoms associated with isoxazole derivatives. Therefore withhold it unless the muscarinic effects are serious.

DISORDERS CAUSED BY HALLUCINOGENIC MUSHROOMS (Table 29-5)
Signs and Symptoms
1. With ingestion of 10 mg of the mushroom, moderate euphoria
2. With ingestion of 20 mg, hallucinations and a loss of time sensation
   a. Heightened imagination developing within 15 to 30 minutes of ingestion
   b. Hallucinations lasting 4 to 6 hours
3. Fever and seizures in children

Treatment
1. Place the victim in a quiet, supportive environment.
2. Reserve activated charcoal administration for the victim of a very large ingestion.
3. When necessary, accomplish sedation with benzodiazepines (diazepam 5 mg q15-20min prn in an adult or 0.1 to 0.3 mg/kg in a child), phenobarbital (30 mg qh), or haloperidol (3 to 5 mg q8h in an adult or 0.10 mg/kg/day in equally divided doses q8h in a child).

Table 29-5.

Hallucinogenic Disorders—Causative Mushrooms and Identification	
NAME	**DESCRIPTION**
Members of the *Psilocybe* family (Plate 24)	These are little brown mushrooms with 0.5- to 4-cm (¼- to 1½-inch) broad caps that are smooth and become sticky or slippery when wet. The stalks are slender and 4 to 15 cm (1½ to 6 inches) long. Gills are gray to purple-gray. The flesh of these mushrooms turns blue or greenish when bruised or cut.
Members of the *Panaeolus* family	These little brown mushrooms are about the same size as *Psilocybe.* Gills are dark gray or black with black spores. Unlike *Psilocybe,* the caps are not sticky or slippery when wet.

DISORDERS CAUSED BY PROTOPLASMIC POISONS (Table 29-6)
Gyromitra Toxin
Signs and Symptoms
1. Symptoms delayed for 4 to 50 hours (average 5 to 12 hours) after ingestion
2. Initially, nausea, vomiting, severe diarrhea
3. In some victims: dizziness, weakness, muscle cramps, loss of coordination
4. With severe ingestion: delirium, seizures, coma
5. Hepatic failure developing over several days after ingestion, although hepatic damage is generally mild
6. Severe hepatic failure and death possible

Table 29-6.

Protoplasmic Disorders—Causative Mushrooms and Identification

NAME	DESCRIPTION
***Gyromitra* toxin**	
Gyromitra esculenta (false morel) (Plate 25)	This mushroom grows in the spring near pines and in sandy soil. It is 5 to 16 cm (2 to 6½ inches) in height with a reddish-brown to dark brown, irregularly shaped cap. The cap's surface is curved and folded, resembling a human brain. The stalk is often as thick as the cap. The inside of the cap and the stalk are hollow.
Amatoxin	
Amanita phalloides (death cap) (Plate 26)	This mushroom grows under deciduous trees in the fall and has a white to greenish can 4 to 16 cm (1½ to 6½ inches) in diameter, often with remnants of the veil (warts). The stalk is thick, 5 to 18 cm (2 to 7 inches) long, with a large bulb at the base, often with a volva or cup. A thin ring is usually present on the stalk. Gills are generally free and white to green.
Amanita virosa (Plate 27)	This mushroom resembles *Amanita phalloides,* but the cap is more yellowish or white.

Treatment

1. Administer activated charcoal, although it is of little proven value.
2. For a victim who develops significant neurologic symptoms, give pyridoxine 25 mg/kg up to 25 kg/day PO.

3. Be aware that no specific antidote or treatment is available for fulminant hepatic failure.

Amatoxin (see Table 29-6)

Signs and Symptoms

1. After a latent period of 4 to 16 hours: severe nausea, vomiting, abdominal cramps, diarrhea; gastrointestinal symptoms abating over the next 12 to 24 hours
2. Hepatic failure between 48 and 72 hours after ingestion in most victims
3. Endocrinopathies possible, including severe hypoglycemia, hypocalcemia, and decreased thyroid function
4. Greater toxicity and higher mortality in children

Treatment

1. Administer activated charcoal (1 g/kg) PO q4-6h.
2. Administer IV NS solution to correct dehydration.
3. Administer benzyl penicillin (penicillin G) 300,000 to 1 million U/kg/day IV in divided doses.
4. Give silibinin (milk thistle), if available, IV 20 to 40 mg/kg/day in divided doses.
5. Administer cimetidine 4 to 10 g IV in an adult for 3 days.
6. Experimental—Try hyperbaric oxygen treatment (dives to 2 atmospheres for 30 minutes once or twice a day).

CHAPTER 30

Animal Attacks and Zoonoses

WOUND CARE

1. Irrigate the wound using, in order of preference, NS solution, boiled or disinfected drinking water, tap water, or filtered fresh (stream) water.
   a. Do not use seawater or brackish water.
   b. Do not soak the wound.
2. If possible, add a germicidal agent to the irrigating solution. In order of preference, use 1% povidone-iodine solution (not "scrub"), benzalkonium chloride, or ordinary hand (camping) soap. In a heavily contaminated wound, a 5% to 10% solution may be used.
3. Complete the irrigation with a germicide-free solution (e.g., plain water) to rinse all irritating chemicals from the wound. Use benzalkonium chloride to cleanse wounds inflicted by animals suspected of being rabid (see Rabies).
   a. Perform the irrigation technique at approximately 10 psi. This can be achieved by attaching a 19-gauge needle or plastic IV catheter to a 35-ml syringe; a pressure of 20 psi, to dislodge adherent debris, can be achieved by attaching a 19-gauge needle or plastic IV catheter to a 12-ml syringe.

b. Use 100 to 200 ml of irrigating solution for a wound a few inches long.

4. Clean the wound, if necessary, by swabbing with a soft clean cloth or sterile gauze. Follow with a repeat irrigation.

5. If the wound edges are macerated, crushed, or extremely contaminated, perform sharp débridement.

6. If the wound must be closed to control bleeding, to allow dressing, or to facilitate evacuation, do so in a manner that allows drainage. Use tape, surgical adhesive strips, or loose approximating sutures or staples in preference to a tight closure. It is not necessary and may be harmful to shave the skin around the wound.

a. Do not suture bite wounds of the hand. These should be irrigated, débrided, and initially left open.

b. Immobilize the hand with a bulky mitten dressing in an elevated position, and start the victim promptly on an antibiotic. If the wound is a human bite, choose amoxicillin/clavulanate, cephalexin, or penicillin *and* dicloxacillin.

7. Cover the wound with a sterile dressing or a clean dry cloth. You can use a topical antiseptic ointment, such as mupirocin, for abrasions and shallow wounds.

8. Apply a splint if appropriate to restrict motion.

9. If the wound is of the high-risk type (see following features) or treatment is hours away, administer a prophylactic antibiotic (e.g., cephalexin, amoxicillin/clavulanate, ciprofloxacin, trimethoprim-sulfamethoxazole [co-trimoxazole]). Dicloxacillin, tetracycline, and erythromycin cannot be relied on to offer coverage against *Pasteurella multocida*. High-risk wounds have the following features:

a. Location: hand, wrist, or foot; scalp or face in infants; over a major joint (possible perforation); through-and-through wound of cheek

b. Type of wound: puncture; tissue crush; carnivore bite over a vital structure (artery, nerve, or joint)

    c. Victim risk factor: older than 50 years; asplenic; chronic alcoholic; immunosuppressed; diabetic; has peripheral vascular insufficiency; receiving chronic corticosteroid therapy; has prosthetic or diseased cardiac valve; has prosthetic or seriously diseased joint

    d. Animal species: domestic cat; large cat; human bite wound to hand; primate; pig

WOUND INFECTION

The causative organisms in a wound infection after animal attack are most often *Staphylococcus* or *Streptococcus*, but you must consider signs and symptoms consistent with an anaerobic infection. Less common pathogens, such as *Pasteurella* or *Eikenella,* are usually sensitive to and effectively treated with most common antibiotics, such as amoxicillin/clavulanate 500 mg PO bid, azithromycin (not yet proven), cefixime, cefuroxime 500 mg PO bid, ciprofloxacin 500 mg PO bid, and cotrimoxazole DS tablet bid. For a human bite of the hand, a reasonable approach is dicloxacillin 500 mg PO qid *plus* ampicillin 500 mg PO qid or cefuroxime 500 mg PO bid.

SPECIFIC ANIMAL CONSIDERATIONS
Dog

1. If a dog's large teeth cause facial or scalp wounds in a small child, particularly an infant, be alert for the possibility of an underlying skull or facial bone fracture.

2. For a bite made by a large dog or any other animal with large teeth, when the bite is close to a major vessel, examine the wound for absent or diminished pulse, sensory or motor deficit, large or expanding hematoma, or extremely active bleeding. Any of these may indicate an arterial injury.

316

Field Guide to Wilderness Medicine

Cat

1. Do not suture a cat bite puncture because it has a high likelihood of becoming infected.
2. *P. multocida* causes an infection that may follow a cat bite. The appropriate prophylactic antibiotic is cefuroxime, amoxicillin/clavulanate, cefixime, trimethoprim-sulfamethoxazole, or ciprofloxacin. *Pasteurella* infection is optimally treated with penicillin.
3. With bites from large cats, suspect deep penetration, even with a seemingly trivial surface wound.

Porcupine

1. Be aware that porcupine quills not only penetrate human skin but also can migrate up to 25 cm (10 inches). The quills are barbed, and their cores are spongy, allowing them to absorb body fluid and expand, which makes removal even more difficult.
2. Pull the quill straight out. In deep penetrations, you may need to make a small nick in the skin to allow egress of the entrapped barb.

Skunk

1. The skunk sprays its victim with musk from anal sacs. The musk causes skin irritation, keratoconjunctivitis, temporary blindness, nausea, and occasionally seizures and loss of consciousness. The chief component of the musk is butylmercaptan.
2. Neutralize the butylmercaptan with a strong oxidizing agent, such as sodium hypochlorite in a 5.25% solution (household bleach), further diluted 1:5 or 1:10 in water. Then cleanse the area with tincture of green soap, followed by a dilute bleach rinse. Tomato juice as a shampoo has been advocated for deodorizing hair, which should then be washed and can be mildly bleached or cropped short.

■   ZOONOSES   ■

DEFINITION

Zoonoses are disorders resulting from exposure to animals.

DISORDERS
Rabies

In the United States the most common rabid animals are skunks, raccoons, bats, and foxes. Overseas, additional animals are wolves, jackals, mongooses, weasels, and raccoon dogs. Woodchucks and cattle may be rabid. In the United States, rodents; urban cats and dogs; and domestic ferrets, rodents, rabbits, and hares are currently considered at low risk. The rabies virus ascends to the central nervous system by traveling along peripheral nerves. The farther the bite is from the brain, the more time the victim has to develop antibodies in response to a course of vaccination. Rabies is transmitted in saliva.

Signs and Symptoms

1. Incubation period: 9 days to more than 1 year, usually (in humans) 2 to 16 weeks
2. Initial symptoms nonspecific
   a. Malaise, fatigue, anxiety, agitation, irritability, insomnia, depression, fever, headache, nausea, vomiting, sore throat, abdominal pain, anorexia
   b. Early pain or paresthesias at the site of the bite in approximately half of victims
3. Neurologic symptoms after prodromal period, which lasts approximately 2 to 10 days; may be in the form of furious or paralytic (dumb) rabies
4. *Furious rabies:* increasing agitation, hyperactivity, seizures, and episodes in which the victim may thrash about, bite, and become aggressive, alternating with periods of relative calm
   a. Hallucinations possible
   b. Severe laryngeal spasm or spasm of respiratory

muscles possible when the victim attempts to drink, or even looks at, water (hydrophobia)
  c. Pharyngeal spasm possible when air is blown on the victim's face
5. *Paralytic (dumb) rabies:* progressive lethargy, incoordination, ascending paralysis

Postbite Treatment

1. Capture the offending animal.
   a. If not obviously diseased or acting abnormally, the domestic cat or dog should be quarantined for a 10-day period.
   b. Rabies prophylaxis can be started and discontinued if the animal remains well for 10 days.
   c. If the animal dies or develops neurologic symptoms within 10 days, the animal's brain should be examined.
   d. Any wild animal that bites a person should be killed immediately and the brain sent for diagnostic laboratory studies.
2. Swab the wound thoroughly with 2% benzalkonium chloride or 20% soap solution. Simple flushing is not sufficient; the wound should be physically swabbed. After a few minutes' contact time, irrigate the chemical agent from the wound (see Wound Care). If nothing else is available, scrub the wound vigorously with soap and water.
3. Infiltrate the wound edges with procaine hydrochloride 1%.
4. Administer rabies antiserum.
   a. The drug of choice is human rabies immune globulin, administered as a single dose of 20 IU/kg of the victim's body weight.
   b. Infiltrate half the dose around the bite wound. If the wound is in a small site, such as the finger, inject as much as feasible in that area.
   c. Inject the remainder IM in the upper outer quadrant of the buttocks in an adult or the anterolateral aspect of the thigh in a small child.

    d. Give the antiserum at the same time that active immunization is started, as described next. If human rabies immune globulin is not administered when active immunization is started, it can be given up to 7 days after the first vaccine dose.

5. Administer human diploid cell vaccine. The vaccine is given as a 1-ml dose regardless of the victim's age on days 0, 3, 7, 14, and 28. Inject it IM into the deltoid in an adult and into the thigh muscles in an infant or small child. Do not give the vaccine in the same syringe as human rabies immune globulin, and do not give it into the buttock.

6. A person who has undergone preexposure immunization with human rabies immune globulin should receive booster doses on days 0 and 3.

7. After immunization, antirabies titers should show a titer of at least 0.5 IU/ml at a 1:25 dilution by rapid fluorescent focus inhibition test (RFFIT) 2 to 4 weeks after the immunization series is completed. If the response is inadequate, an additional booster dose of rabies vaccine can be given each week until a satisfactory response is obtained.

Prevention

1. Obtain preexposure immunization in humans by administering either human diploid cell vaccine or rabies vaccine adsorbed in three injections on days 0, 7, and 21 or 28.

2. Check the antirabies titer, and give a booster dose of vaccine if the titer drops below 0.5 IU/ml at a 1:5 dilution by the RFFIT.

Cat-scratch Disease

Cat-scratch disease has been linked to the organism *Rochalimaea henselae*. Most cases are caused by scratches from cats, but dog and monkey bites, as well as thorns and splinters, have been implicated. Most cases occur in children, with an average incubation period of 3 to 10 days.

Signs and Symptoms
1. Characteristic feature: regional lymphadenitis, usually involving lymph nodes of the arm or leg
   a. May affect only one lymph node
   b. Nodes often painful and tender, and about 25% suppurate
2. Raised, red, slightly tender, and nonpruritic papule with a small central vesicle or eschar that resembles an insect bite at the site of primary inoculation
3. Mild systemic symptoms, including fever (usually less than 39° C [102.2° F]), chills, malaise, anorexia, and nausea
4. Evanescent morbilliform and pleomorphic skin rashes lasting up to 48 hours
5. *Parinaud's oculoglandular syndrome:* conjunctivitis and ipsilateral, enlarged, tender preauricular lymph node
6. Rarely, encephalopathy, seizures, transverse myelitis, arthritis, splenic abscess, optic neuritis, or thrombocytopenic purpura

Treatment
1. Cat-scratch disease usually resolves spontaneously in weeks to months. In approximately 2% of victims (usually adults) the course is prolonged and involves systemic complications.
2. Antibiotics that may help shorten the course of illness include co-trimoxazole and ciprofloxacin. Antibiotics not thought to be of benefit include amoxicillin/clavulanate, erythromycin, dicloxacillin, cephalexin, and tetracycline.

Leptospirosis
Leptospirosis is caused by *Leptospira interrogans,* which infects many wild and domestic animals. Dogs are the most common vectors. The organism is shed in the urine. Humans come in contact with contaminated water or soil.

Signs and Symptoms

1. After incubation period (average 7 to 12 days, range 1 to 26 days), initial phase of abrupt high fever, headache, prostration, myalgias, and prominent conjunctival suffusion without exudate; nausea, vomiting, and abdominal pain possible
2. Nonproductive cough, chest pain, bradycardia, calf/thigh/lumbar muscle tenderness, neck stiffness
3. Maculopapular, petechial, or purpuric rash, with or without pharyngitis
4. Apparent recovery for a few days, followed by return of less dramatic fever associated with relentless headache with meningeal signs; severe cases initially interpreted as septic meningitis, infectious hepatitis, or fever of unknown origin (FUO)
5. *Weil's syndrome* (icteric form): jaundice, petechial hemorrhages, renal insufficiency

Treatment

1. The treatment of choice is doxycycline 100 mg PO bid for 7 days. Tetracycline 20 mg/kg/day PO in four divided doses for 14 days is an alternative. Another choice is procaine penicillin G 3 million U/day IM in four divided doses for 7 to 10 days.
2. A Jarisch-Herxheimer reaction may be seen within a few hours of initial treatment.

Rat-bite Fever

Rat-bite fever is an acute illness caused by *Streptobacillus moniliformis* or *Spirillum minus,* which are part of the oral flora of rodents, including squirrels. It may also result from bites by weasels, dogs, cats, and pigs.

Signs and Symptoms

1. Streptobacillary rat-bite fever:
   a. Incubation period of 1 to several weeks; disease transmitted by contaminated food, milk, or water or by simply playing with pet rats, without a history of bite or injury

b. Initial symptoms: fever, chills, cough, malaise, headache, and, less frequently, lymphadenitis; followed by a nonpruritic morbilliform or petechial rash, which frequently involves the palms and soles
c. Migratory polyarthritis in 50% of victims
d. Centralized lymphadenitis; absence of meningeal signs

2. Spirillary rat-bite fever:
a. Incubation period 7 to 21 days, during which the bite lesion heals
b. Onset heralded by chills, fever, lymphadenitis, and dark-red macular rash
c. Myalgias common, but arthritis absent, which helps in the differentiation from streptobacillary rat-bite fever
d. Disease episodic and relapsing, with a 24- to 72-hour cycle

Treatment
1. Administer procaine penicillin 600,000 units IM bid for 7 to 10 days. Alternative drugs for penicillin-allergic persons are tetracycline 30 mg/kg/day PO in four divided doses, or streptomycin 15 mg/kg/day IM in two divided doses.
2. Note that erythromycin is not effective.

Tularemia
Tularemia represents a variety of syndromes caused by *Francisella tularensis*. This bacterium is a common parasite of rabbits, rodents, hares, moles, beavers, muskrats, squirrels, rats, and mice. The primary mode of transmission to humans is via a bloodsucking arthropod, such as a tick, or by skin or eye inoculation resulting from skinning, dressing, or handling a diseased animal.

Signs and Symptoms
1. Abrupt onset of fever, often with chills and temperature up to 41.5° C (106° F)

2. Headache, which may mimic meningitis in severity
3. Hepatomegaly, splenomegaly
4. Six clinical presentations
   a. Ulceroglandular form (most common)
      (1) Typical skin lesion beginning as red papule or nodule that indurates and ulcerates
      (2) Frequently painful and tender
      (3) Ulcers associated with handling infected animals usually located on the hand, with associated lymphadenopathy in the epitrochlear or axillary area
      (4) Infection transmitted by tick bite, usually initiated on the lower extremity and associated with inguinal or femoral lymphadenopathy
   b. Oculoglandular form
      (1) Unilateral conjunctivitis in and around a nodular lesion on the conjunctiva, extreme ocular pain, photophobia, itching, lacrimation, mucopurulent eye discharge
      (2) Enlargement of the ipsilateral preauricular lymph node
   c. Glandular form: enlarged, tender lymph nodes without an associated skin lesion
   d. Typhoidal form: fever, chills, debility
   e. Oropharyngeal form
      (1) Exudative pharyngitis associated with cervical lymphadenitis
      (2) Also may be seen with typhoidal or oculoglandular form
   f. Pneumonic form: pneumonia, with cough, chest pain, shortness of breath, sputum production, and hemoptysis

Treatment

1. Streptomycin is the drug of choice; administer in a dose of 30 to 40 mg/kg/day IM in two divided doses for 3 days, followed by half the dose for another 4 to 7 days. Alternative antibiotics include IV gentamicin or oral tetracycline or chloramphenicol. The latter

two drugs are given as 50 to 60 mg/kg/day in four divided doses for 14 days. Relapse may occur with the oral drugs. If no other antibiotic is available, give ciprofloxacin or norfloxacin.

Brucellosis

Brucella organisms are carried chiefly by swine, cattle, goats, and sheep. They are usually transmitted to humans by direct skin contact or from the ingestion of contaminated milk products. The incubation period in humans is 1 to 15 weeks.

Signs and Symptoms
1. No specific symptoms or signs; thus the nickname "mimic" disease
2. Most characteristic clinical manifestation: undulating fever
3. Chills, weakness, malaise, headache, muscle and joint pains, backache, weight loss

Treatment
1. Administer tetracycline 50 mg/kg/day PO in four divided doses for 21 days. In severe cases, add streptomycin 20 to 40 mg/kg IM qd for 1 week. In the next week, continue streptomycin at a dose of 15 mg/kg.

Trichinosis

Trichinosis is an infection caused by nematodes of the genus *Trichinella*. The infection is acquired by ingesting larvae encysted in skeletal muscle, usually raw or undercooked pork. It can also be acquired from wild game, such as bear, raccoon, horse, and wild swine.

Signs and Symptoms
1. Nausea, vomiting, and abdominal pain approximately 5 days after ingestion of infective meat; diarrhea or fever possible; gastrointestinal symptoms persisting for 4 to 6 weeks

2. Larvae invading skeletal muscle as early 7 days after ingestion
   a. Capillary damage during larval migration, which appears as facial (especially periorbital) edema, photophobia, blurred vision, diplopia, and complaints of pain associated with eye movements
   b. Splinter hemorrhages in the nail beds, along with cutaneous petechiae and hemorrhagic lesions in the conjunctivae
   c. Fever up to 41° C (105° F)
3. After 2 weeks: cough, dyspnea, pleuritic chest pain, hemoptysis, meningitic symptoms, headache
4. After 3 weeks: myalgias, muscle stiffness

Treatment
1. Be aware that no satisfactory, safe, and effective drug is available for the elimination of larvae.
2. Thiabendazole 25 mg/kg bid for 5 days, maximum 3 g/day, is effective against adult worms in the intestine, but its efficacy against larvae is questionable. Mebendazole is still considered investigational, and neither albendazole nor flubendazole is commercially available in the United States.
3. Use prednisone 30 to 60 mg/day PO for 10 to 30 days for relief from severe inflammatory manifestations.

Hantavirus Pulmonary Syndrome
Hantavirus pulmonary syndrome is a severe respiratory illness predominantly transmitted through a rodent vector, such as the deer mouse. Other small mammals may be infected, such as brush mice and western chipmunks. The animals shed virus in saliva, urine, and feces for weeks.

Signs and Symptoms
1. Prodrome of fever, myalgia, and variable respiratory symptoms, which may include cough and shortness of breath; then rapid onset of acute respiratory distress

2. Headache, chills, abdominal pain, nausea, vomiting; possible hemorrhage related to thrombocytopenia
3. Rapid deterioration, including respiratory failure and hypotension

Treatment
Note that therapy is supportive and based on symptoms. Ribavirin is being used on protocol as an investigational agent.

Prevention
1. Eliminate rodents, and reduce the availability of food sources and nesting sites used by rodents inside the home.
2. Keep food and water covered and stored in rodent-proof metal or thick, plastic containers.
3. Dispose of clutter.
4. Remove food sources that might attract rodents.
5. Spray dead rodents, nests, and droppings with a general-purpose disinfectant before handling. Always wear rubber or plastic gloves.
6. Avoid contact with rodents and rodent burrows. Do not disturb dens.
7. Do not use cabins or other enclosed shelters that are rodent infested until they have been appropriately cleaned and disinfected.
8. Do not pitch tents or place sleeping bags in areas close to rodent feces or burrows or near possible rodent shelters (garbage dumps, wood piles).
9. If possible, do not sleep on bare ground.
10. Burn or bury all garbage promptly.
11. Use only bottled water or water that has been disinfected for oral consumption, cooking, washing dishes, and brushing teeth.

Plague
Plague is a bacterial illness caused by *Yersinia pestis*. Plague is carried by various rodent reservoirs and transmitted by fleas. Carnivorous mammals can acquire

plague by ingesting infected rodents or by being bitten by their fleas. Plague in cats is a serious problem.

Signs and Symptoms
Bubonic plague

1. Incubation period of 2 to 6 days, then appearance of enlarged, tender lymph nodes (buboes) proximal to the point of percutaneous entry
2. Inguinal nodes most often involved because fleas usually bite humans on the legs; axillary buboes from skinning an animal as the mode of transmission
3. High fever, chills, malaise, headache, myalgias
4. Cardiovascular collapse with shock and hemorrhagic phenomena possible, with blackened, hemorrhagic skin lesions

Septicemic plague

1. Fever, chills, malaise, headache, abdominal pain, nausea, vomiting, diarrhea
2. Eventual cardiovascular collapse with disseminated intravascular coagulation (DIC)

Pneumonic plague. Acute, fulminant disease, characterized by symptoms of pneumonia, including tachypnea and bloody sputum

Treatment for all types of plague
1. Initiate treatment if there is any suspicion that the disease may be present.
2. The drug of choice is streptomycin 30 mg/kg/day IM in four divided doses for 5 days. A less preferred alternative is gentamicin 5 mg/kg/day IV in four divided doses, reduced to 3 mg/kg/day after clinical improvement. Tetracycline is often used concurrently with streptomycin. The loading dose is 15 mg/kg PO up to 1 g total dose. Follow this with 40 to 50 mg/kg in six divided doses on the first day. Thereafter, ad-

minister 30 mg/kg PO in four divided doses for 10 to 14 days. An alternative to tetracycline is chloramphenicol, administered in a loading dose of 25 mg/kg PO up to 3 g total, followed by 50 to 75 mg/kg PO in four divided doses for 10 to 14 days. If none of the above drugs is available, give co-trimoxazole (320 mg trimethoprim and 1600 mg sulfamethoxazole) PO 2 or 3 times a day for 14 days.

Prevention
1. The greatest risk of contagion is by aerosol transmission from victims with pneumonic plague. Therefore keep them in strict quarantine and isolation for a minimum of 48 hours after antibiotic therapy is begun (suspected case) or 4 days after beginning antibiotic therapy (obvious case).
2. Treat individuals directly exposed to pneumonic plague prophylactically with tetracycline 500 mg PO q6h for 6 days (adults) or co-trimoxazole (otitis media dose) for children.

CHAPTER 31

Traveler's Diarrhea and Intestinal Protozoa

■ DEFINITIONS ■

Traveler's diarrhea is a syndrome and not a specific disease. Although a large percentage of cases are caused by strains of *Escherichia coli*, traveler's diarrhea can be caused by any number of water-borne or food-borne enteric pathogens, including the following:

1. Viruses, such as rotavirus and Norwalk virus
2. Enteric bacteria, such as enterotoxigenic *E. coli*, *Shigella*, *Campylobacter*, *Aeromonas*, *Salmonella*, and *Vibrio*
3. Intestinal protozoa, including *Giardia lamblia*, *Entamoeba histolytica*, and *Cryptosporidium*

The risk of traveler's diarrhea is high among short-stay travelers in the developing tropical regions of Latin America, southern Asia, and Africa. The enteric pathogens that cause traveler's diarrhea are usually spread by fecal-oral contamination. Water and food are the most common vehicles.

■ **DISORDERS** ■

TRAVELER'S DIARRHEA
Signs and Symptoms
1. Acute diarrhea, possibly accompanied by nausea, loss of appetite, abdominal cramps, low-grade fever, and malaise (Table 31-1)
2. Symptoms beginning as early as 8 to 12 hours after contaminated food or water has been ingested
3. Watery diarrheal stools
4. Dysentery in 10% to 15% of cases, particularly with *Shigella, C. jejuni* or *Salmonella* as cause
   a. Passage of bloody stools
   b. Fever up to 40° C (104° F)

Table 31-1.

Pathophysiologic Syndromes in Diarrheal Disease	
SYNDROME	AGENT
Acute watery diarrhea	Any agent, especially the toxin-mediated diseases (e.g., enterotoxigenic *Escherichia coli*)
Febrile dysentery	*Shigella, Clostridium jejuni, Salmonella;* less commonly, invasive *E. coli, Aeromonas* spp., *Vibrio* spp., *Yersinia enterocolitica, Entamoeba histolytica,* inflammatory bowel disease
Vomiting (as predominant symptom)	Viral agents, preformed toxins of *Staphylococcus* or *Bacillus cereus*
Persistent diarrhea (>14 days' duration)	Protozoa, especially *Giardia lamblia;* small-bowel bacterial overgrowth; invasive enteropathogens; when longer than 30 days: small-bowel injury, inflammatory bowel disease, irritable bowel syndrome

    c. Often associated with abdominal colic, tenderness, and tenesmus

5. With persistent diarrhea (longer than 14 days' duration), possible infection with intestinal protozoan, such as *G. lamblia, E. histolytica,* or *Cryptosporidium* (see later discussions), or less common entities, including:

    a. Pseudomembranous enterocolitis *(Clostridium difficile)* after recent antibiotic use

    b. Lactase deficiency induced by small-bowel pathogens

    c. Viral enteropathogens, such as rotavirus or Norwalk virus

    d. Small-bowel bacterial overgrowth syndrome

    e. Other less common enteric parasites, such as *Strongyloides stercoralis* or *Trichuris trichiura*

    f. Postinfective malabsorption syndrome

    g. Tropical sprue

    h. Inflammatory bowel disease

    i. Others

Treatment

1. Be aware that traveler's diarrhea typically runs a self-limited course of less than 1 week. Recovery without antimicrobial treatment is the norm in healthy adults. However, most travelers choose to avoid the inconvenience and discomfort of diarrhea by seeking medical treatment (Table 31-2).

2. Severe watery traveler's diarrhea can cause life-threatening fluid loss. Treating serious dehydration is an urgent priority, especially in elderly persons, young children, and infants.

3. Fluid replacement is the cornerstone of therapy.

    a. Treating dehydration often significantly decreases malaise.

    b. Make sure the victim drinks oral fluids to approximate fluid losses in the stools.

       (1) Generally, any fruit juice alternated with bottled or disinfected water can be used for

Table 31-2.

Empiric Therapy for Traveler's Diarrhea

CLINICAL SYNDROME	PHARMACOLOGIC AGENT	DOSE AND DURATION
Mild diarrhea without fever or dysentery	Symptomatic treatment	Loperamide 4 mg initially, then 2 mg after each unformed stool, not to exceed 16 mg/d (prescription dose) or 8 mg/d (over-the-counter dose); or bismuth subsalicylate 30 ml (or 2 tabs) q30min for eight doses; both can be given for 2 days
Moderate to severe diarrhea*	Antimicrobial therapy	Trimethoprim/sulfamethoxazole (160 mg/800 mg) bid for 3 days for travel to interior of Mexico in summer; for other areas and times, use one of the following: norfloxacin PO 400 mg bid, ciprofloxacin PO 500 mg bid, ofloxacin PO 300 mg bid, or fleroxacin PO 400 mg qd for 3 days
Vomiting as predominant symptom	Bismuth subsalicylate	Dose given above

*If victim has a fever, the antimicrobial treatment is given alone. If there is no fever and stools do not contain blood or mucus, loperamide may be combined with the antimicrobial for faster relief. Antimicrobials are advised with the passage of the third unformed stool in 24 hours.

oral rehydration in mild to moderate diarrhea.

(2) Packets of oral rehydration salts produced according to World Health Organization (WHO) guidelines can be reconstituted to make oral rehydration solution (see following discussion). These packets are increasingly available in pharmacies throughout the world.

(3) Sports electrolyte solutions also provide adequate fluid replacement if diluted to about half their strength. Full-strength sports drinks are hypertonic and delay gastric absorption.

(4) Maximum gastrointestinal absorption of water occurs when the consumed drink has a glucose concentration of 2.5%. Highly sweetened drinks, such as undiluted apple juice, soft drinks, and undiluted Gatorade, have glucose concentrations of 6% or higher.

c. Urine frequency, color, and volume can serve as markers of adequate rehydration and should be monitored qualitatively.

4. To make an oral rehydration solution (ORS), the following methods generally are used:

a. Method 1:

1 tsp salt

2-3 tbsp sugar or honey

1 L clean or disinfected water

(This formula lacks bicarbonate and potassium.)

b. Method 2:

8-oz cup orange, apple, or other fruit drink

3 cups clean or disinfected water

1 tsp salt

(This formula lacks potassium.)

c. Method 3: half-strength athletic drink, such as Gatorade

d. Method 4:

Starch-based ORS solutions, such as Ricelyte and Cera-Lyte

These are excellent, containing rice starch, which decreases osmotic load and enhances absorption, and electrolytes. Unfortunately, these solutions are not always available.

e. Method 5:

Use a WHO formula ORS packet (usually available and inexpensive in most developing countries).

Add the packet to 1 L clean or disinfected water. WHO ORS is equivalent to:

Sodium chloride	3.5 g
Potassium chloride	1.5 g
Sodium bicarbonate	2.5 g
Glucose	20 g

f. Method 6—Make a WHO-ORS solution:

½ tsp salt

¼ tsp salt substitute (potassium chloride)

½ tsp baking soda (bicarbonate)

2-3 tbsp table sugar or 2 tbsp honey or Karo syrup

1 L clean or disinfected water

5. Use an antiperistaltic drug, such as the over-the-counter agents loperamide (Imodium) or diphenoxylate plus atropine (Lomotil), to offer relief to victims with watery diarrhea and cramps.

a. Of the two drugs, loperamide is better tolerated and has fewer central opiate effects.

b. Avoid antiperistaltic drugs if blood or mucus is present in the stool or if victim has signs of serious illness (high fever, recurrent vomiting, severe abdominal pain) because the inhibition of gut motility may facilitate intestinal infection by invasive bacterial enteropathogens.

c. Be aware that these drugs can be valuable for long bus rides or summit bids where social constraints make frequent rest stops impractical.

d. Know that they can also be important for controlling fluid balance in a victim with profuse diarrhea who is unable to tolerate sufficient oral fluids to maintain a positive balance.

  e. The dose for loperamide is 4 mg for the initial dose and 2 mg after every loose stool, up to a total dose of 8 mg/day.

  f. The combination of loperamide plus an antibiotic is a potentially effective single-dose treatment (see no. 9).

6. Give bismuth subsalicylate (BSS). In large doses (30 ml BSS liquid or 2 BSS tablets PO q30min, maximum eight doses in 24 hours), BSS often improves both diarrhea and cramps. This is a reasonable alternative to starting antibiotic therapy in a victim with mild diarrhea.

7. Most diarrhea in travelers is self-limited, so mild episodes can be treated conservatively with the therapeutic modalities already noted. In more severe cases, give antibiotic treatment.

  a. Because of increasing resistance of bacterial enteropathogens (e.g., *Shigella, Campylobacter*) to trimethoprim/sulfamethoxazole (TMP/SMX, cotrimethoxazole, Bactrim, Septra), ciprofloxacin (Cipro) 500 mg (or another antibiotic) PO bid for 3 days is preferred for empiric treatment of traveler's diarrhea.

  b. Other antibiotics include ofloxacin (Floxin) 200 mg, norfloxacin (Noroxin) 400 mg, and TMP/SMX (160 mg/800 mg DS tablet; it is less effective).

8. Resistance to quinolone antibiotics can develop during the treatment of *C. jejuni* infections. Azithromycin (Zithromax) 250 mg tablets, 1 tablet bid for 3 days, may be used for quinolone-resistant *Campylobacter* infections.

9. Loperamide 4 mg plus ciprofloxacin (Cipro) 750 mg may be sufficient as a single-dose treatment for traveler's diarrhea.

10. An individual with a more severe diarrheal syn-

drome (frequent profuse stools) will often experience relief within hours of beginning empiric antibiotic therapy. Despite the drug's rapid effect, the individual should continue to take the antibiotic for a total of 3 days to prevent relapse.

11. If the victim has begun initial treatment of diarrhea with BSS therapy, at least 8 hours must elapse before optimum antibiotic therapy can occur because BSS impairs the absorption of oral antimicrobial agents.

12. If blood or mucus is present in the stool, advise the victim to take an antibiotic as described earlier but to refrain from using antiperistaltic medication.

13. If the victim is ill with what appears to be a resistant bacterial pathogen, a viral or parasitic infection, or a toxin-induced gastroenteritis (food poisoning), be aware that antibiotic therapy will not alter the course of the diarrhea.

14. Advise any victim who does not respond to empiric antibiotic treatment or who has diarrhea for more than 1 week to obtain clinical follow-up that includes a complete workup for bacterial and parasitic pathogens.

Prevention

1. **Take dietary precautions.** The risk of illness is lowest when most of a traveler's meals are self-prepared and eaten in a private home, highest when food is obtained from street vendors, and intermediate when food is consumed at public restaurants. Unfortunately, many studies evaluating risk have found little correlation between routine precautions and illness.

   a. Dietary recommendations to decrease the potential for transmission of fecal pathogens through food and water are as follows:

      (1) Avoid tap water and ice made from untreated water (most enteric organisms can survive freezing).

      (2) Low-quality bottled water may be contaminated; inquire about the best brands.

(3) Bottled and carbonated drinks, beer, and wine are probably safe.

(4) Boiled or disinfected water is safe.

(5) Alcohol in mixed drinks does not disinfect.

(6) Homemade beverages cannot be guaranteed.

(7) Ice in block form is often handled with unsanitary methods.

(8) Avoid unpasteurized cheese and dairy products.

(9) Avoid raw vegetables and salads, which may be contaminated by fertilization with human waste or washing with contaminated water.

(10) Anything that can be peeled or have the surface removed is generally safe.

(11) Fruits and hearty vegetables can be disinfected by immersion and washing in iodinated water or by exposure to boiling water for 30 seconds.

(12) Avoid raw seafood and fish.

(13) Avoid raw meat because adequate cooking kills all microorganisms and parasites; however, if the meat is left at room temperature and recontaminated, cooked food can incubate pathogenic bacteria.

b. Be aware that safe foods usually include the following:

(1) Well-cooked foods served steaming hot

(2) Baked foods (e.g., bread)

(3) Foods with high sugar content (e.g., syrups, jellies)

(4) Peeled fruits (if you are the peeler)

2. **Use prophylactic medications to prevent traveler's diarrhea.**

a. Of the nonantibiotic drugs, only BSS (Pepto-Bismol) has been shown by controlled studies to offer reasonable protection and safety. The current recommended dose of BSS (for prevention) is 2 tablets 4 times per day. Mild side effects include constipation, nausea, and blackened tongue or stools. BSS taken concurrently with antibiotics should be avoided because of the potential binding of BSS to the antibiotic, which prevents absorption.

b. Do not give BSS to someone with a history of aspirin allergy.

c. Give BSS with caution to small children; people with gout or renal insufficiency; and those taking probenecid, methotrexate, anticoagulants, or products containing aspirin.

3. **Give antimicrobial prophylaxis for traveler's diarrhea.**

a. A broad-spectrum antibiotic taken during travel can effectively prevent illness, but resolution of traveler's diarrhea within a few hours can usually be obtained after oral antibiotic therapy with a quinolone. Thus it is probably unnecessary for the average traveler to ingest an antibiotic for the full duration of a trip. Travelers wanting to avoid illness can initiate empiric antibiotic therapy immediately after the onset of symptoms.

b. Antimicrobial prophylaxis of traveler's diarrhea might be a reasonable strategy for residents of a low-risk country going to a high-risk area for less than 5 weeks with one or more of the following:

   (1) Underlying illness, such as acquired immunodeficiency syndrome (AIDS), inflammatory bowel disease, or a cardiac, renal, or central nervous system disorder

   (2) An itinerary that is so rigid and critical that a person cannot tolerate any inconvenience caused by signs and symptoms; such travelers include competitive athletes, politicians, sales representatives, and people going to special events

c. Antibiotics recommended to prevent traveler's diarrhea include the following (prophylactic dose of 1 tablet a day, used for up to 2 weeks):

   (1) Ciprofloxacin (Cipro) 500 mg

   (2) Ofloxacin (Floxin) 400 mg

(3) Norfloxacin (Noroxin) 400 mg
      (4) TMP/SMX (Bactrim, Septra) 160 mg/800 mg
          DS tablets (less effective)
  d. Despite its dramatic protection against diarrhea, the routine use of antimicrobial prophylaxis by travelers is not recommended because of the following:
      (1) Potential for adverse side effects
      (2) Alteration of normal bacterial flora
      (3) Tendency to "lower one's guard:" Travelers taking prophylactic antibiotics may relax their vigilance, which can increase their risk of acquiring other nonbacterial infections.

FOOD POISONING

Food poisoning results when toxins produced by bacteria are found in foods in concentrations sufficient to produce symptoms. This is not an infection, but a true poisoning. Most food poisoning is caused by *Staphylococcus aureus* or *Bacillus cereus*.

Signs and Symptoms
1. Diarrhea that develops within 6 to 12 hours after a suspicious meal, most likely caused by ingesting a preformed toxin
2. Preceded by severe nausea and vomiting
3. Symptoms usually limited to 24 hours
4. Physical examination nonspecific

Treatment
1. Be aware that treatment is directed toward fluid and electrolyte replacement and the control of nausea.
2. Note that no specific antibiotic therapy exists.

INFECTION CAUSED BY INTESTINAL PROTOZOA

All intestinal protozoa are transmitted by the fecal-oral route. Protozoa typically cause subacute or chronic gastrointestinal symptoms but may also invade the bowel wall and cause severe dysentery with an acute presentation.

Giardia lamblia

G. lamblia is a flagellate protozoan with a life cycle that involves two forms. Trophozoites are responsible for symptomatic illness. They are rarely infective because they die quickly outside of the body. Some trophozoites encyst and are passed in the stools of infected hosts. Cysts are typically the form passed through fecal-oral contact and cause infection. Cysts are very hardy in the external environment and retain viability in cold water for as long as 2 or 3 months. The infective dose of *Giardia* for humans is 10 to 25 cysts.

Giardiasis is a zoonosis with cross-infectivity from animals to humans. Animals that have been implicated as carriers include beavers, cattle, dogs, cats, rodents, sheep, and deer. In North America, *Giardia* is transmitted primarily through drinking water. Worldwide, person-to-person transmission may be more common.

Signs and Symptoms
1. Average incubation period 1 to 3 weeks
2. Sometimes abrupt onset of explosive, watery diarrhea accompanied by abdominal cramps, foul flatus, vomiting, fever, and malaise; typically lasts 3 to 4 days before transition to more common subacute syndrome
3. Onset usually insidious, with symptoms that wax and wane
4. Stools becoming mushy and malodorous
5. Watery diarrhea alternating with soft stools and even constipation
6. Middle and upper abdominal cramping, substantial burning acid indigestion, sulfurous belching, nausea, bowel distention, early satiety, foul flatus
7. Dysenteric symptoms (blood and pus in the stool) *not* features of giardiasis; fever and vomiting infrequent except during initial onset

8. May develop into a chronic process associated with malabsorption and weight loss

Treatment

1. Be aware that treatment in the wilderness is typically initiated empirically.
2. Note that a cure can be achieved with one of several drugs. However, no drug is effective in all cases. In resistant cases, longer courses of two drugs taken concurrently may be effective.
3. Understand that relapse may occur up to several weeks after treatment, which requires a second course of the same medication or an alternative drug.
4. The three groups of drugs currently used are as follows:
    a. *Nitromidazoles,* such as metronidazole (Flagyl) 250 mg tid for 7 to 10 days, or tinidazole (Tiniba, Fasgyn) 2 g as a single dose qd for 2 days; for children, 50 mg/kg as a single PO dose for 2 days with maximum dose of 2 g; note that tinidazole is not currently available in the United States.
    b. *Nitrofuran derivatives,* such as furazolidone (Furoxone) 6 mg/kg/day in four divided doses for 7 days. Furazolidone is available in suspension and is convenient for small children.
    c. *Acridine compounds,* such as quinacrine (Atabrine) 100 mg tid for 7 days. For children the dose is 7 mg/kg/day in three divided doses for 7 days.
5. Serious infection during pregnancy presents a special problem. When possible, withhold treatment until after delivery because none of the treatment options is considered completely safe.

Entamoeba histolytica

E. histolytica is found worldwide. Approximately 10% of the world's population carry the parasite. The prevalence in tropical countries is 30% to 50%. Amebiasis accounts for fewer than 1% of cases of traveler's diarrhea.

As with *Giardia,* the life cycle of *E. histolytica* involves two forms and one host. When a cyst is ingested through fecal contamination of food or water or via person-to-person contact, it divides and produces trophozoites. The trophozoites are the reproductive form, residing in the host and causing illness. The trophozoite cannot survive the external environment and is unlikely to transmit infection. Encystment occurs in the gut, and cysts pass in the stool. The cysts are typically infectious when they are passed. Extraintestinal disease sometimes occurs by hematogenous spread. Abscesses develop primarily in the liver but may also involve the brain and lungs.

Nondysenteric disease

Signs and Symptoms
From 80% to 99% of infections result in an asymptomatic carrier state. In individuals who develop illness, the following may be noted:

1. Most often, colonic inflammation without dysentery, causing lower abdominal cramping and altered stools
2. Weight loss, anorexia, nausea
3. Subacute infection developing into a nondysenteric bowel syndrome with symptoms of intermittent diarrhea, abdominal pain, weight loss, and flatulence

Dysenteric disease

Signs and Symptoms
1. Dysentery developing suddenly or after a period of mild symptoms
2. Symptoms developing in as few as 8 to 10 days, but more often after weeks to months
3. Ill appearance, with frequent bloody stools, tenesmus, moderate to severe abdominal pain and tenderness, and fever (considerable variation in severity)

4. Rarely, significant fever
5. Complications in 1% to 4% of victims: bowel perforation, toxic megacolon, strictures, or an ameboma (inflammatory lesion containing trophozoites that develops in the colon)
6. Amoebic liver abscess acutely or years after infection
7. In the wilderness, diagnosis considered in any victim with dysentery who is not responding to an appropriate antibiotic
8. Asymptomatic cyst shedding and active gastrointestinal illness that persist for years if amebiasis is not treated

Treatment
1. Be aware that, in general, treatment is effective for invasive infections but disappointing for luminal infections (no regimen is completely effective in eradicating intestinal infection).
2. Treatment is based on the location of the infection and the degree of symptoms (Table 31-3).
3. Medications are divided as follows:
   a. *Tissue amebicides,* which are well absorbed and combat invasive amebiasis in the bowel and liver
   b. *Luminal drugs,* which are poorly absorbed and act primarily within the gut
4. Treat invasive disease with a tissue-active drug followed by a luminal agent.
5. For oral therapy, note that high-dose metronidazole (Flagyl) is the drug of choice (750 mg tid for 10 days).
6. Given the luminal-acting drug iodoquinol (diiodohydroxyquin, Yodoxin) 650 mg tid for 21 days.
7. The dose for children is metronidazole 50 mg/kg/day in three divided doses, followed by iodoquinol 40 mg/kg/day in three divided doses for 21 days.
8. Tinidazole (Tiniba, Fasgyn), which is not currently available in the United States, can be given 600 mg bid for 5 days or 2 g qd as a single dose for 3 days.

Table 31-3.

Therapy for Parasitic Infections

ETIOLOGIC AGENT	INDICATION	DRUG AND DURATION
Giardia lamblia	Proven disease	Quinacrine* 100 mg tid for 7 days for adults, 7 mg/kg/day in three divided doses for 7 days for children
	Infants	Furazolidone 1.5 mg/kg qid for 7 days
	Empiric (unproven)	Metronidazole 250 mg tid for 7 days for adults, 15 mg/kg/day in three divided doses for 7 days for children
Entamoeba histolytica	Carrier/no symptoms	Iodoquinol (diiodohydroxyquin) 650 mg tid for 10 days for adults and 40 mg/kg/day in three divided doses for 7 days for children
	Intestinal disease	Metronidazole 750 mg tid for 5-10 days *plus* iodoquinol 650 mg tid for 21 days for adults *or* metronidazole 50 mg/kg/day in three divided doses for 10 days *plus* iodoquinol 40 mg/kg/day in three divided doses for 21 days

*If available; otherwise use tinidazole or metronidazole.

Table 31-3.

Therapy for Parasitic Infections—cont'd		
ETIOLOGIC AGENT	INDICATION	DRUG AND DURATION
Dientamoeba fragilis or *Balantidium coli*	Intestinal disease	Tetracycline 250-500 mg qid for 7-10 days *or* iodoquinol 650 mg tid for 20 days for adults
Entamoeba polecki	Intestinal disease	Metronidazole 750 mg tid for 10 days followed by diloxanide furoate 500 mg tid for 10 days for adults
Blastocystis hominis	Intestinal disease	Iodoquinol 650 mg tid for 20 days *or* metronidazole 750 mg tid for 10 days for adults
Cryptosporidium parvum	Intestinal disease	Paromomycin 500 mg tid for 5-7 days for adults
Isospora belli	Intestinal disease	Trimethoprim/ sulfamethoxazole 160 mg/800 mg bid for 3-4 weeks
Cyclospora or *Sarcocystis*	Intestinal disease	Uncertain

Cryptosporidium

Cryptosporidium has attracted renewed interest recently because of an increase in reported cases. Ingestion of untreated surface water, well water, or raw milk has been implicated as methods of transmission. Food-borne transmission is also suspected.

Signs and Symptoms
1. Syndrome generally mild and self-limited
2. Definitive diagnosis by stool examination or serologic techniques
3. Watery diarrhea (without blood or pus), abdominal cramps, nausea, flatulence; vomiting, low-grade fever

Treatment
1. Note that no clearly effective treatment has been found.
2. Be aware that paromomycin (Humatin) may be effective in eradicating the infection in immunocompetent individuals.

Cyclospora cayetanensis

Cyclospora is a protozoan parasite found in the ground water of developing countries. It was first discovered as a cause of diarrhea among travelers visiting Nepal.

Signs and Symptoms
1. Protracted watery diarrhea that can persist for weeks
2. Definitive diagnosis made by finding the microorganism in a stool sample treated with a modified acid-fast stain

Treatment
1. Unfortunately, *Cyclospora* is resistant to usual water disinfection methods (iodine, chlorine, or filtration).
2. It is best killed by bringing drinking water to a boil.
3. Treatment in adults consists of TMP/SMX (Bactrim, Septra) 160 mg /800 mg DS tablets, 1 tablet PO q12h for 7 days.

CHAPTER 32

Field Water Disinfection

DEFINITION

Water disinfection is the removal of all enteric pathogens from drinking water.

HEAT

1. Enteric pathogens, including cysts, bacteria, viruses, and parasites, can be killed at a temperature well below boiling.
2. Thermal death is a function of both time and temperature; therefore lower temperatures are effective with longer contact times (Box 32-1).
3. The 10-minute boiling rule is for the *sterilization* of water, including the destruction of heat-resistant bacterial spores, which are generally not enteric pathogens. *Disinfection* of water requires less than 10 minutes. *Pasteurization* of food and beverages is accomplished at 65° C (150° F) for 30 minutes or at 71° C (160° F) for 1 to 5 minutes. The majority of the time required to raise the temperature of water to the boiling point works toward disinfection, so water is safe to drink by the time it has reached a full boil. For an extra margin of safety, keep the water covered and hot for several minutes after boiling, or boil for 1 full minute.

Box 32-1.

Thermal Death Points

> ❖ *Giardia lamblia, Entamoeba histolytica* cysts: 60°
>   C (140° F) for 2 to 3 minutes
> ❖ *Cryptosporidium* oocysts: 65° C (150° F) for 2
>   minutes
> ❖ Enteric viruses: within seconds at 80° to 100° C
>   (176° to 212° F)
> ❖ Enteric bacteria: within seconds at 100° C (212°
>   F)

4. The boiling point decreases with the lower atmospheric pressure present at high elevations (Table 32-1). However, elevation should not make a difference. A pressure cooker saves time and fuel at all elevations (Table 32-1).

FILTRATION AND CLARIFICATION
Filtration

1. Field filters that rely solely on the mechanical removal of microorganisms may be adequate for cysts and bacteria but may not reliably remove viruses, which are a major concern in water where high levels of fecal contamination are present (e.g., in developing countries).
2. Most viruses adhere to larger particles or clump together into larger aggregates that may be removed by a filter. However, filtration is not an adequate method to eliminate viruses because the infectious dose of an enteric virus may be quite small. Filters are often expensive and can add considerable weight and bulk to a backpack.
3. The filter pore size required to remove microorganisms effectively is difficult to determine. Microorganisms possess elasticity and deform under pressure,

Table 32-1.

Boiling Points at Various Elevations	
ELEVATION	**BOILING POINT**
10,000 ft (3048 m)	194° F (90° C)
14,000 ft (4267 m)	187° F (86° C)
19,000 ft (5791 m)	178° F (81° C)

Table 32-2.

Average Maximal Pore Size for Removal of Specific Microorganisms	
MICROORGANISM	**PORE SIZE (μm)**
Parasite eggs and larvae	20
G. lamblia, E. histolytica	5
Cryptosporidium	3
Enteric bacteria	0.4
Viruses	0.01 (too small for filtration)

making it possible for them to squeeze through filter pores. Most field filters are depth filters with maze-like passageways that trap particles and organisms smaller than the average diameter of a passage.

4. It is more useful and important to be familiar with the functional removal rate of certain organisms rather than with the rated pore size of the filter. Good testing data are needed to back claims, but objective, comparative data are not generally available (Table 32-2).

Clarification

Clarification of cloudy water can be achieved as follows:

1. Large particles settle by gravity over 1 to 2 hours in *sedimentation*. Although filters remove particu-

late debris, thus improving the appearance and taste of "dirty" water, they clog quickly if the water contains large particles.

2. Smaller suspended particles can be removed by coagulation-flocculation (C-F). This is accomplished in the field by adding alum (aluminum potassium sulfate) (Box 32-2). Alum is used in the food industry as a pickling powder and is nontoxic. C-F will remove contaminants that cause an unpleasant color and taste, some dissolved metals, and some microorganisms.

Charcoal Resins

1. *Granular activated charcoal* (GAC) removes organic pollutants, chemicals, and radioactive particles by absorption. This improves the color, taste, and smell of the water. Although some microorganisms adhere to GAC or become trapped in charcoal filters, GAC does not remove *all* microorganisms, so it does not disinfect.

2. GAC can be used to remove halogens (iodine, chlorine) after disinfection.

3. If GAC is used to remove iodine or chlorine, wait until after the required contact time for disinfection be-

Box 32-2.

Water Clarification Using Alum

1. Add a pinch of alum to each gallon of water.
2. Mix well, stir occasionally for 30 minutes, and then allow 30 to 60 minutes for settling.
3. The water should clear; if it does not, add another pinch of alum.
4. Decant or pour the water through a paper filter to remove clumps of flocculate.

fore running water through charcoal or adding charcoal to the water.

4. Filters that use iodine resins, followed by GAC, rely on a different dynamic for disinfection.
   a. Although residual-free iodine is largely removed by GAC, iodine is thought to remain bound to microorganisms following the resin pass-through and GAC pass-through phases.
   b. The necessary contact time for iodine resins is not absolutely determined, but it is clearly less than that required with standard iodine solutions.

Halogens

Halogens (chlorine and iodine) are effective disinfectants that are active against bacteria, viruses, *Giardia,* and cysts of amebae, excluding *Cryptosporidium.* They are readily available and inexpensive.

Concentration and Demand

1. Disinfection with halogens depends on both the concentration of halogen and the amount of time the halogen is in contact with the water (contact time). An increase in one allows a decrease in the other.
2. Minor factors affecting this method include the water temperature (cold slows reaction time) and the presence of organic contaminants in the water, which react with halogen and decrease its disinfectant action.
3. In cold water the contact time or dose should be increased, and in polluted water, the dose must be increased.
4. Use 4 parts per million (ppm) as a target concentration for surface water and allow extra contact time, especially if the water is cold.
5. In cloudy water that will not settle out by sedimentation, the halogen dose should be at least 8 ppm to account for the greater halogen demand that results from the presence of organic material. Ideally, use C-F to clarify the water before halogenation, then use a smaller amount of halogen.

Pathogen Sensitivity

1. Bacteria are extremely sensitive to halogens.
2. Viruses and *Giardia* require higher concentrations or longer contact times.
3. *Cryptosporidium* cysts are extremely resistant to halogens.
4. Certain parasite eggs, such as *Ascaris,* are resistant but are not usually spread by water. These types of resistant cysts and eggs are susceptible to heat or filtration.
5. Although *Cryptosporidium* oocysts have been found in surface water and have been identified as the etiologic agent in cases of traveler's diarrhea and municipal water-borne outbreaks, it is unclear how much risk they pose in pristine wilderness waters.

Chlorine vs. Iodine

1. Compared with chlorine, iodine is less affected by pH or nitrogenous wastes, and it tastes better.
2. Chlorine (Table 32-3) and iodine (Table 32-4) are available in either liquid or tablet form.
3. Concern surrounds the physiologic activity of iodine.
   a. At levels used for water disinfection, iodine is safe for most people, even when used for a prolonged period.
   b. Despite iodine's relative safety, however, some alteration in thyroid function can be measured, and some persons experience magnification of existing thyroid problems.
   c. Hypersensitivity reactions to iodine can occur.
   d. Iodine use is not recommended for persons with unstable thyroid disease or a known iodine allergy.
   e. Iodine should not be used during pregnancy for more than several weeks because of the risk of neonatal goiter.
   f. Caution dictates not using iodine for more than several months at a time.

Table 32-3.

Experimental Data for 99.9% Kill With Chlorine			
CONCENTRATION	TIME	pH	TEMPERATURE
G. LAMBLIA (CONSISTENT WITH ENTAMOEBA HISTOLYTICA)			
0.5 mg/L	6-24 hr	6-8	3°-5° C (37°-41° F)
4.0 mg/L	60 min	6-8	3°-5° C (37°-41° F)
8.0 mg/L	30 min	6-8	3°-5° C (37°-41° F)
3.0 mg/L	10 min	6-8	15° C (59° F)
1.5 mg/L	10 min	6-8	25° C (77° F)
ENTERIC VIRUSES			
0.5 mg/L	40 min	7.8	2° C (35.6° F)
0.3 mg/L	30 min	7.8	25° C (77° F)
E. COLI			
0.03 mg/L	5 min	7.0	2°-5° C (35.6°-41° F)

4. Iodine resins may reduce toxicity concerns because they leave low concentrations of dissolved iodine in the water. They also allow for the complete removal of iodine residual with GAC. Iodine resins have been incorporated into many different filter designs now available for field use.

5. Halogens can be applied with equal ease to large and small quantities of water.

Table 32-4.

Experimental Data for 99% Kill With Iodine

CONCENTRATION	TIME	pH	TEMPERATURE
GIARDIA AND AMEBAE CYSTS			
3.0 mg/L	15 min	7.0	20° C (68° F)
7.0 mg/L	30 min	7.4	3° C (37.4° F)
POLIOVIRUS			
20 mg/L	1.5 min	7.0	25° C (77° F)
E. COLI			
1.0 mg/L	1 min	6.5-8.5	2°-5° C (35.6°-41° F)

Problems
1. The taste of the water can be unpleasant when the halogen concentration exceeds 4 to 5 mg/L.
2. The potency of some products (tablets, solutions) decreases with time and is affected by prolonged exposure to moisture or heat (tablets) and air (e.g., iodine crystals).
3. Liquids are corrosive and can stain clothes and equipment.
4. The actual concentration (after halogen demand) is not known.

Improving the taste of water disinfected with halogens

1. Add flavoring to the water after adequate contact time. Iodine will react with sugar additives, thereby reducing the free iodine available for disinfection.

2. Use charcoal (GAC) to remove halogen after contact time.
3. Reduce the concentration and increase the contact time in clean water. For a small group of people, use a collapsible plastic container to disinfect water with low doses of iodine during the day or overnight.
4. Iodine and chlorine taste and iodine color can be removed by chemical reduction. In addition, a higher halogen dose (shorter contact time) can be used if followed by chemical reduction.

Chemical reduction. To remove iodine and chlorine taste and iodine color, add a few granules per liter of ascorbic acid (vitamin C, available in powder or crystal form) or sodium thiosulfate (nontoxic) after the required contact time. These chemicals reduce iodine or chlorine to iodide or chloride, which has no taste or color. Ascorbic acid leaves behind a slightly tart taste. Iodide still has physiologic activity, which means that a person with unstable thyroid disease or known iodine allergy or a pregnant woman should continue to exercise caution.

CHOOSING THE PREFERRED TECHNIQUE

1. The best technique for disinfection for either an individual or a group depends on the number of persons, space and weight available, quality of source water, personal taste preferences, and availability of fuel.
2. Unfortunately, optimal protection for all situations may require a two-step process of filtration or C-F and halogenation because halogens do not kill *Cryptosporidium,* and filtration misses some viruses.
3. Heat works as a one-step process, but it will not improve the taste and look of water if it is cloudy or tastes poor initially.
4. An iodine resin, combined with microfiltration to remove resistant cysts, is also a viable one-step process for all situations.

Alpine Camping

1. For alpine camping where a high-quality water source is available, heat, mechanical or iodine resin filtration, or a low-dose halogen can be used.
2. Heat is limited by fuel supply.
3. Filtration has the advantage of imparting no taste and requiring no contact time.

Agricultural Runoff and Discharge From Upstream Towns

1. Treat water with agricultural runoff or sewage plant discharge from an upstream town or city with heat or a two-step process of filtration to remove *Cryptosporidium*, then with a halogen to ensure destruction of all viruses.
2. You can also use an iodine resin filter with microfiltration. A filter containing a charcoal element has the added advantage of removing many chemicals, such as pesticides.

Surface Water in Undeveloped Countries

1. View all surface water in undeveloped countries, even if visually clear, as highly contaminated with enteric pathogens.
2. Heat is effective for disinfection, but simple mechanical filtration is not adequate because of the potential for enteric viruses.
3. A halogen is reasonable but will miss *Cryptosporidium* and parasite eggs.
4. A two-stage process offers added protection.

Cloudy Water in Developed or Undeveloped Countries

1. Pretreat cloudy water in developed or undeveloped countries that does not clear with sedimentation with C-F, then disinfect with heat or a halogen.
2. Note that filters can clog rapidly with silted or cloudy water.

Table 32-5.

Water Disinfection Techniques

IODINATION TECHNIQUE (ADDED TO 1 L OR QT OF WATER)	AMOUNT FOR 4 ppm	AMOUNT FOR 8 ppm
Iodine tablets (tetraglycine hydroperiodide, EDWGT, Potable Aqua, Globaline)	½ tablet	1 tablet
2% iodine solution (tincture)	0.2 ml 5 gtt (drops)	0.4 ml 10 gtt
10% povidone-iodine solution	0.35 ml 8 gtt	0.70 ml 16 gtt
Saturated iodine crystals in water	13 ml	26 ml
Saturated iodine crystals in alcohol	0.1 ml	0.2 ml

CHLORINATION TECHNIQUES (ADDED TO 1 L OR QT OF WATER)	AMOUNT FOR 5 ppm	AMOUNT FOR 10 ppm
Household bleach 5% (sodium hypochlorite)	0.1 ml 2 gtt	0.2 ml 4 gtt
AquaClear (sodium dichloroisocyanurate)		1 (17-mg) tablet
AquaCure, AquaPure, Chlor-floc (chlorine plus flocculating agent)		8 ppm/tablet

EDWGT, Emergency drinking water germicidal tablet.
NOTE: Measure with a dropper (1 drop = 0.04 to 0.05 ml) or tuberculin syringe. A povidone-iodine solution releases free iodine in levels adequate for disinfection, but scant data are available.

Table 32-6.

Halogen Doses

HALOGEN CONCENTRATION (ppm)	CONTACT TIME (MIN) AT VARIOUS WATER TEMPERATURES*		
	5° C (41° F)	15° C (59° F)	30° C (86° F)
2	240	180	60
4	180	60	45
8	60	30	15

*Recent data indicate that very cold water requires prolonged contact time with iodine or chlorine to kill *Giardia* cysts. These contact times in cold water have been extended from the usual recommendations to account for this and for the uncertainty regarding residual concentrations of active halogen.

Systems Where Water Will Be Stored

1. Halogens have a distinct advantage in locations where the water will be stored for a time, such as on a boat or in a home without running water.
2. Note that when only heat or filtration is used before storage, the water can become recontaminated and bacterial regrowth can occur. Superchlorination-dechlorination is particularly useful in this situation, because a high level of chlorination can be maintained for a long period.
   a. When ready to use the water, pour it into a smaller container and dechlorinate it.
   b. If another means of chlorination is used, maintain a minimum residual of 3 to 5 mg/L in the water.
3. Iodine will work for short-term storage, but it should not be used when long-term storage is a possibility because iodine is a poor algicide.
4. On a long-distance, ocean-going boat where water

must be desalinated during the voyage, a reverse osmosis membrane filter is necessary.

Techniques and Halogen Doses

Table 32-5 summarizes the various techniques used in water disinfection. Table 32-6 lists recommended halogen doses.

CHAPTER 33

Travel-Acquired Illnesses

The major travel-acquired illnesses that occur in the wilderness are yellow fever, hepatitis, typhoid and paratyphoid fevers, meningococcal disease, Japanese B encephalitis, and malaria. Each of these disorders can be prevented if the traveler takes specific precautions or prophylactic agents.

■ DISORDERS ■

YELLOW FEVER

Yellow fever is caused by a single-stranded ribonucleic acid (RNA) flavivirus that is transmitted by mosquitoes. The liver is the principal target organ. All recent cases of American yellow fever were acquired in the jungle environment; however, urban transmission continues to occur in Africa.

Signs and Symptoms
1. May appear as an undifferentiated viral syndrome
2. Specific diagnosis in the wilderness extremely difficult; clinical suspicion based on immune status, geographic distribution of the disease, travel history, and characteristic triphasic fever, as follows:
   a. Headache, fever, and malaise often accompanied by bradycardia and conjunctival suffusion

b. After 3 to 4 days, brief remission
c. Within 24 hours, intoxication phase: jaundice, fever, prostration, and, in severe cases, hypotension, shock, oliguria, and obtundation; hemorrhage usually manifested as hematemesis, but bleeding from multiple sites possible

Treatment

1. Perform a careful physical examination. Be aware that the diagnosis requires thick and thin blood smears to rule out malaria and blood cultures for bacterial pathogens; both of these necessitate evacuation to a qualified medical facility. If the victim's condition progresses to the intoxication phase, arrange for immediate evacuation to an intensive care unit (ICU).
2. Note that no effective antiviral treatment is available for yellow fever.
3. Supportive care includes the following:
   a. Control fever with acetaminophen (do not use salicylates).
   b. Give IV fluids and oral rehydration fluids.
   c. Transfer the victim to a hospital as quickly as possible.

Prevention

1. Give yellow fever vaccine (more than 95% of those vaccinated achieve significant antibody levels). Be aware that repeat vaccinations are recommended every 10 years.
2. Avoid the causative organism through mosquito protection measures in endemic areas, including repellent and proper netting.

Dengue

Dengue virus is a single-stranded RNA flavivirus that is transmitted by the day-biting urban mosquito *Aedes aegypti* or the jungle mosquito *Aedes albopictus*. *A. aegypti* is the principal vector for dengue viruses worldwide.

Viral transmission is maintained through a mosquito-human cycle without a major animal reservoir.

Signs and Symptoms
1. Clinically, may range from undifferentiated viral symptoms with fever and mild respiratory/GI symptoms to DHF (see below)
2. Incubation period 5 to 8 days
3. Early prodromal symptoms of nausea and vomiting common, followed by high fever lasting for days (mean 5 days)
4. Headache and lymphadenopathy common, as well as myalgias ("breakbone fever")
5. After several days, often maculopapular or morbilliform rash spreading outward from chest
6. In more severe cases, referred to as *dengue hemorrhage fever* (DHF) or *dengue shock syndrome* (DSS); with severe DHF/DSS, may progress to circulatory failure with shock; spontaneous bleeding from almost any site
7. After infection, extreme fatigue persisting for weeks or months
8. DHF/DSS unlikely in traveler not previously infected with dengue
9. Awareness of the local epidemiology of DHF/DSS important in establishing the diagnosis, with definitive diagnosis of all forms requiring serology (antibody identification) or viral isolation from serum

Treatment
1. Know that treatment is symptomatic.
2. In DHF/DSS, administer acetaminophen for fever and myalgias (do not use salicylates).
3. Vigorously maintain hydration.
4. Be aware that severe DHF or any DSS is a medical emergency and requires immediate evacuation and hospitalization.
5. Note that no specific therapy exists for any form of dengue.

HEPATITIS
Hepatitis A

Hepatitis A virus (HAV) is transmitted mainly through the fecal-oral route, either by person-to-person contact or by ingestion of contaminated food or water. Occasional cases are associated with exposure to nonhuman primates. HAV is endemic worldwide, but underdeveloped regions have a significantly higher prevalence. In most instances, resolution of the acute disease is permanent, but rare cases of relapse have been noted. Death from HAV is rare. After natural infection, HAV antibodies confer immunity. HAV patients are infectious for approximately 2 weeks before the onset of symptoms. Viral shedding declines with the onset of jaundice. The victim is typically not infectious 1 to 2 weeks after the onset of clinical disease.

Signs and Symptoms
1. Incubation period ranging from 2 to 7 weeks
2. Infection asymptomatic or mild
3. Classic syndrome: early onset of anorexia, followed by nausea, vomiting, fever, and abdominal pain
4. Symptoms possibly accompanied by hepatosplenomegaly
5. Jaundice after GI syndrome by several days to a few weeks; resolution of jaundice lasting another 3 to 4 weeks
6. Although rare, sometimes (0.5% to 1%) follows a fulminant course, resulting in hepatic necrosis, hepatic encephalopathy, and often death
7. Clinical presentation often milder than with other types of viral hepatitis, but not distinctive enough to allow clinical differentiation

Treatment
1. Be aware that no specific therapy exists for HAV.
2. Instruct affected persons concerning enteric precautions to avoid transmission to others (compulsive handwashing).

3. Although infectivity drops sharply soon after the onset of jaundice, to be safe, continue enteric and blood-drawing precautions for 2 weeks.

Prevention
1. See discussion of HAV vaccine in the Chapter 34.
2. See discussion of dietary precautions in Chapter 31.

Hepatitis B

Hepatitis B (HBV) is transmitted through the exchange of blood, semen, or, rarely, saliva from infected people. Although spread is possible from persons with acute disease, in most cases chronic carriers spread the disease. In many areas of the developing world, chronic carriers are 10% to 20% of the total population. The risk is much higher among persons regularly exposed to body fluids, including medical personnel and those who engage in sexual contact abroad. Victims with HBV infection may be infectious within 1 to 2 weeks after inoculation, well before any clinical symptoms develop.

Signs and Symptoms
1. Range of incubation period 7 to 22 weeks
2. Manifestations similar to those of HAV: fever, anorexia, nausea, vomiting, abdominal pain
3. Additional prodrome of rash, arthralgias, or arthritis and fever in up to 20% of HBV patients (rare in HAV)
4. Jaundice developing a short time after GI symptoms
5. With self-limited disease, recovery complete by 6 months
6. With fulminant (1% to 3%) course, hepatic necrosis, hepatic encephalopathy, often death
7. Other possibilities:
   a. Asymptomatic chronic carrier state
   b. Chronic active hepatitis
   c. Chronic progressive hepatitis
8. Definitive diagnosis requires antigen and antibody tests

Treatment

1. Be aware that no specific therapy exists for HBV.
2. Instruct affected persons concerning enteric precautions to avoid transmission to others (compulsive handwashing).
3. Note that prolonged and sometimes persistent viremia makes blood and body fluid precautions necessary until antigen and antibody testing show noninfectivity.

Prevention

Prophylaxis is indicated for those travelers at high risk, specifically, medical workers or those anticipating sexual contact with local inhabitants in endemic areas (see Chapter 34).

Other Forms of Hepatitis

Hepatitis C

Previously "non-A, non-B hepatitis," hepatitis C is similar to HBV in both transmission and clinical course.

Hepatitis D

Formerly the "delta agent," active hepatitis D is found only in individuals who are positive for hepatitis B surface antigen (Hb_sAg).

Hepatitis E

Formerly "enterically transmitted non-A, non-B hepatitis," hepatitis E is similar to HAV in both transmission and clinical course.

Treatment

No specific vaccine exists for these forms. Immunity to hepatitis D is conferred with immunity to HBV. As with other types of hepatitis, the best method of prevention is avoidance of infected body fluids and prudent selection of food and water when traveling.

TYPHOID AND PARATYPHOID FEVER (ENTERIC FEVERS)

Typhoid fever occurs worldwide, but its prevalence and attack rates are much higher in undeveloped countries. Humans are the only host for *Salmonella typhi*, the most common cause of the typhoid fever syndrome. Nearly all cases are contracted through the ingestion of contaminated food and water. The risk of transmission is relatively high in Mexico, Peru, India, Pakistan, Chile, Sub-Saharan Africa, and Southeast Asia.

Salmonella species are gram-negative enteric bacilli. *S. typhi* is the prime cause of typhoid fever, but other species may cause a typhoid fever–like syndrome. The term *enteric fever* is used to describe a severe systemic infection with *S. paratyphi* (paratyphoid fever). The clinical appearance of S. *paratyphi* infection is similar to that seen with typhoid (see next), but typically *S. paratyphi* infection runs a shorter course.

Signs and Symptoms
1. Onset of illness usually 10 to 14 days after exposure to the pathogen
2. Gastroenteritis possible early in the course of the disease; abdominal pain or diarrhea with classic typhoid fever
3. Fever
   a. Usually the first sign of the disease
   b. May be accompanied by bradycardia
   c. Increases slowly over several days and remains constant for 2 to 3 weeks, after which defervescence begins
4. Headaches, malaise, anorexia
5. "Rose spots" (2- to 4-mm maculopapular blanching lesions) classically described on the trunk, although not seen in most victims
6. Hepatomegaly, splenomegaly in many patients
7. Uncomplicated, untreated typhoid fever usually resolving spontaneously in 3 to 4 weeks

8. Life-threatening complications:
   a. Intestinal perforation leading to peritonitis
   b. GI hemorrhage
   c. Pneumonia
   d. Multisystem failure with myocardial involvement
9. Definitive diagnosis possible by bacterial culture
10. Possible for victims to remain asymptomatic carriers and continue to shed organisms for years

Treatment
1. Give antibiotics:
   a. Chloramphenicol 50 mg/kg/day in four divided doses for 2 weeks; some resistance has been noted
   b. Ampicillin 100 mg/kg/day in four divided doses for at least 2 weeks
   c. Co-trimethoxazole: 80 mg trimethoprim plus 400 mg sulfamethoxazole/day in two divided doses for at least 2 weeks
   d. Ciprofloxacin 500 mg bid for 2 weeks
2. Make sure that the victim has adequate nutrition and food support.
3. Be aware that relapse can occur after 2 weeks of therapy and necessitates re-treatment with the same regimen.

Prevention
1. Because typhoid vaccine does not ensure protection, tell vaccinated persons to avoid potentially contaminated food and drink (see Chapter 31).
2. See discussion of typhoid fever vaccine in Chapter 34.

MENINGOCOCCAL DISEASE
Meningococcal disease is caused by *Neisseria meningitidis,* a gram-negative diplococcus. Meningococcal meningitis classically attacks children and young adults and is often seen in epidemic form. Despite effective antibiotic therapy and immunization, this disease remains problematic in many parts of the world.

Epidemic situations pose the greatest health problem to both travelers and resident populations. Since 1970, large outbreaks have occurred in Brazil; China; the Sahel region of Sub-Saharan Africa; New Delhi, India; and Nepal.

Transmission of the organism occurs through respiratory secretions, so close contact is believed to be important in the spread of the disease.

Signs and Symptoms
1. Variety of forms, including but not limited to the following:
   a. Bacteremia with septic shock
   b. Meningitis, often with bacteremia
   c. Pneumonia
2. Sustained meningococcemia: may lead to severe toxemia with hypotension, fever, and DIC
3. Meningitis caused by *N. meningitidis:* classic triad of fever, headache, and stiff neck; also possibly accompanied by bacteremia and any of several skin manifestations, including petechiae, pustules, or maculopapular rash
4. Severe meningitis: may progress to mental status deterioration, hypotension, congestive heart failure, DIC, and death
5. Presumptive diagnosis in epidemic based on clinical presentation
6. Definitive diagnosis: culture of organism from cerebrospinal fluid or blood

Treatment
1. Be aware that meningococcal meningitis, or sepsis, is a medical emergency, with victims suspected requiring **immediate** evacuation to an appropriate medical facility.
2. Note that, fortunately, the organism remains sensitive to many antibiotics, such as the following:
   a. Penicillin G 300,000 U/kg/day (up to 24 million U/day) IV in divided doses q2h for 7 to 10 days for serious disease.

   b. Ceftriaxone 2 g q12h IV
   c. Chloramphenicol 12.5 mg/kg q6h IV
3. Give supportive care, including close monitoring for hypotension and cardiac failure (necessitates ICU technology) and IV fluid support.
4. Be aware that dexamethasone may be of value for victims in coma or with evidence of increased intracranial pressure.
5. Make sure that contacts receive prophylaxis to eradicate the organism (rifampin 600 mg PO q12h for four doses).

Prevention
See discussion of meningococcal vaccine in Chapter 34.

JAPANESE B ENCEPHALITIS
Japanese encephalitis is a viral infection transmitted by *Culex* mosquitoes. Transmission takes place year-round in tropical and subtropical areas and during the late spring, summer, and early fall in temperate climates.

   Encephalitis is caused by a neurotropic flavivirus. After initial replication near the mosquito bite, viremia occurs and, if prolonged, may seed infection to the brain. The virus causes central nervous system nerve cell destruction and necrosis.

   Most infections in endemic areas involve children, but this disease may occur in any age-group. At present, Japanese B encephalitis transmission is most likely in India, Southeast Asia, China, Korea, Indonesia, the far western Pacific region, eastern Russia, and Japan.

Signs and Symptoms
1. No clinical illness in most infections
2. Encephalitis (about 1 in 300 infections)
3. Mild undifferentiated febrile illness (encephalitis victims often with a similar prodrome)
4. Headache, lethargy, fever, confusion; possible tremors or seizures
5. Reported mortality with clinical encephalitis: 10% to 50%

6. Encephalitis syndrome not easily distinguished from other arboviral encephalitis
7. Definitive diagnosis: serologic testing

Treatment
1. Be aware that no specific therapy exists for this disease.
2. Note that supportive care often requires an ICU.
3. Practice blood and body fluid precautions.

Prevention
1. An effective inactivated vaccine is recommended for travelers to endemic areas in the transmission season who will be staying for longer than a month.
2. See discussion of Japanese encephalitis vaccine in Chapter 34.

Malaria
Malaria is a mosquito-transmitted blood-borne parasitic infection present throughout tropical and developing areas of the world. Parasites are transmitted by the female *Anopheles* mosquito, which tends to bite between dusk and dawn. Estimated worldwide incidence is 280 million cases per year. Malaria infection causes a severe febrile illness that is potentially fatal.

Four species of malaria typically cause disease in humans, as follows:

1. *Plasmodium vivax* (worldwide distribution)
2. *Plasmodium falciparum* (worldwide distribution)
3. *Plasmodium ovale* (West Africa)
4. *Plasmodium malariae* (worldwide distribution)

Signs and Symptoms
1. Clinical manifestations first evident 1 to 2 weeks after entry into endemic area (sooner if infected blood obtained through transfusion or shared needles)
2. No pathognomonic signs, but common symptoms (Table 33-1)

Table 33-1.

Common Symptoms and Their Incidence in Malaria

SYMPTOM	INCIDENCE (%)
Fever	97
Chills	97
Headaches	94
Nausea/vomiting	62
Abdominal pain	56
Myalgia	50
Backache	9
Dark urine	3

3. Paroxysms of chills followed by high fever and sweating
   a. May last several hours and occur every 2 to 3 days
   b. Classic periodic attacks often not observed in severe *P. falciparum* malaria; fever possibly constant
4. Abdominal cramps, diarrhea
5. Cerebral malaria (associated with high levels of *P. falciparum* parasitemia), characterized by high fevers, confusion, and eventually coma and death
6. Acute renal failure, pulmonary edema
7. Definitive diagnosis only by the presence of parasite-containing red blood cells (detected on thick and thin blood smears)
8. Clinical attacks during the first 4 to 8 weeks after return from the area of exposure
9. Prolonged latent incubation times (up to 3 years) reported

Treatment

If treatment is required, this implies failure of malaria chemoprophylaxis. Taking prophylactic medications does not exclude the possibility of becoming infected because no current drug or drug regimen can be considered to provide 100% protection against malaria.

1. Be aware that "stand-by" therapy (self-treatment) is recommended for travelers to chloroquine-resistant *P. falciparum* (CRPF) areas who meet the following qualifications:
   a. Unable to take mefloquine
   b. Using an antimalarial agent with suboptimal efficacy
   c. Going to remote areas where access to medical care is limited
2. Note the drugs used for stand-by therapy (Table 33-2). Have the victim take a treatment dose of one of the following antimalarial agents when signs and symptoms suggest an acute attack and prompt medical attention is not available:
   a. Sulfadoxine plus pyrimethamine (Fansidar)
   b. Halofantrine (Halfan)
   c. Mefloquine (Lariam) (World Health Organization)
3. Be aware that most victims can be treated with oral medications. If vomiting occurs within 30 minutes, repeat the full oral dose after giving the victim an antiemetic, such as metoclopramide (Reglan) 10 mg PO, IM, or IV.

Prevention
Chemoprophylaxis: general principles

1. Determine the risk of malaria infection for a geographic location.
2. Select an antimalarial drug regimen based on the risk of CRPF malaria (Tables 33-3 and 33-4).
   a. Consider toxicity and contraindications in choosing a regimen for chemoprophylaxis of CRPF malaria.
   b. Be aware that resistance to multiple antimalarial drugs has made prevention and treatment of

Table 33-2.
Malaria Drugs for Standby Treatment

DRUG	ADULT DOSE	PEDIATRIC DOSE
Pyrimethamine 25 mg/sulfadoxine 500 mg (Fansidar)	3 tablets PO as single dose	2-11 mo: ¼ tablet 1-3 yr: ½ tablet 4-8 yr: 1 tablet 9-14 yr: 2 tablets >14 yr: 3 tablets PO as single dose
Mefloquine 250 mg (Lariam)	2 tablets as single dose, followed by 2 tablets after 8-12 hr; reduce 2nd dose to 1 tablet for adults <60 kg	15 mg/kg PO as single dose (do not use in infants <15 kg)
Halofantrine 250 mg (Halfan)	2 tablets in one dose + 2 tablets after 6 hr + 2 tablets after 6 more hr (total dose 6 tablets in 12 hr); *repeat therapy in 7 days in nonimmune patients*	

From Jong EC, White NJ: *The travel and tropical medicine manual*, ed 2, Philadelphia, 1995, WB Saunders.

Continued

Table 33-2.

Malaria Drugs for Standby Treatment—cont'd

DRUG	ADULT DOSE	PEDIATRIC DOSE
Halofantrine 2% suspension (Halfan)		8 mg/kg PO × 3 doses, each dose 6 hr apart; *repeat therapy in 7 days in non-immune patients*
Quinine sulfate tablet	650 mg tid for 3 days (continue for 7 days in Southeast Asia)	10 mg/kg tid for 3 days (continue for 7 days in Southeast Asia)
Plus tetracycline	250 mg qid for 7 days	>8 yr: 5 mg/kg PO qid for 7 days
Or plus doxycycline	100 mg PO bid for 7 days	>8 yr: 2 mg/kg PO bid for 7 days
Or plus clindamycin	10 mg/kg tid for 5 days	10 mg/kg tid for 5 days
Or plus Fansidar	Fansidar dose above	Fansidar dose above

From Jong EC, White NJ: *The travel and tropical medicine manual,* ed 2, Philadelphia, WB Saunders.

Table 33-3.

Malaria Chemoprophylaxis Based on Geographic Risk

GEOGRAPHIC AREA	DRUG OF CHOICE	ALTERNATIVE
CHLOROQUINE-SENSITIVE AREAS LOCATED WITHIN:		
Mexico	Chloroquine	Standby*
Caribbean	Chloroquine	Standby*
Central America (west of Panama Canal)	Chloroquine	Standby*
Middle East (Egypt, Turkey, Iraq, Syria, United Arab Emirates)	Chloroquine	Standby*
CHLOROQUINE-RESISTANT AREAS LOCATED WITHIN:		
Central America (east of Panama Canal)	Mefloquine	Chloroquine + standby*
South America	Mefloquine	Chloroquine + standby*
South America (Amazon Basin)	Mefloquine	Doxycycline
Middle East	Mefloquine	Chloroquine + standby*
Africa (sub-Saharan)	Mefloquine	Doxycycline (or C+P+SB)†
Southeast Asia	Mefloquine	Doxycycline
Thailand (border areas near Cambodia and Burma)	Doxycycline	Proguanil + sulfa or dapsone
Oceania	Mefloquine	Doxycycline

From Jong EC, White NJ: *The travel and tropical medicine manual,* ed 2, Philadelphia, WB Saunders.
*Standby malaria treatment: take a treatment dose of the antimalarial drug when experiencing signs and symptoms of malaria and if prompt medical attention is not available:
1. Pyrimethamine plus sulfadoxine (Fansidar) *or*
2. Halofantrine (Halfan)
†*C+P+SB,* Chloroquine plus proguanil (Paludrine) plus carry standby malaria treatment.

Table 33-4.

Malaria Chemoprophylaxis

DRUG	DOSE
ADULTS	
Chloroquine phosphate (Aralen)	250 mg, 2 tab/wk
	500 mg, 2 tab/wk
Mefloquine (Lariam)	250 mg, 1 tab/wk
Doxycycline (Vibramycin)	100 mg, 1 tab/wk
Proguanil (Paludrine) (in addition to weekly chloroquine)	100 mg, 2 tab/day
Pyrimethamine-dapsone (Maloprim)	12.5 mg pyrimethamine, 100 mg dapsone, 1 tab/wk
CHILDREN	
Chloroquine phosphate	8.3 mg/kg/wk
Hydroxychloroquine sulfate	6.5 mg/kg/wk
Proguanil	<2 yr: 50 mg/day
	2-6 yr: 100 mg/day
	7-10 yr: 150 mg/day
	>10 yr: 200 mg/day
Pyrimethamine-dapsone	<2 yr: ¼ tab/wk
	3-10 yr: ½ tab/wk
	>10 yr: 1 tab/wk
Mefloquine (not FDA approved)	15-19 kg: ¼ tab/wk
	20-30 kg: ½ tab/wk
	31-40 kg: ¾ tab/wk

From Jong EC, White NJ: *The travel and tropical medicine manual,* ed 2, Philadelphia, WB Saunders.

P. fal ciparum malaria a major problem in some endemic areas.

3. Start administration of the antimalarial drug 1 to 2 weeks before departure to allow time to accomplish the following:
   a. Become familiar with any drug side effects.
   b. Switch to an alternative drug if necessary.
   c. Habituate to the timing of doses.
   d. Build up to steady-state drug levels.
4. Maintain the antimalarial drug dosing schedule during exposure.
5. Continue the antimalarial drug regimen for 4 weeks after leaving the area of malaria infection.

Malaria chemoprophylaxis: specific agents

1. Chloroquine (Aralen) has decreasing efficacy in areas of CRPF.
   a. Once-weekly dosing
   b. Relatively inexpensive
   c. Drug of choice for chemoprophylaxis against *P. vivax, P. malariae,* and *P. ovale;* also drug of choice where *P. falciparum* still chloroquine sensitive
   d. Relatively safe
   e. Contraindicated in persons receiving chloroquine therapy for other conditions, those with psoriasis, and those with retinal degeneration
   f. Pruritus possible in black patients
   g. Rare reports of neuropsychiatric side effects
   h. Safe during pregnancy
   i. Safe use for period of 5 to 6 years
2. Mefloquine (Lariam) is the drug of choice for chemoprophylaxis for travel in CRPF areas.
   a. Once-weekly dosing
   b. Relatively expensive
   c. Contraindicated in persons taking certain chronic medications that affect cardiac conduction (i.e., beta-blocker drugs, antiarrhythmia drugs, anticonvulsive drugs)

d. Probably safe during pregnancy and for children weighing less than 15 kg (33 lb)
e. Reported neuropsychiatric side effects; use with caution for drivers, pilots, etc.
f. Probably safe use for up to 3 years
g. Resistance demonstrated in strains of CRPF in Thailand along Cambodian and Burmese borders

3. Doxycycline (Vibramycin) is an effective chemoprophylaxis against CRPF and multidrug-resistant *P. falciparum* malaria.
   a. Daily dosing
   b. Inexpensive
   c. Contraindicated during pregnancy and lactation and for children under 8 years of age
   d. Phototoxicity a potentially serious side effect
   e. GI intolerance in many patients
   f. May predispose females to vaginal candidiasis
   g. May be less effective against *P. vivax* malaria in Indonesia and Papua New Guinea

4. Chloroquine (Aralen) plus proguanil (Paludrine) may be an effective combination.
   a. Weekly chloroquine plus daily proguanil a complex regimen, which may affect compliance
   b. Relatively inexpensive
   c. Less effective than weekly mefloquine
   d. Not efficacious in Asia against CRPF malaria
   e. Not recommended unless traveler going to CRPF areas cannot tolerate mefloquine or doxycycline
   f. Both drugs considered safe during pregnancy
   g. Side effects of proguanil: mouth ulcerations, GI upset, hair loss

5. Pyrimethamine (12.5 mg) plus dapsone (100 mg) (Maloprim) combination may be considered.
   a. Once-weekly dosing
   b. Used in Africa and Asia against CRPF malaria
   c. Resistance developed in some CRPF strains
   d. Less efficacious than weekly mefloquine or daily doxycycline against both CRPF and *P. vivax* malaria
   e. Relatively inexpensive

f. Possibility of dose-related bone marrow suppression (monthly complete blood counts obtained if used longer than 1 month)

    g. Not safe during pregnancy

Other malaria prevention strategies

1. Apply behavioral modification strategies.
    a. Limit exposure to mosquitoes (i.e., time spent outdoors).
    b. Use physical barriers, such as screens, doors, nets, and curtains
    c. Wear protective clothing (long sleeves and long pants when possible, sprayed or impregnated with insecticide).
    d. Use mosquito bed-nets (sprayed or impregnated with insecticide).
2. Insect repellents and insecticides are highly recommended as adjuncts to malaria chemoprophylaxis. They provide additional protection from insect-transmitted infections that have no vaccines or chemoprophylaxis. The most effective insect repellent for skin application contains diethyltoluamide (DEET). Examples include the following:
    a. Ultrathon Insect Repellent: 35% DEET in polymer formulation; provides up to 12-hour protection against mosquitoes; also effective against ticks, biting flies, chiggers, fleas, and gnats (3M, Minneapolis, Minn)
    b. DEET plus Insect Repellent: 17.5% DEET with 2.5% R 326; apply q4h for mosquitoes, q8h for biting flies (Sawyer Products, Safety Harbor, Fla)
    c. Skedaddle Insect Protection for Children: 10% DEET using molecular entrapment technology (Little Point Corp., Cambridge, Mass)
3. Permethrin-containing spray insecticide is effective for external clothing and mosquito nets. Examples include the following:
    a. Permanone Tick Repellent (Coulston International Corp., Easton, Penn)

    b. Duranon Tick Repellent: permethrin in a formula lasting up to 2 weeks; repels ticks, chiggers, and mosquitoes (Coulston International Corp., Easton, Penn)

    c. Peripel: permethrin liquid for soaking bed-nets (Burroughs Welcome, Great Britain)

4. Partial immunity can be stimulated by repeated infections in residents of malaria-endemic areas; however, this immunity is gained at the expense of chronic anemia and is lost when residents go abroad for work or study.

5. Malaria vaccines are being developed and will most likely become available in the future.

CHAPTER 34

Immunizations for Travel

ROUTINE IMMUNIZATIONS

Travelers should have **all** current immunizations recorded in *The International Certificates of Vaccination* (the "little yellow booklet"), as approved by the World Health Organization (WHO). Table 34-1 provides routine immunization schedules and booster intervals. Routine immunizations are those customarily given in childhood and updated in adult life, including the following:

1. **Tetanus and diphtheria.** Booster doses of tetanus/diphtheria (Td) vaccine given at 10-year intervals throughout life are recommended to maintain immunity. If the person has no record or recollection of immunization, it is advisable to obtain this vaccine before traveling.
2. **Pertussis.** Immunization is acquired in childhood.
3. **Measles.** Individuals born after 1956 who have not received a measles booster should obtain this before traveling. This is an attenuated live virus and should be avoided 3 months before and during pregnancy.
4. **Mumps.** Immunization is acquired in childhood.
5. **Rubella.** Immunization is acquired in childhood.
6. **Poliovirus.** Poliomyelitis vaccine is usually not

Table 34-1.

Dosage Schedules for Routine Immunizations

VACCINE	PRIMARY SERIES	BOOSTER INTERVAL
Diphtheria and tetanus toxoids and pertussis vaccine adsorbed (DTP) (use in children <7 yr old)	4 doses* IM of vaccine: first 3 doses given 4-8 wk apart; dose 4 given 6-12 mo after dose 3	Booster at 4-6 yr of age
Haemophilus B conjugate (Hib conjugate vaccines are not considered interchangeable for the primary immunization series)		
PRP-HbOC	3 doses* IM or SC at 2, 4, 6 mo	Booster at 15 mo
PRP-OMP	2 doses* IM or SC at 2, 4 mo	Booster at 15 mo
PRP-D, PRP-HbOC, or PRP-OMP	1 dose* IM or SC at ≥15 mo up to 5th birthday	None
Hepatitis B (Engerix B) (accelerated schedule)	3 doses at 0, 30, 60 days (1 ml IM in deltoid area)	4th dose recommended at 12 mo if still at risk for hepatitis B exposure
Hepatitis B (Engerix B) (standard schedule)	3 doses at 0, 1, 6 mo (1 ml IM in deltoid area)	Need for booster not determined

From Jong EC: Immunizations for international travelers. In *The travel medicine advisor,* Atlanta, 1993, American Health Consultants.
*See manufacturer's package for recommendations on dosage.

Table 34-1.

Dosage Schedules for Routine Immunizations—cont'd

VACCINE	PRIMARY SERIES	BOOSTER INTERVAL
Hepatitis B (Recombivax) (standard schedule)	3 doses at 0, 1, 6 mo (1 ml IM in deltoid area)	Need for booster not determined
Influenza virus	1 dose* IM or SC annually	
Measles/ mumps/ rubella (MMR)†	1 dose* SC at 15 mo of age or older	Boost measles vaccine at 12 yr old; boost measles vaccine *once* in adult life before international travel for people born after 1957 and before 1980
Pneumococcus (23-valent)	1 dose* SC	None
Poliomyelitis, enhanced inactivated (e-IPV) (killed vaccine, safe for all ages)	Give doses* 1 and 2 SC or IM 4-8 wk apart; give dose 3 at 6-12 mo after dose 2; give dose 4 to children 4-6 yr of age	Give dose *once* to people before travel in areas of risk

†May be contraindicated in patients with any of the following conditions: pregnancy; leukemia; lymphoma; generalized malignancy; or immunosuppression from HIV infection or treatment with corticosteroids, alkylating drugs, antimetabolites, or radiation therapy.

Continued

Table 34-1.

Dosage Schedules for Routine Immunizations—cont'd

VACCINE	PRIMARY SERIES	BOOSTER INTERVAL
Poliomyelitis, oral (OPV) (attenuated live virus)†	Give doses* 1 and 2 PO 6-8 wk apart; give dose 3 at 6 wk after dose 2 (customarily at 8-12 mo after dose 2); give dose 4 to children 4-6 yr of age	Give dose *once* to people less than 18 yr before travel in areas of risk
Tetanus and diphtheria toxoids ad-sorbed (Td) (for children >7 yr of age and for adults)	3 doses (0.5 ml SC or IM): doses 1 and 2 given 4-8 wk apart, dose 3 at 6-12 mo later	Routine booster dose every 10 yr

From Jong EC: Immunizations for international travelers. In *The travel medicine advisor,* Atlanta, 1993, American Health Consultants, PO Box 740056, Atlanta, GA 30374, 800-688-2421.

boosted after childhood in the United States except for anticipated high-risk exposure through work or travel to areas where polio is endemic. The attenuated live-virus oral polio vaccine (OPV) is recommended for a primary immunization series given before 18 years of age. The enhanced inactivated (killed) virus polio vaccine (e-IPV) is recommended for primary immunization and for booster doses in people 18 years of age and older because of a higher risk of complications associated with OPV in older persons.

7. *Haemophilus influenza* type B (Hib). Immunization is acquired in childhood. Groups at risk include children less than 6 years of age, Native Americans, and persons with asplenia, sickle-cell disease, Hodgkin's disease, or antibody deficiency disease.

8. **Hepatitis B.** Hepatitis B vaccine is now recommended as a routine immunization for children in the United States; however, adults at high risk should also receive immunization (see later discussion).

Additional Routine Immunizations

1. **Influenza vaccine** is recommended for all health care workers and for international travelers because prolonged air travel and exposure to crowded or extreme environments create a predisposition to infection. Other considerations are based on conventional recommendations regarding underlying health and age (e.g., all people over 65 years of age and those with chronic lung, heart, or kidney disease or with impaired immunity).

2. **Pneumococcal vaccine** is recommended for all persons over 65 years of age and those with chronic lung, heart, or kidney disease or with impaired immunity.

RECOMMENDED TRAVELER'S VACCINES

Specific recommendations are based on the following:

✣ Geographic destination(s)
✣ Duration of trip
✣ Style of travel
✣ Purpose of trip
✣ Underlying health of traveler
✣ Access to medical care during trip

Cholera

Cholera vaccine is not highly efficacious and is no longer endorsed by WHO as a requirement for entry into any country. Some countries still require cholera vaccine for travelers arriving from a cholera-endemic area. The primary series consists of two doses given a week or more apart. However, a single cholera dose should meet entry requirements. Travelers going to cholera-endemic or cholera-epidemic areas should follow food and water precautions to prevent all forms of traveler's diarrhea. Persons with underlying gastric conditions, such as achlorhydria or partial gastric resection, may benefit from immunization in view of the increased susceptibility to infection.

An oral live cholera vaccine is now available in Europe and Canada. This vaccine is effective as a single dose and confers immunity for 3 years. Adverse reactions are uncommon.

Typhoid Fever

Oral and injectable types of typhoid fever vaccines are available. Even if a typhoid fever vaccine is administered before travel, it is essential to follow routine precautions related to the ingestion of food and water because efficacy of vaccination is only 40% to 80%.

Injectable Vaccine
1. Contains heat-phenol-inactivated whole-cell typhoid
2. Requires two doses given 4 weeks apart and a booster dose after 3 or more years
3. Associated with side effects, including low-grade fever, malaise, soreness at injection site, and headache
4. New form now available: Typhoid Vi polysaccharide; safe for children 2 years of age and older and given as a single dose; relatively few side effects

Oral vaccine
1. Licensed in the United States since 1989
2. Contains live attenuated *Salmonella typhi*

3. Given as a series, taken every other day for four doses
4. Booster interval of 5 years
5. Better tolerated than the injectable form; minimal side effects, including gastrointestinal upset, fever, or headache
6. Not recommended for children younger than 6 years of age
7. Liquid formulation taken with a buffer more effective than capsules; also easily administered to young children, but not yet licensed in the United States

Hepatitis A

Up to 60% of adults over 40 years of age from industrialized countries may have natural immunity to hepatitis A. Most travelers under 40 years of age are susceptible. Prophylaxis is recommended for persons traveling to developing countries if they anticipate eating in and visiting areas with poor sanitation.

If time allows, a screening test for hepatitis A antibody should be performed for the following groups:

✤ Frequent travelers
✤ Travelers over 40 years of age
✤ Travelers of foreign birth

Choices for prophylaxis include conventional immune globulin (IG) or one of the newer vaccines, HAVRIX and VAQTA. For frequent travelers, HAVRIX or VAQTA is preferred to eliminate the need for repeated IG injections.

Immune Globulin (Human IG)
1. Effective for both preexposure and postexposure prophylaxis
2. Recommended dose: 0.02 ml/kg body weight by IM injection if the stay is less than 3 months; for longer periods, 0.06 ml/kg
3. For a person having intimate contact (household or

sexual) with an infected individual: 0.02 ml/kg IM if it can be given within 2 weeks of exposure

Hepatitis B

Hepatitis B vaccine is now recommended as a routine immunization for children in the United States. Only adults at high risk need to receive immunization.

Immunization should be considered for travelers staying 6 or more months in Asia, Africa, or other endemic areas. In addition, immunization is recommended for travelers at high risk, such as medical workers or those anticipating sexual contact with locals in endemic areas. Two vaccines are available, Recombivax and Engerix B. Both are recombinant vaccines containing killed virus.

Vaccine Summary

1. Standard adult dose: 1.0 ml IM at 0, 1, and 6 months, with a booster at 5 to 7 years or if measured antibody titer is less than 10 IU/ml
2. Engerix B
   a. Also approved on an accelerated dosage schedule of 0, 1, and 2 months
   b. Booster recommended at 12 months if risk of infection continues
3. For children less than 11 years old: 0.25 ml Recombivax or 0.5 ml Engerix B
4. For children age 11 to 19 years: 0.5 ml Recombivax or 1.0 ml Engerix B
5. Expected efficacy greater than 80% for recombinant purified protein vaccines

Meningococcus

Meningococcal vaccine is recommended for people trekking in Nepal, traveling to Tanzania or Burundi, and living or working in Sub-Saharan Africa or Brazil. The vaccine is required for travel to Saudi Arabia in the late spring.

It is prudent to check with local and federal health

officials to determine current recommendations for vaccination because epidemic areas are not geographically fixed and previously uninvolved areas may experience epidemics.

Vaccine Summary
1. Adult recommended dose: single 0.5 ml injected SC
2. Clinical efficacy greater than 65%, but duration of immunity not established; revaccination recommended for adults every 3 years if high risk continues
3. Vaccine efficacy variable in young children; second dose recommended for children after 2 to 3 years if risk continues
4. Contraindicated in children under 3 months of age

Japanese Encephalitis Virus
Japanese encephalitis is a viral infection transmitted by *Culex* mosquitoes in mainland Asia and Southeast Asia. Transmission is year-round in tropical and subtropical areas and during the late spring, summer, and early fall in temperate climates. Japanese encephalitis is not considered a risk for short-term travelers visiting tourist destinations in urban and developed resort areas.

The risk of infection can be greatly decreased by personal measures that prevent mosquito bites (e.g., protective clothing, insect repellents, bed-nets). Vaccine should be offered to the following groups:

- ✤ Travelers who anticipate prolonged stays in *rural* endemic areas
- ✤ Travelers planning to *live* in an endemic area (e.g., expatriate workers, students)

Vaccine Summary
1. Recommended dose for persons over 3 years of age: 1.0 ml SC in three doses at 0, 7, and 30 days, with the third dose given on day 14 if required

2. Recommended dose for children less than 3 years of age: 0.5 ml SC; no data for infants less than 1 year of age
3. Booster recommended every 2 to 3 years
4. Expected efficacy greater than 90%
5. Hypersensitivity reaction possible, so the Centers for Disease Control and Prevention (CDC) recommends that vaccine recipients do the following:
   a. Be directly observed for 30 minutes after injection of Japanese encephalitis virus vaccine
   b. Not depart on their journey until 10 days after the last dose because of the possibility of delayed adverse reactions

Rabies

See Chapter 30.

Plague

Plague is a bacterial disease caused by *Yersinia pestis*. It is transmitted to humans by fleas or direct contact with infected animals. Person-to-person spread is common through respiratory secretions.

International travelers going on standard tourist itineraries to countries where plague is reported are unlikely to be at high risk. Persons at risk of exposure include field biologists and those who will reside or work in rural areas, where avoidance of rodents and fleas is difficult. It is recommended that travelers at risk avoid flea bites by using topical insect repellents containing DEET and permethrin insecticides on clothing and bed nets (see Chapter 33).

Vaccine Summary
1. A killed bacterial vaccine with poorly documented protective efficacy
2. Primary series of three injections recommended, with first two doses given 4 or more weeks apart and third dose given 3 to 6 months later

3. Boosters given every 6 months for as long as exposure present
4. Both local and systemic side effects possible, including mild pain, redness, and induration at the injection site; with repeated doses, malaise, fever, and headache with increasing severity possible
5. Alternative to plague vaccine: use of prophylactic oral tetracycline (500 mg qd) or doxycycline (100 mg bid) during periods of active exposure to plague-infected animals or humans (unproved as yet by controlled clinical studies)

Tick-borne Encephalitis

Tick-borne encephalitis (TBE) is a viral disease spread by ticks in parts of Europe and the Commonwealth of Independent States (the former Soviet Union). It is transmitted to humans by bites from infected ticks, primarily *Ixodes ricinus,* usually found in forested areas of endemic regions from April through August. A similar TBE is caused by *I. persulcatus.* This TBE results in systemic infection after ingestion of unpasteurized dairy products from infected cows, goats, or sheep.

The infection rate for TBE is very low, even in endemic areas. Vaccination against TBE is not available in the United States. Travelers planning outdoor activities in endemic areas need to rely on personal measures (DEET on exposed areas of skin and permethrin-based insecticide on clothing) to avoid tick attachment and bites. All travelers to endemic areas should avoid the ingestion of unpasteurized dairy products.

Vaccine Summary
1. Available in Europe: a three-dose SC injection series given over 6 months; made by Immuno (Vienna, Austria); not recommended by the CDC for travelers to endemic Western Europe
2. No vaccine generally obtained by most travelers

from North America to endemic areas because of lack of availability and long immunization schedule

Tuberculosis (BCG Vaccine)

BCG (bacillus Calmette-Guérin) vaccine is widely used worldwide for childhood immunization against tuberculosis. In the United States the CDC does not routinely recommend BCG. No consensus exists on the efficacy of BCG vaccine, but the vaccine is approved for use in children who will live where tuberculosis is prevalent or where exposure to adults with active or recently arrested tuberculosis is likely. It is also recommended for children of infected mothers. Vaccination may be appropriate for purified protein derivative (PPD) skin test–negative health care personnel who are going to work in areas of high endemic prevalence and who will have access to medical diagnosis and treatment.

Vaccine Summary

1. A live attenuated vaccine contraindicated in persons with immunosuppression; pregnancy a relative contraindication
2. Emergence of multidrug-resistant strains of the organism in the United States, along with a dramatic increase in incidence of tuberculosis
3. Trends also seen abroad, especially in areas with a high incidence of acquired immunodeficiency syndrome (AIDS)

Yellow Fever

Yellow fever is a viral infection transmitted by *Aedes aegypti* mosquitoes in equatorial South America and Africa. The vaccine for yellow fever is highly immunoprotective.

Vaccine Summary

1. Vaccine strain an attenuated live virus and well tolerated
2. Administered as single injection (0.5 ml SC)

3. Significant antibody levels achieved in more than 95% of persons vaccinated
4. Booster interval every 10 years, although persistent antibody titers have been detected 30 to 40 years after vaccination
5. Not recommended for infants less than 9 months of age because of postvaccination encephalitis
6. Not recommended during pregnancy unless risk of yellow fever thought to be greater than risk of adverse effects from vaccine
7. Other contraindications: immunosuppression or history of severe allergy to eggs
8. Other means of reducing risk of yellow fever (or any mosquito-borne disease): liberal use of mosquito repellent and netting in endemic areas

CHAPTER 35

Near Drowning and Cold Water Immersion

GENERAL EVALUATION

1. Assume an underlying cause for the event. Anticipate cervical spine fracture or a significant head injury. Other common causes include hypoglycemia (with or without diabetes), seizure disorder, and acute myocardial infarction.
2. Initiate resuscitation whenever possible until a reliable core temperature can be measured.

GENERAL TREATMENT
Minimally Symptomatic Victim

1. If the victim is short of breath, observe closely for deterioration for at least 6 hours.
2. Administer oxygen 4 to 6 L/min by face mask; increase the flow to 8 to 10 L/min if the victim continues to be short of breath.
3. Keep the victim warm and dry.

Moderately to Severely Symptomatic Victim

1. Examine for signs of distress.
   a. Tachypnea
   b. Dyspnea

c. Persistent cough
d. Tachycardia or unexplained hypertension
e. Increasing anxiety
f. Pallor or cyanosis, first acral, then central

2. If distress is present, administer high-flow oxygen (12 to 15 L/min by nonrebreathing face mask or demand valve).
3. Keep the victim warm and dry.
4. Anticipate vomiting.
5. *Anticipate that the victim's condition will deteriorate. Begin to plan transport or evacuation.*

Victim in Cardiopulmonary Arrest

1. Manage the airway. Perform endotracheal intubation or administer high-flow oxygen by bag-valve-mask.
2. Position the victim on the side to allow water to drain from the mouth. Proper positioning must be balanced with consideration given to an obvious or occult cervical or thoracic spine injury.
3. Do not perform the Heimlich maneuver unless the abdomen is rigidly distended (presumably with water) and mechanical ventilation is deemed to be otherwise **impossible.** *Forced emesis achieved with this maneuver may cause the victim to aspirate and worsen the pulmonary injury.*

Cold Water Immersion
See also Chapter 2.

1. Anticipate systemic hypothermia.
2. Protect the victim of moderate (core temperature below 28° C, or 82° F) or severe hypothermia from vigorous physical activity to avoid inducing ventricular fibrillation.
3. Continue to resuscitate the victim until he or she is warm or the rescue is no longer feasible.

Termination of Resuscitation

1. The victim has sustained an obviously fatal injury (e.g., limb loss with severe hemorrhage).
2. The victim displays normal body temperature and absent vital signs with or without postmortem lividity after 30 minutes of resuscitative efforts.
3. The victim displays rigor mortis.
4. The victim is hypothermic, and without signs of life after rewarming.
5. The victim is hypothermic and the rescue effort must be discontinued because of rescuer fatigue.

CHAPTER 36

Scuba Diving-Related Disorders

The disorders related to scuba diving include those caused by dysbarism, nitrogen narcosis, contaminated breathing gas, and decompression sickness.

■ DISORDERS ■

DYSBARISM

Dysbarism encompasses all the pathologic changes caused by altered environmental pressure. At sea level, atmospheric pressure is 14.7 lb/in². Each 10-m (33-foot) descent under water increases the pressure by 1 atmosphere. Gas in enclosed spaces obeys Boyle's law, which states that the pressure of a given quantity of gas when its temperature remains unchanged varies inversely with its volume.

Mask Squeeze

An air space is present between the face and the glass of a scuba (self-contained underwater breathing apparatus) diving mask. If nasal exhalations do not maintain air pressure within this space during descent, the volume of air contracts, creating negative pressure. This leads to capillary rupture, which is potentially dangerous after keratotomy because of the slow healing rate of corneal incisions.

Signs and Symptoms
1. Skin ecchymoses in mask pattern
2. Conjunctival hemorrhage similar to strangulation injury

Treatment
No treatment is needed because the manifestations are self-limited.

Ear Canal Squeeze
A tight-fitting wet suit hood, ear plugs, exostoses, or cerumen impaction can trap air in the external auditory canal. On descent, this air contracts in the enclosed space between the tympanic membrane and the (occluded) external opening of the ear.

Signs and Symptoms
1. Pain, swelling, erythema, and petechiae or hemorrhagic blebs of external ear canal wall
2. Hemorrhage possible
3. In severe cases, tympanic membrane rupturing outward

Treatment
1. If a remediable occlusion exists, correct it.
2. If inflammation of the external canal occurs without tympanic membrane rupture, instill eardrops suitable for the treatment of otitis externa (containing a steroid component) as directed for 2 to 3 days.
3. If the tympanic membrane is perforated, seek otolaryngologic evaluation. Do not allow further diving until the membrane has healed.

Middle Ear Squeeze (Barotitis Media)
If air cannot enter the middle ear via the (contracted or blocked) eustachian tube during an underwater de-

scent, the existing air in the middle ear space contracts, creating a relative vacuum and pulling the tympanic membrane inward (Fig. 36-1).

Signs and Symptoms
1. Initially, slight pain that progresses to severe pain with further underwater descent
2. Hemorrhage in the tympanic membrane revealed on

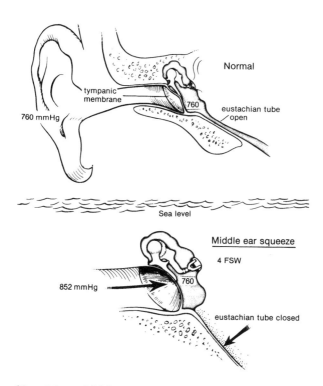

Fig. 36-1. Middle ear trauma. Symptoms include feeling of "fullness" and pain caused by stretching of tympanic membrane.

otoscopy; ranges from erythema over the malleus to gross blood throughout the tympanic membrane; blood around the mouth and nose and hearing loss also possible

3. If the tympanic membrane ruptures:
   a. Sudden severe pain, accompanied by vertigo as water rushes into the middle ear
   b. Total hearing loss in the affected ear

Treatment

1. Before tympanic membrane rupture, administer an oral decongestant and a long-acting topical decongestant nasal spray, such as oxymetazoline.
2. For tympanic membrane rupture, administer an antibiotic, such as amoxicillin/clavulanate, for 7 days. Suspend all diving activities until the tympanic membrane is fully healed or has been surgically repaired and eustachian tube function allows easy autoinflation.

Barosinusitis

Barosinusitis, or "sinus squeeze," results from an inability to inflate a paranasal sinus during descent, at which time contraction of the trapped air creates a relative vacuum. This damages the sinus wall mucosa, which ultimately hemorrhages. Less often, a "reverse sinus squeeze" can occur on ascent in the water because the expanding air cannot be vented from the sinus.

Signs and Symptoms

1. Pain in and over the affected sinus, with radiation similar to that seen with sinusitis (e.g., into the upper teeth with maxillary involvement)
2. May be accompanied by epistaxis

Treatment

1. Give oral and topical decongestants (mucosal vasoconstrictors), such as pseudoephedrine and oxymetazoline.
2. Administer an analgesic as appropriate.

3. If an episode of sinus squeeze has occurred, particularly with epistaxis, and the victim subsequently develops symptoms of sinusitis (pain, fever, tenderness over the affected sinus, nasal discharge), administer an appropriate antibiotic, such as amoxicillin/clavulanate or azithromycin.

Barodontalgia

Barodontalgia, or "tooth squeeze," is caused by entrapped gas in the interior of a tooth or in the structures surrounding a tooth. The confined gas develops either positive or negative pressure relative to the ambient pressure, which places force on the surrounding sensitive dental structures.

Signs and Symptoms
1. Tooth pain, with normal referral pathways
2. Expulsion of a filling or crown; "exploding" or cracked tooth
3. Imploded tooth

Treatment
1. Supply symptomatic and supportive therapy for the specific type of dental trauma.
2. Administer an analgesic.

Labyrinthine Window Rupture

Labyrinthine window rupture affects the inner ear, with possible injury to the cochleovestibular system. This may lead to permanent deafness or vestibular dysfunction.

Signs and Symptoms
1. Roaring tinnitus, vertigo, hearing loss
2. Feeling of "fullness" in or blockage of the affected ear
3. Nausea, vomiting, nystagmus, pallor, diaphoresis, disorientation, ataxia
4. Symptoms of inner ear barotrauma developing immediately or delayed for hours

Treatment
1. Allow the victim to rest in bed, with the head elevated 30 degrees.
2. Make sure the victim avoids strenuous activities.
3. Suspend all diving activities until the victim is cleared by an otolaryngologist.

Alternobaric Vertigo

Alternobaric vertigo usually occurs with ascent and is caused by the sudden development of unequal middle ear pressure.

Signs and Symptoms
1. Asymmetric vestibular stimulation and resultant pronounced vertigo
2. Vertigo usually transient but may last for several hours or days

Treatment
1. Allow the victim to rest in a supine position, with the head elevated 30 degrees.
2. Make sure the victim avoids strenuous activities.
3. If labyrinthine window rupture is suspected, suspend all diving activities until the victim is cleared by an otolaryngologist.

Lung Squeeze

Lung squeeze is observed in a breath-holding diver who descends to a depth at which total lung volume is reduced to less than residual volume, which causes transpulmonic pressure to exceed intraalveolar pressure. This produces the transudation of fluid or blood (from rupture of pulmonary capillaries) into the alveoli.

Signs and Symptoms
1. Shortness of breath, cough, hemoptysis
2. In severe cases, pulmonary edema

Treatment
1. Administer oxygen 5 L/min by nonrebreather face mask
2. Suspend all diving activities.

Pulmonary Barotrauma of Ascent (Pulmonary Overpressurization Syndrome)

Pulmonary barotrauma of ascent results from expansion of gas trapped in the lungs, which ruptures alveoli or is forced across the pulmonary capillary membrane.

Signs and Symptoms
1. History of rapid and uncontrolled ascent to the surface before onset of symptoms
2. Pneumomediastinum: gradually increasing hoarseness or "brassy" voice, neck fullness, substernal chest pain several hours after diving
3. Subcutaneous emphysema (crepitus) possible
4. In severe cases, possible chest pain, dyspnea, bloody sputum, dysphagia
5. Syncope possible
6. Pneumothorax
   a. Pleuritic chest pain, breathlessness, dyspnea
   b. With tension pneumothorax, progressive respiratory difficulty, cyanosis, distended neck veins, hyperresonant chest percussion, tracheal shift, absent or diminished breath sounds

Treatment
1. For pneumomediastinum, administer supplemental oxygen 5 L/min by nonrebreather mask. Have the victim rest.
2. For pneumothorax, administer supplemental oxygen 5 L/min by nonrebreather mask.
   a. Observe the victim closely for worsening condition.
   b. Be prepared to insert a thoracostomy (chest) tube or a decompression flutter valve.

Arterial Gas Embolism

Arterial gas embolism results from air bubbles entering the pulmonary venous circulation from ruptured alveoli. Gas bubbles are showered into the heart, from which they may be distributed to the coronary and carotid arteries. Arterial gas embolism typically develops immediately after a diver surfaces.

Signs and Symptoms

Sudden loss of consciousness on surfacing from a dive should be considered to indicate air embolism until proved otherwise.

1. Cardiac: chest pain related to myocardial ischemia, arrhythmias, or cardiac arrest
2. Neurologic
   a. Possibly confusing pattern, as showers of bubbles randomly embolize cerebral circulation
   b. Manifestations often typical of acute stroke (cerebrovascular accident), although hemiplegia infrequent
   c. Most often observed signs: loss of consciousness, monoplegia or asymmetric multiplegia, focal paralysis, paresthesias or other sensory disturbances, convulsions, aphasia, confusion, blindness or other visual field defects, vertigo, dizziness, headache
   d. Rare signs: sharply circumscribed areas of glossal pallor

Treatment

1. Transport the victim for recompression treatment in a hyperbaric (oxygen) chamber.
   a. If an aircraft is used, do not expose the victim to significant cabin altitude. Ideally, the aircraft will be pressurized to sea level.
   b. In an unpressurized aircraft, maintain the flying altitude as low as possible, not to exceed 300 m (1000 feet) above sea level.

2. Maintain the victim in a supine position.
3. Administer oxygen 5 to 10 L/min by nonrebreather face mask.
4. Begin an IV infusion of isotonic solution to maintain urine output at 1 to 2 ml/kg/hr.
5. Obtain help with the treatment of dive-related incidents 24 hours a day by calling the Divers Alert Network at Duke University (919-684-8111).
6. Although experimental proof of their efficacy is lacking, high-dose parenteral corticosteroids have been widely recommended as an adjunct to recompression treatment. Administer hydrocortisone hemisuccinate 1 g or methylprednisolone sodium succinate 125 mg, followed by dexamethasone 4 to 6 mg q6h for 72 hours.

NITROGEN NARCOSIS

Nitrogen narcosis is the increasing development of anesthesia or intoxication as the partial pressure of nitrogen in inspired compressed air increases at depth.

Signs and Symptoms

1. Usually becomes apparent at depths between 21 and 30 m (70 and 100 feet)
2. Lightheadedness, loss of fine sensory discrimination, giddiness, euphoria
3. Progressively worsening symptoms at deeper depths
   a. When deeper than 45 m (150 feet): severe intoxication, manifested by increasingly poor judgment and impaired reasoning, overconfidence, and slowed reflexes
   b. At depths of 75 to 90 m (250 to 300 feet): auditory and visual hallucinations, feeling of impending blackout
   c. By 120 m (400 feet): loss of consciousness

Treatment

Have the victim ascend to a shallower depth for symptoms to resolve.

CONTAMINATED BREATHING GAS

The pressurized air within a scuba tank may be contaminated with oil or carbon monoxide.

Signs and Symptoms
1. With oil contamination: cough, shortness of breath, oily taste in mouth
2. With carbon monoxide contamination: headache, nausea, dizziness during the dive
   a. Examination at the surface: lethargy, mental dullness, nonspecific neurologic deficits
   b. May be confused with those accompanying decompression sickness (see next) or air embolism (see earlier)

Treatment
Administer oxygen 5 to 10 L/min by nonrebreather face mask.

DECOMPRESSION SICKNESS

Decompression sickness is caused by the formation of bubbles of inert gas (e.g., nitrogen) within the intravascular and extravascular spaces after a reduction in ambient pressure.

Signs and Symptoms
1. Symptoms developing in the first hour after surfacing from a dive, with some victims noticing symptoms within 6 hours after diving; rarely, symptoms not noted until 24 to 48 hours after diving
2. Musculoskeletal decompression sickness or "limb bends": periarticular joint pain most common symptom
   a. Shoulders and elbows most often affected
   b. Pain usually described as dull ache deep within the affected joint, but also characterized as sharp or throbbing
   c. Pain worse with joint movement, or "grating" sensation

d. Vague area of numbness surrounding the affected joint

    e. Palpable tenderness

    f. Variably present diagnostic feature: pain temporarily relieved by inflation to 150 to 250 mm Hg of sphygmomanometer cuff placed around the joint

3. Neurologic decompression sickness: back pain, girdling abdominal pain, extremity heaviness or weakness, paresthesias of extremities, anal sphincter weakness or fecal incontinence, loss of bulbocavernosus reflex, bladder distention and urinary retention, paralysis, hyperesthesia or hypoesthesia, paresis, scotomata, headache, dysphagia, confusion, visual field deficit, spotty motor or sensory deficits, disorientation, mental dullness

4. Fatigue

5. Cutaneous: pruritus, mottling, local or generalized hyperemia, marbled skin

6. "Chokes": dyspnea, substernal pain made worse on deep inhalation, nonproductive cough, cyanosis, tachypnea, tachycardia

7. Vasomotor decompression sickness: weakness, sweating, unconsciousness, hypotension, tachycardia, pallor, mottling, decreased urine output

Treatment

Transport the victim for recompression treatment in a hyperbaric (oxygen) chamber.

If an aircraft is used, do not expose the victim to significant cabin altitude. Ideally, the aircraft will be pressurized to sea level.

In an unpressurized aircraft, maintain the flying altitude as low as possible, not to exceed 300 m (1000 feet) above sea level.

Maintain the victim in a supine position.

Administer oxygen 5 to 10 L/min by nonrebreather face mask.

Begin an IV infusion of isotonic solution to maintain urine output at 1 to 2 ml/kg/hr.

Obtain help with the treatment of dive-related incidents
24 hours a day by calling the Divers Alert Network at
Duke University (919-684-8111).

Although experimental proof of their efficacy is lacking,
high-dose parenteral corticosteroids have been
widely recommended as an adjunct to recompression
treatment. Administer hydrocortisone hemisuccinate
1 g or methylprednisolone sodium succinate 125 mg,
followed by dexamethasone 4 to 6 mg q6h for 72
hours.

CHAPTER 37

Injuries From Nonvenomous Aquatic Animals

Sharks, barracuda, moray eels, needlefish, and coral present dangers to those venturing into the ocean. The injuries inflicted range from bites or stings to cuts and abrasions.

GENERAL TREATMENT
Wound Management

1. Irrigate all wounds with a sterile diluent, preferably NS solution. Seawater is not recommended because it carries a hypothetic risk of infection. Use disinfected tap water if saline solution is not available.
   a. Note that proper irrigation technique involves using a 19-gauge needle or 18-gauge plastic IV catheter attached to a syringe to deliver a pressure of 10 to 20 psi.
   b. Flush 100 to 250 ml of irrigant through each wound.
   c. If the wound was caused by a stingray, warm the irrigant to 45° C (113° F) (see Chapter 38).
2. Add an antiseptic to the irrigation fluid. Use povidone-iodine in a concentration of 1% to 5% with a contact time of 1 to 5 minutes. After antiseptic irri-

gation, thoroughly irrigate the wound with NS solution.

3. Scrub the area to remove debris that cannot be irrigated from the wound.

4. Remove any crushed or devitalized tissue using sharp dissection.

5. In the field, perform wound closure using the technique that is least constrictive and prone to contain bacteria, which could initiate a wound infection. Unless a wound preparation equivalent to that achieved in a hospital is undertaken, it is often better to approximate the wound edges with adhesive strips or loosely placed sutures than perform a tight approximation of the margins.

6. At the earliest sign of wound infection, release sufficient fasteners to allow prompt and thorough drainage from the wound.

Antibiotic Therapy

The following recommendations are based on the malignant potential of soft tissue infections caused by *Vibrio* or *Aeromonas* species.

1. Be aware that minor abrasions or lacerations (e.g., coral cuts, superficial sea urchin puncture wounds) do not require prophylactic antibiotics in the normal host. However, for persons who are chronically ill (e.g., diabetes, hemophilia, thalassemia), are immunologically impaired (e.g., leukemia, AIDS, chemotherapy, or prolonged corticosteroid therapy), or have serious liver disease (e.g., hepatitis, cirrhosis, hemochromatosis), particularly those with elevated serum iron levels, immediately begin a regimen of oral ciprofloxacin, trimethoprim/sulfamethoxazole (co-trimethoxazole), or tetracycline. Note that penicillin, ampicillin, amoxicillin, and erythromycin are not acceptable alternatives. Although other quinolones have not been extensively tested against *Vibrio* species, they may be useful alternatives.

2. Note that the appearance of an infection indicates the need for prompt débridement and antibiotic therapy. If an infection develops, choose antibiotic coverage that will also be efficacious against *Staphylococcus* and *Streptococcus* species.

3. From an infection perspective, consider the following as serious injuries: large lacerations, extensive or deep burns, deep puncture wounds, and a retained foreign body.

   a. These injuries may be caused by shark or barracuda bites, stingray spine wounds, any spine puncture that enters a joint space, and full-thickness coral cuts.

   b. If the victim will require hospitalization for any of these serious injuries and IV antibiotics are accessible, know that the recommended drugs for prophylaxis include gentamicin, tobramycin, amikacin, co-trimethoxazole, cefoperazone, cefotaxime, and ceftazidime.

4. Manage infected wounds with antibiotics as noted earlier, with the addition of imipenem-cilastatin for severe, progressive infections and sepsis.

INJURIES CAUSED BY SHARKS AND BARRACUDA

Treatment

1. Manage abrasions caused by contact with sharkskin as if they were second-degree burns. Cleanse the wound thoroughly, then apply a thin layer of mupirocin (Bactroban) ointment or silver sulfadiazine cream under a sterile dressing.

2. Control all active hemorrhage with pressure, if possible. If necessary, ligate large disrupted vessels.

3. Insert at least two large-bore IV lines.

4. Keep the victim well oxygenated and warm.

5. Transport the victim to a proper emergency facility equipped to handle major trauma and appropriate surgical management of the wounds.

6. If the wound is more than minor, administer a prophylactic antibiotic (see earlier).

MORAY EEL INJURY

Morays are forceful and vicious biters that can inflict severe puncture wounds with their narrow and viselike jaws, which are equipped with long, sharp, retrorse, and fanglike teeth.

Treatment

1. Explore each wound to locate any retained teeth.
2. Irrigate each wound copiously.
3. Because the risk for infection is high, do not suture any puncture wounds unless it is necessary temporarily to control hemorrhage.
4. If the wound is extensive and more linear in configuration (resembling a dog bite), débride the wound edges and loosely approximate them with nonabsorbable sutures or staples.
5. Administer a prophylactic antibiotic (see earlier).

NEEDLEFISH INJURY

The pointed snout (teeth) of a needlefish that leaps from the water can penetrate into a human victim, creating a stab wound with a residual foreign body (the fish).

Signs and Symptoms

Stab wound that may contain a foreign body

Treatment

1. Be aware that the major risk is wound infection caused by the retained organic material.
2. Cleanse the wound thoroughly, then débride and dress it.
3. If the wound is more than superficial, administer a prophylactic antibiotic (see earlier).

CORAL CUTS AND ABRASIONS

Signs and Symptoms

1. Initial reactions: stinging pain, erythema, pruritus
2. Break in skin surrounded within minutes by erythematous wheal, which fades over 1 to 2 hours
3. Red raised welts and local pruritus accompanied by

low-grade fever and malaise, known as "coral poisoning"
4. Progresses to cellulitis with ulceration and tissue sloughing
5. Healing over 3 to 6 weeks, with prolonged morbidity
6. Lymphangitis and reactive bursitis also seen

Treatment
1. Promptly and vigorously scrub the wound with soap and water, then irrigate copiously to remove all foreign material.
2. Use hydrogen peroxide to bubble out tiny particles of organic material deposited from the surface of the coral.
3. If a stinging sensation is prominent, be aware that envenomation may have occurred. Briefly rinse the area with diluted (half-strength or 2.5%) household vinegar to diminish discomfort. Follow with a thorough NS solution or tap water irrigation.
4. If a coral-induced laceration is severe, close it with adhesive strips rather than sutures, if possible, because the margins of the wound are likely to become inflamed and necrotic. Be aware that serial débridement may become necessary.
5. To achieve a bed of healing tissue, apply twice-daily sterile wet-to-dry dressings, using NS solution or a dilute antiseptic (e.g., povidone-iodine 1% to 5%). Alternatively, use a nontoxic topical antiseptic ointment (e.g., bacitracin, mupirocin, polymixin B-bacitracin-neomycin) sparingly, and cover the wound with a nonadherent dressing.
6. Be aware that despite the best efforts at primary irrigation and decontamination, the wound may heal slowly, with moderate to severe soft tissue inflammation and ulcer formation. Débride all devitalized tissue regularly using sharp dissection. Continue this regimen until healthy granulation tissue is formed.
7. Treat any wound that appears infected with an antibiotic (see earlier).

CHAPTER 38

Envenomation by Marine Life

Interactions with various forms of marine life can result in anaphylactic reactions or envenomation.

■ DISORDERS ■

ANAPHYLAXIS

Signs and Symptoms
For signs and symptoms typical of anaphylactic reactions, see Chapter 8.

Treatment
1. Maintain the airway and administer oxygen.
2. Obtain IV access. Administer lactated Ringer's (LR) or NS solution to support the blood pressure to 90 mm Hg systolic.
3. Administer epinephrine.
   a. Begin with aqueous epinephrine 1:1000 SC in the deltoid region.
   b. The dose for adults is 0.3 to 0.5 ml and for children 0.01 ml/kg.
   c. An alternative is to inject the contents of an EpiPen or EpiPen Jr. IM into the lateral thigh region. Repeat in 20 minutes if relief is partial.
   d. If the reaction is limited to pruritus and urticaria,

there is no wheezing or facial swelling, and the victim is older than 45 years, administer an antihistamine and reserve epinephrine for a worsened condition.

4. If the reaction is life threatening and there is no response to SC epinephrine, administer IV epinephrine.

   a. Give an adult a 0.1-mg bolus of 1:1000 aqueous epinephrine (0.1 ml) diluted in 10 ml of NS solution (final dilution 1:100,000) infused over 10 minutes.

   b. Prepare a mixture for continuous infusion by adding 1 mg 1:1000 aqueous epinephrine (1 ml) to 250 ml of NS solution, to create a concentration of 4 $\mu g/ml$. This infusion should be started at 1 $\mu g/min$ (15 minidrops/min) and increased to 4 to 5 $\mu g/min$ if the clinical response is inadequate.

   c. In infants and children, starting dose is 0.1 $\mu g/kg/min$ up to a maximum of 1.5 $\mu g/kg/min$, noting that infusion rates in excess of 0.5 $\mu g/kg/min$ may be associated with cardiac ischemia and arrhythmias.

5. Relieve bronchospasm by administering micronized albuterol or metaproterenol by hand-held metered-dose inhaler (MDI).

6. Administer antihistamines.

   a. For a mild reaction, give diphenhydramine 50 to 75 mg IV, IM, or PO. The dose for children is 1 mg/kg.

   b. Nonsedating antihistamines, such as fexofenadine 60 mg or cimetidine 300 mg, are adjuncts.

7. Administer corticosteroids.

   a. If the reaction is severe or prolonged, or if the victim is regularly medicated with corticosteroids, administer hydrocortisone 200 mg, methylprednisolone 50 mg, or dexamethasone 15 mg IV with a 10-day oral taper to follow. The parenteral dose of hydrocortisone for children is 2.5 mg/kg.

b. With PO therapy, administer prednisone 60 to 100 mg for adults and 1 mg/kg for children.

REACTION TO SPONGES

Sponges are stationary animals that attach to the sea floor or coral beds. Embedded in their connective tissue matrices are spicules of silicon dioxide or calcium carbonate. Other chemical toxins and secondary coelenterate (stinging) inhabitants contribute to the skin irritation and systemic manifestations that result from dermal contact.

Signs and Symptoms

1. Within a few hours after contact: burning and itching of the skin, possibly progressing to local joint swelling and stiffness, soft tissue edema, blistering
   a. Skin becoming mottled or purpuric
   b. If untreated, subsidence of minor reaction in 3 to 7 days
2. With involvement of large areas of skin: fever, chills, malaise, dizziness, nausea, muscle cramps, formication
   a. Bullae becoming purulent
   b. Surface skin desquamation after 10 days

Treatment

1. Gently dry the skin.
2. To remove embedded microscopic spicules, apply sticky adhesive tape, a commercial facial peel, or a thin layer of rubber cement, then peel away the adherent spicules.
3. Apply a 5% acetic acid (vinegar) soak for 10 to 30 minutes 3 or 4 times a day. If vinegar is not available, use isopropyl alcohol 40%. Do not use a topical steroid preparation as the primary (initial) decontaminant because this may worsen the reaction.
4. After decontamination and at least two vinegar applications, use a mild emollient cream to soothe the skin.

5. If the allergic component is mild, apply a topical steroid preparation. If the allergic component is severe, as manifested by weeping, crusting, and vesiculation, administer a systemic corticosteroid (e.g., prednisone 60 to 100 mg, tapered over 14 days).
6. Perform frequent follow-up wound checks because significant infections sometimes develop. Culture infected wounds and administer antibiotics (see Chapter 37).

Prevention
1. Ensure that all divers and net handlers wear proper gloves.
2. Do not allow sponges to be broken, crumbled, or crushed with bare hands.
3. Be aware that dried sponges may remain toxic.

JELLYFISH STINGS (ALSO FIRE CORAL, HYDROIDS [Plate 28], AND ANEMONES)
These creatures sting with a variation of the microscopic stinging cell, the nematocyst, which is stimulated to fire its venom-bearing injector into the victim by physical contact, hypotonicity, or chemical stimulation. An encounter with a single long-tentacled creature (Plate 29) can simultaneously trigger thousands of stinging cells.

Signs and Symptoms
1. Skin irritation: stinging, pruritus, paresthesias, burning, throbbing, redness, tentacle prints, impression patterns, blistering, local edema, petechial hemorrhages, skin ulceration (Plate 30), necrosis, secondary infection
2. Neurologic: malaise, headache, aphonia, diminished touch and temperature sensation, vertigo, ataxia, spastic or flaccid paralysis, mononeuritis multiplex, parasympathetic dysautonomia, plexopathy, peripheral nerve palsy, delirium, loss of consciousness, coma

3. Cardiovascular: anaphylaxis, hemolysis, hypotension, small artery spasm, bradycardia, tachycardia, congestive heart failure, ventricular fibrillation
4. Respiratory: rhinitis, bronchospasm, laryngeal edema, dyspnea, cyanosis, pulmonary edema, respiratory failure
5. Musculoskeletal: abdominal rigidity, myalgia, muscle cramp/spasm, arthralgia, arthritis
6. Gastrointestinal: nausea, vomiting, diarrhea, dysphagia, hypersalivation, thirst
7. Ocular: conjunctivitis, chemosis, corneal ulcer, iridocyclitis, elevated intraocular pressure, lacrimation
8. Other: chills, fever, acute renal failure, nightmares

Treatment

1. For systemic reactions:
   a. Maintain the airway and administer oxygen.
   b. Obtain IV access. Administer LR or NS solution to support the blood pressure to 90 mm Hg systolic.
   c. Treat anaphylaxis if present (see Chapter 8).
   d. If the sting is from the box jellyfish (*Chironex fleckeri*) or severe and from the sea wasp (*Chiropsalmus quadrigatus*), consider immediate administration of *C. fleckeri* antivenin (Fig. 38-1). Administer this in a dose of 1 ampule (20,000 U/ampule) IV diluted 1:5 to 1:10 in isotonic crystalloid. A large sting in an adult may require the initial administration of 2 ampules. Alternatively, administer this in a dose of 3 ampules IM into the thigh. Antivenin administration may be repeated once or twice every 2 to 4 hours until there is no further worsening of the reaction (skin discoloration, pain, or systemic effects).
   e. Some authorities in Australia now recommend the pressure-immobilization technique (see Chapter 26) to treat a box jellyfish sting, preferably after application of vinegar (see 2d below).
2. For dermatitis:
   a. *If possible, apply a topical decontaminant immediately (see step d). If more than 1 or 2 minutes will elapse*

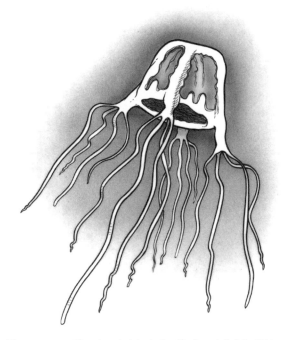

Fig. 38-1. The dreaded Indo-Pacific box jellyfish *(Chironex fleckeri).*

before the application of the decontaminant, rinse the wound with seawater. Do not rinse gently with fresh water; if fresh water is to be used, the stream must be forceful (e.g., jet stream from a shower). Do not immerse the wound in hot water.
b. Apply dry (nonmoist) cold (insulated ice) packs.
c. *Do not rub or abrade the wound.*
d. If these have been done, apply a topical decontaminant. The efficacy may vary depending on the stinging species.
   (1) Acetic acid 5% (vinegar) is the decontaminant of choice with a box jellyfish *(C. fleckeri)* sting.

(2) For other stings, diminish the pain using vinegar, isopropyl (rubbing) alcohol 40%, sodium bicarbonate (baking soda), papain (papaya latex or nonseasoned meat tenderizer, the latter in a brief [less than 15 minutes] application), or dilute household ammonia. Urinating on the sting may be helpful, as may the application of sugar or olive oil.

(3) *Do not apply a solvent* (e.g., formalin, ether, gasoline).

(4) Perfume, aftershave, or high-proof liquor may worsen the skin reaction.

e. After decontamination, remove the adherent nematocysts. Apply shaving cream or a paste of soap or baking soda, flour, or talc, and shave the area with a razor or other sharp edge.

f. Apply a local anesthetic ointment or mild steroid preparation to soothe the skin.

g. If the reaction is severe, administer a systemic corticosteroid (e.g., prednisone 60 to 100 mg, tapered over 14 days).

h. Inspect the wound regularly for ulceration and the onset of infection.

Prevention

1. Give all jellyfish a wide berth when swimming or diving.
2. Wear a "stinger suit" when immersed in jellyfish-infested water.
3. When diving, scan for surface concentrations of stinging animals.
4. If "stinger enclosures" are present, do not venture beyond their confines.

SEA BATHER'S ERUPTION

Sea bather's eruption (Plate 31), commonly termed "sea lice," predominantly involves covered areas of the body and has been attributed to stings from the microscopic larvae of jellyfish and anemones.

Signs and Symptoms

1. Stinging of the skin while still in the water or immediately on exiting; may be intensified by the application of fresh water
2. Skin redness, papules, urticaria, and blisters minutes to 12 hours after exposure
   a. Most common areas: buttocks, genitals, and under breasts (women)
   b. Individual lesions resembling insect bites
   c. Also seen under bathing caps and swim fins and along the edge of the cuffs of wet suits
3. Fever, chills, headache, fatigue, malaise, vomiting, conjunctivitis, and urethritis

Treatment

1. Apply a topical decontaminant. Acetic acid 5% (vinegar) seems to be less effective than papain. Otherwise, scrub thoroughly with soap and water.
2. After decontamination, apply calamine lotion with 1% menthol to control itching. A topical corticosteroid preparation may be of benefit.
3. If the reaction is severe, administer a systemic corticosteroid (e.g., prednisone 60 to 100 mg, tapered over 14 days).

STARFISH PUNCTURE

The most common venomous starfish have glandular tissue interspersed underneath the epidermis that covers the rigid spines, which may attain a length of 4 to 6 cm (1½ to 2½ inches). The envenomation occurs when a spine punctures the skin.

Signs and Symptoms

1. Intense pain, moderate bleeding, local soft tissue edema
2. With multiple stings: paresthesias, nausea, vomiting, lymphadenopathy, muscular paralysis

Treatment

1. Immerse the wound into nonscalding hot water to tolerance (45° C [113° F]) for 30 to 90 minutes or until there is significant pain relief.
2. Remove any obvious spine fragments. Do not attempt to crush remaining fragments.
3. Observe closely for subsequent wound infection.
4. *Consider* prophylactic antibiotics (see Chapter 37).

SEA URCHIN SPINE PUNCTURE OR ENVENOMATION BY PEDICELLARIAE

Sea urchins envenom their victims in one of two ways: (1) puncture wound by sharp, venom-bearing spine(s) or (2) inoculation of venom via the venom gland in the base of flowerlike, stalked pincer organs (globiferous pedicellariae) (Fig. 38-2).

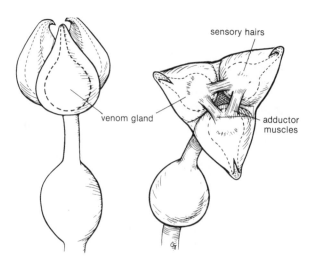

Fig. 38-2. Globiferous pedicellaria of sea urchin used to hold and envenom prey.

Signs and Symptoms

1. Intense pain, burning, local muscle aching, erythema, soft tissue edema, black or purple tattoos (Plate 32) at sites of spine punctures
2. Malaise, weakness, arthralgias, aphonia, dizziness, syncope, generalized muscular paralysis, respiratory distress, hypotension

Treatment

1. Immerse the wound into nonscalding hot water to tolerance (45° C [113° F]) for 30 to 90 minutes or until significant pain relief.
2. Remove any obvious spine fragments. Do not attempt to crush remaining fragments. If spines are felt to remain within the victim near a joint, splint the affected limb.
3. If pedicellariae are attached, apply shaving foam and scrape them away with a razor.
4. Observe closely for subsequent wound infection.
5. *Consider* prophylactic antibiotics (see Chapter 37).

BRISTLEWORM IRRITATION

Certain segmented marine worms have chitinous bristles arranged in soft rows around the body. These are dislodged into the human victim when a worm is handled.

Signs and Symptoms

Burning sensation, raised red urticarial rash, papular dermatitis, soft tissue edema, pruritus

Treatment

1. Remove all large visible bristles using a forceps.
2. Dry the skin gently.
3. To remove embedded spines, apply sticky adhesive tape, a commercial facial peel, or a thin layer of rubber cement, then peel away the adherent spines.
4. Apply acetic acid 5% (vinegar), isopropyl alcohol

40%, dilute ammonia, or a paste of unseasoned meat tenderizer for 10 to 15 minutes to achieve pain relief.
5. Apply a thin layer of a topical corticosteroid preparation.
6. If the reaction is severe, administer a systemic corticosteroid (e.g., prednisone 60 to 100 mg, tapered over 14 days).

CONE SHELL (SNAIL) STING

These cone-shaped shelled mollusks intoxicate their victims by injecting rapid-acting venom by means of a detachable, dartlike radular tooth (Fig. 38-3).

Signs and Symptoms
1. Mild sting (puncture) that resembles bee or wasp sting
2. Alternative initial symptoms: localized ischemia, cyanosis, numbness in area around wound
3. More serious envenomations: paresthesias at wound site, which become perioral and then generalized
4. Dysphagia, nausea, syncope, weakness, areflexia, aphonia, diplopia, blurred vision, pruritus, DIC, generalized muscular paralysis leading to respiratory failure, cardiac failure, and coma

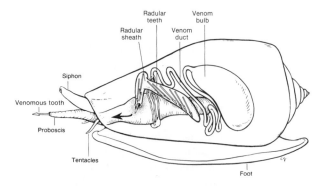

Fig. 38-3.   Venom apparatus of cone shell.

Treatment
1. Apply the pressure immobilization technique for venom sequestration (see Figure 26-2):
2. If practical by virtue of the sting's location, place a cloth or gauze pad approximately 6 to 8 cm (2½ to 3 inches) by 6 to 8 cm by 2 cm (1-inch thickness) directly over the sting, and hold it firmly in place using a circumferential bandage 15 to 18 cm (6 to 7 inches) wide, applied at lymphatic-venous occlusive pressure. If the cloth or gauze pad is not available, a rolled bandage may be used alone.
3. Do not occlude the arterial circulation, as determined by the detection of arterial pulsations and proper capillary refill.
4. Splint the limb, and do not release the bandage until after the victim has been brought to proper medical attention and you are prepared to provide systemic support, or after 24 hours.
5. Check frequently that swelling beneath the bandage has not compromised the arterial circulation.

BLUE-RINGED OCTOPUS BITE
The blue-ringed octopus bite injects the victim with a venom containing tetrodotoxin, a paralytic agent.

Signs and Symptoms
1. Local reaction: one or two puncture wounds characterized by minimal discomfort, described as minor ache, slight stinging, or pulsating sensation
   a. Occasionally, initial numbness at site, followed in 5 to 10 minutes by discomfort that may spread to involve the entire limb, persisting for up to 6 hours
   b. Within 30 minutes: redness, swelling, tenderness, heat, pruritus
   c. Most common local tissue reaction: absence of symptoms, small spot of blood, or tiny blanched area
2. Within 10 to 15 minutes: oral and facial numbness, rapidly followed by diplopia, blurred vision, apho-

nia, dysphagia, ataxia, myoclonus, weakness, sense of detachment, nausea, vomiting, flaccid muscular paralysis, and respiratory failure

Treatment
1. Apply the pressure immobilization technique for venom sequestration (see Fig. 26-2).
2. Be prepared to assist ventilations. Administer oxygen.

STINGRAY SPINE PUNCTURE
The venom organ of stingrays consists of one to four venomous stingers on the dorsum of the whiplike caudal appendage. The cartilaginous spine(s) is covered with venom glands and an epidermal sheath. When the spine(s) enters the victim, the sheath is disrupted and venom extruded, so that the wound is both a puncture/laceration and an envenomation.

Signs and Symptoms
1. Immediate local intense pain with central radiation, soft tissue edema, and dusky (ischemic) discoloration with surrounding erythema
2. Rapid (hours to days) fat and muscle hemorrhage and necrosis
3. Weakness, nausea, vomiting, diarrhea, diaphoresis, vertigo, tachycardia, headache, syncope, seizures, inguinal or axillary pain, muscle cramps, fasciculations, generalized edema (with truncal wounds), paralysis, hypotension, arrhythmias

Treatment
1. Immerse the wound into nonscalding hot water to tolerance (45° C [113° F]) for 30 to 90 minutes or until significant pain relief. No reason exists to add ammonia, magnesium sulfate, potassium permanganate, or a solvent to the soaking solution. *Do not immerse the wound into ice water.*

2. Remove any obvious spine fragments. This may be done during the hot water soak.
3. Administer appropriate pain medications. Consider local or regional anesthetic administration.
4. Administer prophylactic antibiotics if the wound is more than minor or if the victim is immunocompromised (see Chapter 37).
5. Do not suture the wound closed unless bleeding cannot be controlled with pressure or this wound closure method is necessary for evacuation.

SCORPIONFISH SPINE PUNCTURE

Scorpionfish (Plate 33), lionfish (Plate 34), and stonefish (Plate 35) envenom their victims using dorsal, anal, and pelvic spines, which are erected as a defense mechanism (Fig. 38-4). Other venomous fish that sting in a manner similar to scorpionfish include the Atlantic toadfish, European ratfish, rabbitfishes, stargazers, and leatherbacks. Other marine fishes carry spines that envenom to a lesser degree.

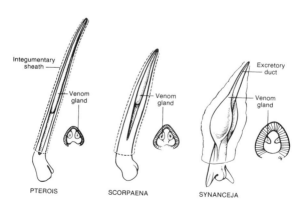

Fig. 38-4. Lionfish, scorpionfish, and stonefish spines with associated venom glands.

Signs and Symptoms

The severity of the envenomation depends on the number and type of stings, species, amount of venom released, and age and underlying health of the victim. In general, the severity is considered to be stonefish > scorpionfish > lionfish.

1. Immediate, intense pain with central radiation
   a. If untreated, pain peaking at 60 to 90 minutes and persisting for 6 to 12 hours (stonefish)
   b. Stonefish pain possibly severe enough to cause delirium and persisting at high levels for days
2. Wound and surrounding area initially ischemic and then cyanotic, with more broadly surrounding areas of erythema, edema, and warmth
   a. Vesicles possible
   b. Tissue sloughing within 48 hours
3. Anxiety, headache, tremors, maculopapular skin rash, nausea, vomiting, diarrhea, abdominal pain, diaphoresis, pallor, restlessness, delirium, seizures, limb paralysis, peripheral neuropathy, lymphangitis, arthritis, fever, hypertension, respiratory distress, pulmonary edema, bradycardia, tachycardia, atrioventricular block, ventricular fibrillation, congestive heart failure, syncope, hypotension

Treatment

1. Immerse the wound into nonscalding hot water to tolerance (45° C [113° F]) for 30 to 90 minutes or until significant pain relief. No reason exists to add ammonia, magnesium sulfate, potassium permanganate, or a solvent to the soaking solution. *Do not immerse the wound into ice water.*
2. Remove any obvious spine fragments. This may be done during the hot water soak.
3. Administer appropriate pain medications. Consider local or regional anesthetic administration.
4. Administer prophylactic antibiotics if the wound is

more than minor or the victim is immunocompromised (see Chapter 37).

5. Give stonefish antivenin in cases of severe systemic reaction from stings of *Synanceja* species. The antivenin is supplied in ampules containing 2 ml (2000 units) of hyperimmune horse serum, with 1 vial neutralizing one or two significant punctures. Administer to the victim with all due anticipation of anaphylaxis associated with the administration of an antivenin product.

CATFISH SPINE STING

The most frequent stinger is the freshwater catfish; the marine coral catfish has also been reported to sting humans. The venom apparatus consists of dorsal and pectoral fin spines. Some catfish generate skin secretions that are toxic.

Signs and Symptoms

1. Instantaneous stinging, throbbing, or scalding pain with central radiation; normally, pain subsiding within 30 to 60 minutes, but possibly lasting up to 48 hours
2. Area around the wound ischemic, with central pallor that grows cyanotic before onset of erythema and edema
3. Local muscle spasm, diaphoresis, fasciculations, weakness, syncope, hypotension, respiratory distress

Treatment

1. Immerse the wound into nonscalding hot water to tolerance (45° C [113° F]) for 30 to 90 minutes or until significant pain relief. No reason exists to add ammonia, magnesium sulfate, potassium permanganate, or a solvent to the soaking solution. *Do not immerse the wound into ice water.*
2. Remove any obvious spine fragments. This may be done during the hot water soak.

3. Administer appropriate pain medications. Consider local or regional anesthetic administration.
4. Administer prophylactic antibiotics if the wound is more than minor or the victim is immunocompromised (see Chapter 37).
5. Be aware that tiny Amazonian catfishes swim up the human urethra and are not easily dislodged. Ingestion of a large quantity of ascorbic acid, which is then excreted in the urine, may soften the spines and allow the fish to be "passed."

WEEVERFISH SPINE STING

The weeverfish is the most venomous fish of the temperate zone. It is found in the Mediterranean Sea, eastern Atlantic Ocean, and European coastal areas. The venom apparatus consists of dorsal and opercular spines associated with venom glands.

Signs and Symptoms
1. Instantaneous burning, scalding, or crushing pain with central radiation
   a. Peak of pain at 30 minutes with subsidence within 24 hours, but can last for days
   b. Possibly of an intensity sufficient to induce irrational behavior and syncope
2. Little bleeding at puncture wound site; often appears pale and edematous initially
   a. Over 6 to 12 hours, wound becoming red, ecchymotic, and warm
   b. Increasing edema for 7 to 10 days, causing the entire limb to become swollen
3. Headache, delirium, aphonia, fever, chills, dyspnea, diaphoresis, cyanosis, nausea, vomiting, seizures, syncope, hypotension, cardiac arrhythmias

Treatment
1. Immerse the wound into nonscalding hot water to tolerance (45° C [113° F]) for 30 to 90 minutes or until significant pain relief. No reason exists to add ammo-

nia, magnesium sulfate, potassium permanganate, or a solvent to the soaking solution. *Do not immerse the wound into ice water.*
2. Remove any obvious spine fragments. This may be done during the hot water soak.
3. Administer appropriate pain medications. Consider local or regional anesthetic administration.
4. Administer prophylactic antibiotics if the wound is more than minor or the victim is immunocompromised (see Chapter 37).

SEA SNAKE BITE

Sea snakes have a venom apparatus consisting of two to four maxillary fangs and a pair of associated venom glands. Most bites do not result in envenomation.

Signs and Symptoms
1. Onset potentially delayed by up to 8 hours
2. No appreciable local reaction to a sea snake bite other than the initial pricking sensation
3. Initially, euphoria, malaise, or anxiety
4. Over 30 to 60 minutes, classic muscle aching and stiffness (particularly of the bitten extremity and neck muscles), along with dysarthria and sialorrhea
5. Within 3 to 6 hours, moderate to severe pain with passive movements of the neck, trunk, and limbs
6. Ascending flaccid or spastic paralysis, beginning in lower extremities
7. Nausea, vomiting, myoclonus, muscle spasm, ophthalmoplegia, ptosis, dilated and poorly reactive pupils, facial paralysis, trismus
8. In severe cases, skin cool and cyanotic, loss of vision, possible coma

Treatment
1. Apply the pressure immobilization technique for venom sequestration (see Fig. 26-2).
2. Be prepared to assist ventilations. Administer oxygen.

3. With any evidence of envenomation, give polyvalent sea snake antivenin. The minimum effective adult dosage is 1 ampule (1000 units). The victim may require 3 to 10 ampules depending on the severity of the envenomation. Administer the antivenin with all due anticipation of anaphylaxis associated with the administration of an antivenin product.

CHAPTER 39

Seafood Toxidromes

The most common toxidromes associated with seafood that may be encountered in the wilderness are ciguatera fish poisoning, clupeotoxin fish poisoning, scombroid fish poisoning, tetrodotoxin fish poisoning, paralytic shellfish poisoning, *Vibrio* fish poisoning, anisakiasis, and domoic acid intoxication.

■ DISORDERS ■

CIGUATERA FISH POISONING

Ciguatera fish poisoning afflicts more than 400 species of bottom-feeding reef fishes. The most frequently affected fish are the jacks, snappers, triggerfishes, and barracudas. All toxins to date have been unaffected by freeze-drying, heat, cold, and gastric acid, and none has any effect on the odor, color, or taste of the fish.

Signs and Symptoms
1. Onset possible within 15 to 30 minutes of ingestion and generally within 1 to 3 hours; increasing severity over ensuing 4 to 6 hours
2. Abdominal pain, nausea, vomiting, diarrhea, chills, paresthesias (particularly of the extremities and circumoral region), pruritus (particularly of the palms and soles after a delay of 2 to 5 days), tongue and throat numbness or burning, sensation of "carbon-

ation" during swallowing, odontalgia or dental dys-esthesias, dysphagia, dysuria, dyspnea, weakness, fatigue, tremor, fasciculations, athetosis, meningis-mus, aphonia, ataxia, vertigo, pain and weakness in the lower extremities, visual blurring, transient blindness, hyporeflexia, seizures, nasal congestion and dryness, conjunctivitis, maculopapular skin rash, skin vesiculations, dermatographia, sialorrhea, diaphoresis, headache, arthralgias, myalgias (par-ticularly in the lower back and thighs), insomnia, bradycardia, hypotension, central respiratory failure, coma

3. Diarrhea, vomiting, and abdominal pain usually seen about 3 to 6 hours after ingestion and possibly per-sisting for 48 hours
4. Tachycardia and hypertension possible
5. More severe reactions in persons previously stricken with the poisoning
6. Pathognomonic symptom: reversal of hot and cold tactile perception, which may result from generalized thermal hypersensitivity or paresthesias
7. Pruritus exacerbated by anything that increases skin temperature (blood flow), such as exercise or alcohol consumption
8. If parrotfish ingested, possible second phase, show-ing locomotor ataxia, dysmetria, and resting or ki-netic tremor

Treatment

1. Be aware that therapy is supportive and based on symptoms.
2. Control nausea and vomiting with an antiemetic (prochlorperazine 2.5 mg IV or promethazine 25 mg IM).
3. Control hypotension with intravenous crystalloid volume replacement or oral rehydration if toler-ated.
4. For arrhythmias, heart block, hypotension, or severe

neurologic symptoms, administer mannitol 1 g/kg body weight IV over 45 to 60 minutes during the acute phase (days 1 to 5).
5. Be aware that bradyarrhythmias respond to atropine (0.5 mg IV, up to 2 mg).
6. For pruritus, administer hydroxyzine 25 mg PO q6-8h. Cool showers may help. Amitriptyline 25 mg PO bid may relieve pruritus and dysesthesias, as well as reactive emotional depression.
7. In the recovery phase, avoid ingestion of fish, fish sauces, shellfish, shellfish sauces, alcoholic beverages, and nuts and nut oils.

CLUPEOTOXIN FISH POISONING
Clupeotoxin fish poisoning involves plankton-feeding fish, which ingest planktonic blue-green algae and surface dinoflagellates. These include herrings, sardines, anchovies, tarpons, bonefishes, and deep-sea slickheads. The poison does not impart any unusual appearance, odor, or flavor to the fish.

Signs and Symptoms
1. Onset abrupt, within 30 to 60 minutes of ingestion
2. Initially, marked metallic taste, xerostomia, nausea, vomiting, diarrhea, abdominal pain
3. Next symptoms: chills, headache, diaphoresis, severe paresthesias, muscle cramps, vertigo, malaise, tachycardia, peripheral cyanosis, hypotension
4. Death can occur within 15 minutes of onset of symptoms

Treatment
1. Know that therapy is supportive and based on symptoms.
2. Because of the severe nature of the intoxication, early gastric emptying is desirable. However, the affliction is so unusual that the victim may die before the diagnosis is suspected.

SCOMBROID FISH POISONING

Scombroid fish (dark fleshed; predominantly tuna) and some nonscombroid fish (e.g., Hawaiian dolphin) are affected with this toxin. Histidine within muscle tissue is decarboxylated to form histamine and similar compounds. Thus the poisoning is also known as "pseudoallergic" fish poisoning. Affected fish typically have a sharply metallic or peppery taste. However, they may be normal in appearance, color, and flavor. Not all persons who eat a contaminated fish become ill, possibly because of an uneven distribution of histamine within the fish.

Signs and Symptoms
1. Onset within 15 to 90 minutes of ingestion
2. Flushing (sharply demarcated, exacerbated by ultraviolet exposure, particularly of the face, neck, and upper trunk), sensation of warmth without elevated core temperature, conjunctival hyperemia, pruritus, urticaria, angioneurotic edema, bronchospasm, nausea, vomiting, diarrhea, epigastric pain, abdominal cramps, dysphagia, headache, thirst, pharyngitis, burning of the gingivae, palpitations, tachycardia, dizziness, hypotension
3. If untreated, resolution of symptoms generally within 8 to 12 hours
4. Reaction much more severe in a person who is concurrently ingesting isoniazid

Treatment
1. Administer an antihistamine (diphenhydramine 25 to 50 mg PO or IV; cimetidine 300 mg or ranitidine 50 mg IV). Alternatives are nizatidine 150 mg PO or famotidine 20 mg PO.
2. If the victim is severely ill with facial swelling indicative of an airway obstruction, hypotension, or significant bronchospasm, treat as for an allergic reaction with epinephrine and inhaled bronchodilators in ad-

dition to antihistamines. Be aware that corticosteroids are of no proven benefit.
3. Control nausea and vomiting that do not remit after antihistamine administration with an antiemetic (prochlorperazine 2.5 mg IV or promethazine 25 mg IM).
4. Treat persistent headache with acetaminophen or an antihistamine.

Prevention
1. Make sure that all captured fish are gutted, cooled, and placed on ice or frozen immediately.
2. Do not consume fish that has been handled improperly or carries the odor of ammonia. Fresh fish generally has a sheen or oily rainbow appearance; avoid "dull" fish.

TETRODOTOXIN FISH POISONING
Tetrodotoxin is a potent nonprotein poison that interferes with central and peripheral neuromuscular transmission. It is found in pufferfish (blowfish, globefish, swellfish, toadfish, balloonfish) and porcupine fish. "Puffers" are prepared as delicacies (fugu) and when ingested may cause paresthesias, a sensation of "floating," flushing of the skin, generalized warmth, and mild weakness with euphoria.

Signs and Symptoms
1. Onset possibly as rapid as 10 minutes or delayed for up to 4 hours
2. Initial symptoms: oral paresthesias, lightheadedness, then general paresthesias
3. Rapidly developing symptoms: hypersalivation, diaphoresis, lethargy, headache, nausea, vomiting, diarrhea, abdominal pain, weakness, ataxia, incoordination, tremor, paralysis, cyanosis, aphonia, dysphagia, seizures, dyspnea, bronchorrhea, bronchospasm, respiratory failure, coma, hypotension

4. When mechanical ventilation maintained and no an-
oxic brain injury present, full mentation maintained
with total flaccid paralysis

Treatment
1. Be aware that the toxin is stable in gastric acid and
partially inactivated in alkaline solutions.
2. Secure the airway and administer oxygen.
3. Perform gastric lavage with 2 L of 2% sodium bicarbonate in 200-ml aliquots, followed by placement of
50 to 100 g of activated charcoal in 70% sorbitol solution (or 30 g of "highly activated" charcoal in sorbitol).
4. Know that further therapy is supportive and based
on symptoms.

PARALYTIC SHELLFISH POISONING
Paralytic shellfish poisoning (PSP) is induced by ingesting toxic filter-feeding organisms, such as clams, oysters, scallops, mussels, chitons, limpets, murex, starfish,
and sandcrabs. The toxins that cause PSP are water
soluble and stable in heat and gastric acid. They inhibit
neuromuscular transmission.

Signs and Symptoms
1. Within minutes to a few hours after ingestion of contaminated shellfish, onset of intraoral and perioral
paresthesias, notably of the lips, tongue, and gums,
that then progress rapidly to involve the neck and
distal extremities
2. Tingling or burning sensation that becomes numbness
3. Lightheadedness, sensation of "floating," disequilib-
rium, incoordination, weakness, hyperreflexia, in-
coherence, dysarthria, sialorrhea, dysphagia, thirst,
diarrhea, abdominal pain, nausea, vomiting, nystagmus, dysmetria, headache, diaphoresis, loss of vision, sensation of loose teeth, chest pain, tachycardia

4. Flaccid paralysis and respiratory insufficiency 2 to 12 hours after ingestion
5. Unless there is a period of anoxia, victim often awake and alert, although paralyzed

Treatment

1. Secure the airway and administer oxygen.
2. Perform gastric lavage with 2 L of 2% sodium bicarbonate in 200-ml aliquots, followed by placement of 50 to 100 g of activated charcoal in 70% sorbitol solution (or 30 g of "highly activated" charcoal in sorbitol).
3. Be aware that further therapy is supportive and based on symptoms.

VIBRIO FISH POISONING

Vibrio organisms can cause gastroenteric disease and soft tissue infections, particularly in immunocompromised hosts. The most common vector is raw oysters, shrimp, or fish. Although some variation in clinical presentation exists depending on the particular *Vibrio* species (e.g., *vulnificus, parahaemolyticus, mimicus*), a general description of the signs and symptoms and an approach to therapy will suffice for the initiation of field therapy. Persons particularly prone to septicemia and rapid demise are those with elevated serum iron levels, achlorhydria, chronic liver disease, diabetes, human immunodeficiency virus (HIV) infection, alcoholism, cancer, and various forms of immunosuppression.

Signs and Symptoms

1. Gastroenteric manifestations
   a. Ingestion of raw or partially cooked seafood products followed in 6 to 76 hours by explosive diarrhea, nausea, vomiting, headache, abdominal pain, fever, chills, and prostration
   b. Blood in stools
   c. Hypotension initially secondary to dehydration

and then, in immunocompromised individuals, to sepsis
2. Soft tissue infection
   a. Ingestion of raw or partially cooked seafood products or direct skin (wound) contact with ocean water followed in 12 to 48 hours by skin erythema, vesiculation, and hemorrhagic or contused-appearing bullae, progressing rapidly to necrotizing fasciitis and tissue necrosis
   b. Hypotension secondary to sepsis

Treatment
1. Treat dehydration and hypotension with intravenous crystalloid fluid replacement.
2. Administer an appropriate antibiotic as soon as a *Vibrio* infection is suspected.
   a. Appropriate antibiotics include imipenem-cilastatin, trimethoprim-sulfamethoxazole, cipro-floxacin, tetracycline, carbenicillin, chloramphenicol, tobramycin, gentamicin, and many third-generation cephalosporins.
   b. For information about antibiotic prophylaxis for marine-acquired wounds, see Chapter 37.

ANISAKIASIS
Anisakiasis is caused by penetration of the *Anisakis* nematode larva through the gastric mucosa. The nematode originates from the muscle tissue of raw fish.

Signs and Symptoms
1. Within 1 hour of ingestion of raw fish: severe epigastric pain, nausea, and vomiting, mimicking acute abdomen
   a. If the worm does not implant, may be coughed up, vomited, or defecated, usually within 48 hours of the meal
   b. If the worm is felt in the oropharynx or esophagus, "tingling throat" sensation
2. Intestinal anisakiasis more often delayed in onset (up

to 7 days after ingestion) and marked by abdominal pain, nausea, vomiting, diarrhea, and fever

Treatment
Unfortunately, no effective field treatment exists. Until the worm is rejected or endoscopically removed, give symptomatic therapy (e.g., an antacid).

DOMOIC ACID INTOXICATION
Shellfish, particularly certain species of mussels, that have concentrated domoic acid generate in humans a syndrome of *amnesic shellfish poisoning.*

Signs and Symptoms
1. In 15 minutes to 38 hours (median 5 hours) after ingestion of contaminated shellfish, rapid onset of arousal, confusion, disorientation, and memory loss
2. Severe headache, nausea, vomiting, diarrhea, abdominal cramps, hiccoughs, arrhythmias, hypotension, seizures, ophthalmoplegia, hemiparesis, mutism, grimacing, agitation, emotional lability, coma, copious bronchial secretions, pulmonary edema

Treatment
1. Be aware that therapy is supportive and based on symptoms.
2. For seizures, administer a potent rapid-acting anticonvulsant, such as diazepam.

CHAPTER 40

Aquatic Skin Disorders

Among the disorders acquired in water that affect the skin are various dermatoses, cutaneous larva migrans, infections, sensitivity to diving equipment, and otitis externa.

■ DISORDERS ■

SEA MOSS DERMATITIS (DOGGER BANK ITCH)

Sea moss dermatitis is caused by a seaweedlike animal colony, usually drawn up within fishing nets.

Signs and Symptoms
1. Irritation, first appearing on the hands
2. Recurrent exposures more severe, characterized by vesiculated and edematous eruption of the hands, arms, legs, and face

Treatment
1. Treat as for mild poison oak dermatitis (see Chapter 28).
   a. Depending on the severity of the reaction, apply calamine lotion or a topical corticosteroid preparation.

b. Give an oral antihistamine to help control itching.
2. Treat a severe reaction with an oral corticosteroid, specifically prednisone 60 to 100 mg for adults and 1 mg/kg body weight for children, with a 2-week taper.

SEAWEED DERMATITIS

The stinging seaweed *Microcoleus lyngbyaceus* is green or olive colored, drab, and finely filamentous. The typical victim does not remove a wet bathing suit for a time after leaving the water.

Signs and Symptoms
1. In minutes to hours after exposure, a pruritic, burning, moist, and erythematous rash developing in bathing suit distribution, followed by bullous escharotic desquamation in the genital, perineal, and perianal regions
2. Oral and ocular mucous membrane irritation, facial rash, conjunctivitis

Treatment
1. Wash the skin vigorously with soap and water.
2. Apply a brief soak of isopropyl alcohol 40%.
3. Apply a topical corticosteroid preparation. This may need to be medium to high potency.
4. Treat a severe reaction with an oral corticosteroid, specifically prednisone 60 to 100 mg for adults and 1 mg/kg for children, with a 2-week taper.

SCHISTOSOMIASIS (CERCARIAL DERMATITIS, "SWIMMER'S ITCH")

Swimmer's itch is caused by penetration of the epidermis by the cercariae of avian, rodent, or ungulate schistosomes. The cercariae are immature larval forms, usually microscopic, of the parasitic flatworms. Although penetration of cercariae may occur in the water, it usually occurs as the film of water evaporates on the skin. The eruption occurs primarily on exposed areas of the body.

Signs and Symptoms
1. Initial symptom: prickling sensation
2. Itching 40 to 60 minutes after the cercariae penetrate the skin, accompanied by erythema and mild edema
3. Subsidence of the initial urticarial reaction over 60 minutes, leaving red macules that become papular and more pruritic over the next 10 to 15 hours
4. Vesicles, which may become pustules, frequently forming within 48 hours and possibly persisting for 7 to 14 days
5. Peak inflammatory response within 3 days and subsidence slowly over 1 to 2 weeks

Treatment
1. In a mild case, apply isopropyl alcohol 40% or equal parts of isopropyl alcohol and calamine lotion to control the itching.
2. For a severe case, give an oral corticosteroid, specifically prednisone 60 to 100 mg for adults and 1 mg/kg for children, with a 2-week taper.
3. Manage secondary bacterial infection, which is frequently caused by *Staphylococcus aureus* or *Streptococcus* species, with a topical antiseptic ointment (mupirocin, bacitracin) or a systemic antibiotic (e.g., erythromycin, dicloxacillin).

Prevention
Obtain some prevention by brisk rubbing with a rough, dry towel immediately on leaving the water to remove moisture that harbors the cercariae. Washing the skin with rubbing alcohol or soap and water is not effective.

SEA BATHER'S ERUPTION
See Chapter 38.

LEECHES
Leeches attach to the skin of the victim with jaws that allow the introduction of an anticoagulant, which causes moderate painless bleeding at the site of removal. Leeches feed until they are engorged, then fall off.

Signs and Symptoms
1. In unsensitized individual, freely bleeding wound that heals slowly
2. In sensitized victim, urticarial, bullous, or necrotic reaction to the bite

Treatment
1. To remove a leech, apply a few drops of brine, alcohol, or strong vinegar, or hold a flame near the site of attachment. Do not rip the leech off the skin because its jaws may remain and induce intense inflammation.
2. After removal of the leech, inspect the wound site closely for retained mouthparts.
3. Hasten hemostasis by the application of a styptic pencil, topical thrombin solution, or oxidized regenerated cellulose absorbable hemostat.
4. Clean wounds several times daily with an antiseptic. Treat any secondary infection that develops with an antibiotic.

SEA "LOUSE" DERMATITIS
Sea "lice" are small, biting marine crustaceans often buried in the sandy bottom that attach to fish, feet, or hands.

Signs and Symptoms
1. Immediate sharp pain, with noticeable punctate hemorrhage
2. Injury resolving over 5 to 7 days

Treatment
1. Clean the acute wound with a brisk soap and water scrub or brief hydrogen peroxide application, then cover lightly with antiseptic ointment.
2. Inspect daily for secondary infection.

CUTANEOUS LARVA MIGRANS
Cutaneous larva migrans ("creeping eruption") is caused by the larvae of various nematode parasites for

which humans are an abnormal final host. The larvae penetrate the epidermis but are unable to penetrate the dermis. The feet and buttocks are most often involved with the superficial serpiginous tunnels.

Signs and Symptoms
1. Thin, wandering, linear or serpiginous, raised, and tunnel-like lesion 2 to 3 mm in width
2. Severe itching
3. Creeping eruption as the larvae move a few millimeters to a few centimeters each day
4. Older lesions that are dry and crusted

Treatment
1. Use cryotherapy with ethyl chloride for a very mild infestation, topical thiabendazole in a more refractory case, and oral thiabendazole (25 to 50 mg/kg) for 2 to 4 days in a more severe case.
2. Secondary infection may occur and require incision and drainage of pustules or furuncles and the use of topical and systemic antibiotics.

SOAPFISH DERMATITIS
The soapfish *Rypticus saponaceus* releases a soapy mucus when handled or disturbed.

Signs and Symptoms
Skin irritation with redness, itching, and mild swelling

Treatment
1. Apply cold compresses of Burow's solution to alleviate the burning and itching.
2. For a severe case, apply a topical steroid preparation.

MYCOBACTERIUM MARINUM INFECTION
Infection occurs after exposure to fresh or salt water. *Mycobacterium marinum* invades skin through a preexisting skin lesion. Most lesions heal spontaneously within 2 to 3 years.

Signs and Symptoms

1. Development of localized area of cellulitis 7 to 10 days after sustaining puncture wound or laceration, particularly of the cooler distal extremity; may progress to localized arthritis, bony erosion, formation of subcutaneous nodules, and superficial desquamation
2. Development of red papule within 3 to 4 weeks after inoculation that transforms into hard purple nodule, with scaling, ulceration, and verrucous appearance; may enlarge to 6 cm in diameter, although 1 to 2 cm more common
3. New lesions developing in pattern that resembles sporotrichosis, with dermal granulomas in linear distribution along the superficial lymphatics

Treatment

Administer minocycline (100 mg PO bid for 2 to 4 months) or tetracycline (2 g qd for 2 to 4 months).

ERYSIPELOTHRIX RHUSOPATHIAE INFECTION

Erysipeloid is commonly known as "speck finger," "fish handlers' disease," or "blubber finger." *Erysipelothrix rhusopathiae* enters the skin through a puncture wound or abrasion, usually on the finger or hand.

Signs and Symptoms

1. Appearance of violaceous, raised area (Plate 36) within 2 to 7 days after inoculation
2. Enlarged area, accompanied by pain and itching
3. Low-grade fever, malaise
4. Hallmark lesion: purplish skin irritation or paronychia, with edema and small amount of purulent discharge
   a. Surrounded by area of relative central fading, in turn surrounded by centripetally advancing, raised, well-demarcated, and marginated erythematous or violaceous ring
   b. Lesion warm and tender, with progression up the

dorsal edge of the finger into the web space and descent along the adjoining finger
5. Infection seldom affecting the palm
6. Regional inflamed lymph nodes
7. Malaise, fever
8. Arthritis

Treatment
1. For skin involvement, administer penicillin VK (250 to 500 mg PO qid), cephalexin (250 mg PO qid), or ciprofloxacin (500 mg PO bid) for 10 days.
2. If arthritis is present, give IV penicillin G.

AEROMONAS HYDROPHILA INFECTION

Aeromonas hydrophila poses a threat to freshwater aquarists in the same manner that *Vibrio* species do to marine aquarists.

Signs and Symptoms
1. Within 24 hours, wound (particularly of puncture variety) that becomes cellulitic, with erythema, edema, and purulent discharge
   a. Most frequently affects the lower extremity
   b. Appearance indistinguishable from streptococcal cellulitis
2. Localized pain, lymphangitis, fever, chills
3. Rapidly advancing gas-forming soft tissue reaction, with bullae formation and necrotizing myositis

Treatment
1. Administer an antibiotic, such as chloramphenicol, gentamicin, tobramycin, tetracycline, trimethoprim/sulfamethoxazole (co-trimethoxazole), ciprofloxacin, cefotaxime, moxalactam, or imipenem.
2. For severe infection, administer IV antibiotics as soon as possible.

VIBRIO SPECIES INFECTION

For information on antibiotic prophylaxis against *Vibrio* species infection, see Chapter 37. For information on antibiotic therapy for established *Vibrio* species infection, see Chapter 39.

REACTIONS TO DIVING EQUIPMENT

Some chemical components in the plastic and rubber used to create masks and mouthpieces can cause irritant or allergic dermatitis.

Signs and Symptoms
1. "Mask burn," which may appear as reddish imprint of the mask on the face or a severe, vesicular, and weeping eruption
2. Glossitis
3. Redness and lichenification over exposed surfaces of the feet (contact with swim fins)

Treatment
1. Treat acute facial dermatitis with cool compresses of Burow's solution.
2. For a severe skin reaction, treat with an oral corticosteroid, specifically prednisone 60 to 100 mg for adults and 1 mg/kg for children, with a 2-week taper.
3. For a serious intraoral reaction, use a twice-daily mouthwash of equal parts of antihistamine (diphenhydramine) elixir and magnesium salts (Milk of Magnesia). Coat individual sores twice daily and at bedtime with triamcinolone acetonide (0.1%) dental paste (Kenalog in Orabase) for 5 to 7 days.

OTITIS EXTERNA (SWIMMER'S EAR)

Otitis externa is inflammation and infection of the external ear canal caused by constant moisture, warm body temperature, and introduction of microorganisms.

Signs and Symptoms
1. Initial symptoms: itching, mild pain; rarely, decreased hearing
2. Possibly sensation of "fullness" in the affected ear
3. Pain that worsens as the inflammation progresses until it is uncomfortable to push on the tragus or pull on the earlobe
4. Severe infections: possible cellulitis, with purulent discharge, occlusion of the ear canal, cervical lymphadenopathy, headache, nausea, fever, and toxemia

Treatment
1. The most important topical therapy is reacidification and desiccation of the ear canal, which can be accomplished with a 50:50 mixture of isopropyl alcohol 40% and acetic acid 5% (vinegar) or with Burow's solution (Domeboro: aluminum sulfate and calcium acetate).
2. Avoid oily solutions.
3. Administer appropriate pain medications
4. For a mild infection (slight pain and discharge), use ear drops, such as nonaqueous acetic acid (VoSol Otic). Colistin sulfate has been recommended to combat *Pseudomonas*. Using acetic acid or acetic acid with hydrocortisone 1% (VoSol Otic HC) avoids sensitization that may occur with neomycin-containing products.
5. If the ear canal is so swollen that drops will not penetrate the debris, place a gauze or foam wick and keep it soaked with the topical solution for 24 to 72 hours.
6. If adenopathy, profuse purulent discharge, or fever is present, give oral co-trimethoxazole or amoxicillin-clavulanate.

Prevention
1. The most important preventive measure is to diminish moisture retention in the external ear canal.
2. Do not use cotton-tipped applicators to extract mois-

ture because they can damage the ear canal lining or press cerumen deeply into the canal.

3. Acidifying and desiccating agents are effective prophylaxis.

4. Achieve prevention by briefly rinsing with common rubbing alcohol, vinegar, or a mixture of these after each entry into the water. Avoid petroleum jelly or other substances intended to form a watertight seal because they may act as a moist trap for debris.

CHAPTER 41

Search and Rescue

DEFINITIONS

Wilderness search and rescue customarily includes the following phases:

1. Preplanning
2. The actual trip or operation
3. Predetermined termination criteria
4. Posttrip critique (including preplanning for the next operation)

During any rescue the following rudiments are essential for a safe and efficient operation:

1. *Provide for the safety of rescuers and victims.* Monitor and mitigate items essential for the survival of the individuals within the group. This must include injury prevention from environmental and rescuer causes; provision of water, shelter, and possibly food; and providing a mechanism for personal hygiene.
2. *Communicate needs and changes during all phases of the operation.* Call for backup at the earliest possible time. Ensure that rescuers are apprised of the activities and needs of the others when there is a need to know. Keep command, base camp, medical control, and incoming rescuers informed. This

may include resources ranging from using people as runners to linking with the latest digital and satellite technology. Communication seems to be the most frequently missed or most poorly managed item.

3. *Locate and reach the victim with medical-rescue personnel and equipment.* Implement organized and methodical procedures for finding the victim as soon as the safety of rescuers and victims has been ascertained. Being aware of limitations allows the rescue party to call for help when needed and reduces risk to the victim and rescue personnel.

4. *Treat and monitor the victim during evacuation.* Be sure to include psychologic and medical aspects of treatment as part of this task. Support basic personal hygiene and physiologic functions. Psychologic support is also essential and may be as basic as hand-holding or verbal encouragement by a familiar and constant voice. Help the victim to feel involved with the rescue by communicating when time allows.

PREPLANNING
Research the Location

Review all geographic and medical concerns specific to the rescue location, identifying any hazards that pose a threat in advance. Determine the topography of the area and potential evacuation routes (and nearest phones) before beginning any travel. Make sure that the location of cached equipment and supplies and the phone numbers of available rescue resources and local hospitals are communicated to each member of the party.

Rescue Resources

1. The outdoor recreation and rescue communities emphasize personal responsibility. Most groups that attempt an activity initially try self-rescue. If the group has the skills and technical abilities to accomplish this task, self-rescue is appropriate. However, the

participants must know their own limitations. If the group lacks the skills necessary for a safe self-rescue, its members must be capable and willing to mobilize local organized rescue resources. Organized rescue is often more expeditious and may reduce the number of participants who are injured or killed.

2. Within the United States, law enforcement agencies are generally the agencies responsible for the command structure and direction of an operation. Mutual aid contracts or interagency agreements may give certain agencies responsibility for specific incidents. Knowing the political structure and agency responsibilities in the United States and foreign countries makes any response run much more efficiently. In addition, the financial cost of rescue in other countries may be extreme. When adventuring outside the United States, always discuss rescue issues (e.g., forms of payment, available resources, notification systems) with the foreign U.S. embassy. In the United States, follow these guidelines:

   a. County sheriffs have jurisdiction in unincorporated county areas and in most Bureau of Land Management (BLM) and U.S. Forest Service (USFS) lands, by congressional mandate.

   b. The city police have jurisdiction on city lands and, in some cases, adjacent watersheds.

   c. Fire districts and city fire department may have jurisdiction over Hazardous Materials or Urban Search and Rescue operations.

   d. Emergency medical services (EMS) usually have jurisdiction over medical care of sick or injured persons.

   e. The National Park Service has jurisdiction over their lands except where otherwise mandated.

Support Services
With regard to support services, any one responsible agency may not have the most efficient means of conducting a rescue operation. It may delegate or request

help from other groups who are more capable of performing the actual rescue, such as the following:

1. Volunteer search and rescue (SAR) and sheriff's SAR groups usually have both responsibility and authority to conduct an operation.
2. Technically specialized volunteer teams, in addition to the regular SAR teams, may be available and may be certified by national organizations. Examples include local ski patrols and the National Ski Patrol (NSP), the National Cave Rescue Commission (NCRC), the Mountain Rescue Association (MRA), and the National Association for Search and Rescue (NASAR).
3. Do not overlook commercial enterprises or professional individuals or teams, even if they are not specifically certified. They often "practice" on a daily basis. Such groups include mountain, river, and bicycle guides, commercial mine rescue teams, and military units (ocean, air, and ground operations).

Personal Preparation

Be aware that rescue operations are inherently dangerous. No amount of preparation can remove these dangers completely. Personal preparation can reduce the impact and the likelihood of an incident becoming a problem for a rescuer. To effect a rescue in the backcountry, the rescue party members must possess personal skills specific to the terrain where they will operate.

Fitness

1. Participate in a regular physical fitness program.
2. Recognize that psychologic fitness includes the following underlying principles:
   a. The victims are responsible for their own predicament.
   b. Rescuers must ensure their own safety during both training and rescue operations.

(1) Have backups available whenever possible.
(2) Use appropriate safety equipment for the environment. Make sure that anchors are secure. Tie in anyone near an edge or precipice. Make sure that helmets are worn by persons exposed to falls or falling objects. Wear personal flotation devices when performing a rescue near or in the water.
(3) Double-check everything.
(4) Practice using all systems before they are needed in an actual rescue operation.

c. Rescuers must be aware of their exposure to such risks as rockfalls, avalanches, dangerous plants and animals, faulty equipment, violent victims, untrained personnel, unrealistic personnel or victims, weather, exposure to falls, and water hazards.

d. Rescuers must be realistic about life and death situations in the backcountry. Victims may die if they are seriously injured and definitive care is far away. The death or significant injury of a friend, trip member, or child may cause profound psychologic impact, such as posttraumatic stress syndrome. It is important to realize that, at times, no action or intervention can affect the outcome. A Critical Stress Debriefing Team may be requested through the local EMS agency or sheriff's office.

Training

1. As a rescuer, participate in wilderness medical and rescue conferences and practice regularly under realistic conditions (e.g., a training session should not necessarily be cancelled because of inclement weather).
2. Basic survival, navigation, and first-aid skills are essential for all team members. Although complete information on these areas is beyond the scope of this field guide, two basic items are essential for survival: procurement of drinking water and maintenance of body temperature.

a. Dehydration is a major problem for both rescuer and victim. Take the following steps to prevent problems:

(1) Drink before you are thirsty, and monitor rescuer and victim hydration status by observing urine output and color (minimum urine output should consist of ⅓ L bottle every 6 hours, and urine should remain light or "straw" colored).

(2) Sterilize or disinfect water (see Chapter 32). In winter, insulate each water bottle with a commercial foam wrap, or cover it with an old sock or Ensolite and duct tape. Use petrolatum (Vaseline) on bottle threads to keep the cap from freezing closed. Melt snow for water (average water:snow yield 1:7). On mild days, spread snow on a dark plastic sheet to melt. Use a straw or piece of IV tubing to access trickles of water under the snow's surface.

(3) Derive electrolytes from food, and maintain fuel stores by eating before you are hungry.

b. Be aware that evaporation and wind can cause significant heat loss. Use garbage bags to create a hasty personal shelter and vapor barrier (carry two for yourself and two for the victim). For an improvised bivouac, place one bag over the legs from the bottom and the other bag over the top, covering the head except for a small area cut out for the face. Use duct tape to join the bags for a complete seal. "Space blankets" (reflective lightweight Mylar tarps) flap in the wind and are not as useful as "space bags," into which the victim can be placed.

Personal Equipment

1. Your pack should be lightweight but rugged. An external frame snags trees and is generally less stable than an internal frame. Remember that the person with the largest pack usually carries the most.

2. Your footwear may be anything from sneakers to

double mountain boots, depending on the environment and situation.

3. Shell material should protect from wind, evaporative heat loss, and external moisture. Because of the moisture and temperature difference (vapor pressure) between the inside and outside, breathable waterproof products work best in cold weather when you will be experiencing little physical exertion. As temperature and physical activity increase, the practical differences between these products and simple coated nylon decrease. Sweating and condensation are uncomfortable but, if minimized, are not dangerous. They can be controlled by venting and modifying work load and pace. Excessive body moisture can cause increased evaporative heat loss, increased conductive heat loss (through wet clothes) and noticeable symptoms of dehydration and hypothermia.

4. Insulation guidelines are as follows:
   a. Layer clothing for easy changing as weather and exertion change.
   b. Avoid materials, such as down or cotton, that lose their insulating qualities when wet. "Water-compatible" materials (e.g., pile, wool, Polypro) absorb less water and lose less loft.

5. Be aware that great amounts of heat can be lost from the uncovered head and neck. Put on or take off your hat, "neck gaiter," or balaclava to compensate for underheating or overheating. Wear a helmet (UIAA approved) for safety. Bring a wide-brimmed hat for sun protection. Remember: a baseball-type hat does not cover the ears or the back of the neck.

6. For hand protection, use water-compatible material with a windproof water-resistant shell as needed.

7. For eye protection, 100% ultraviolet (UV) filtering is suggested for exposure to snow or altitude. Side shields are essential in the snow at high altitude. Make sure that each person is carrying a spare pair of sunglasses.

8. Miscellaneous gear can include the following:
   a. Bivouac ("bivi") and survival gear (garbage bags/

bivi sack, duct tape, whistle, candles and fire source, flares, smoke signal, signal mirror, etc.)

b. Personal care items (hygiene, personal first-aid kit that includes sun block, blister care, etc.)

c. Self-evacuation and rescue equipment. Comprehensive information on these areas is beyond the scope of this field guide. Familiarity and competency with the use of the following items are recommended:

   (1) Tubular webbing (2.5 cm [1 inch] in diameter) for an improvised chest and seat harness

   (2) Kernmantle (5 to 7 mm [⅕ to ⅓ inch] in diameter) rope for lowering or raising if the terrain has a potential for ledges that are too steep or high for a simple climb up or down

   (3) Carabiners to improvise lowering (rappelling), or climbing devices on the ropes

   (4) Tubular webbing (2.5 cm) or 4-mm rope for making improvised breaking devices (e.g., Prusik knot) for use with ropes and carabiners

RESCUE OPERATIONS
Victim Access

1. Be sure that all rescuers are aware of the *fall line*. This virtual line represents the path of travel for rocks, avalanches, or drifting boats and is the direction a rescuer may fall if footing is lost. Always avoid approaching the victim from directly above the fall line when working on loose ground or snow.

2. Accessing the victim usually requires you to have the skills essential for navigation, travel, and survival in the rescue environment.

3. The first person to the victim must have the medical skills required to stabilize the victim's condition.

Victim Evaluation and Treatment at Scene

1. In most cases it takes at least 2 hours for an outside rescue or transport team to arrive. Use the time well. Carefully assess the situation and arrange efficient

packaging. It is difficult to redo systems once an evacuation has begun. If time and circumstances allow, test the system on an uninjured party member before using it on the victim (e.g., "work out the bugs").

2. Reduce the danger and minimize the risks to rescuers first, victims second. Make sure that safety officers (to watch for and halt high-risk activity) and equipment backups (e.g., belay or fixed safety lines) are in place when possible.

3. Perform the initial assessment and treatment essential to salvage or stabilize the victim's condition. This includes the *primary survey:*
   ✤ *Airway* opened
   ✤ *Breathing* restored
   ✤ *Circulation* (severe bleeding controlled and pulse assessed) evaluated
   ✤ *Disability* determined (mental status checked and spine stabilized if any potential for injury)
   ✤ All areas of the victim requiring further evaluation *exposed* (with consideration for environmental factors)

4. Perform a detailed head-to-toe assessment *(secondary survey)* of the victim before litter packaging. Continue to reevaluate the victim throughout the evacuation. Note the following:
   a. *Mechanism of injury or illness (MOI).* Medical conditions, trauma, environmental stress, or any combination of the three mechanisms raises your index of suspicion for a serious injury (e.g., a fall from 3 times the victim's height would mean great potential for head, spine, and internal injuries; chest pain in a 45-year-old man before a snowmobile accident [vs. a tree accident] occurring 12 hours earlier would suggest an MOI for spine, head, and internal injuries, hypothermia, frostbite, and myocardial infarction).
   b. *Victim medical history* (SAMPLE):
      ✤ S = Signs, symptoms, and chief complaint
      ✤ A = Allergies

❖ M = Medications taken regularly
❖ P = Past medical history
❖ L = Last oral intake to suggest fuel or fluid deficiency
❖ E = History of present injury or illness

c. *Initial vital signs,* with subsequent monitoring at regular intervals. Vital sign changes occurring over time, coupled with the victim's mechanism of injury, help to direct treatment.

5. Take time to determine short-term and long-term plans, as well as contingencies for victim management and evacuation. Situations usually change, requiring a dynamic approach to problem solving.

Victim Evacuation and Transportation Needs

Based on the scene and victim assessments, evacuation may be divided into the following four methods:

1. *No evacuation.* Definitive care either is not needed or is available at the scene.
2. *Assisted evacuation.* Definitive therapy is needed, but the victim is ambulatory and needs moderate support. Consider walking assists, with either one or two persons.
3. *Simple carries.* The victim can sit, or the injuries allow positioning other than horizontal. Examples would include a victim with exhaustion and dehydration or an uncomplicated limb fracture.
   a. One-person carries may include the fireman's carry, backpack carry, and webbing piggyback or split-coil (Tragsitz) seat transport (Figs. 41-1 and 41-2).
   b. Two persons may be needed to support the victim or for a belay in steeper terrain.
      (1) Four-hand seat carry, ski pole/sapling pack carry (Fig. 41-3)
      (2) Webbing piggyback or split-coil Tragsitz on-belay (Fig. 41-4)

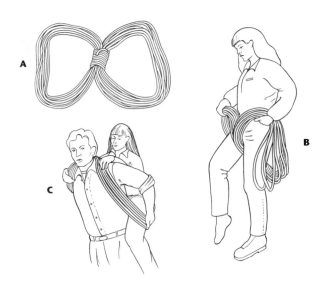

Fig. 41-1. Split-coil knot. **A,** Rope coil is split. **B,** Victim climbs through rope. **C,** Rescuer hoists sitting victim.

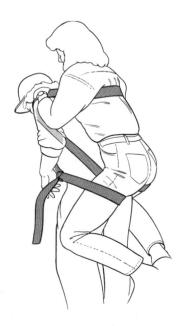

Fig. 41-2. Webbing carry. Webbing crisscrosses in front of victim's chest before passing over rescuer's shoulders.

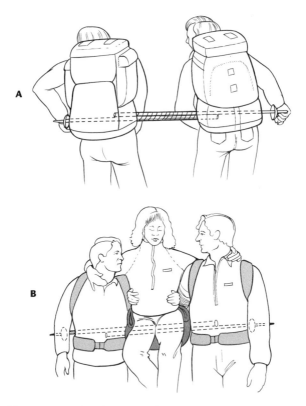

Fig. 41-3. Ski pole seat. **A,** Ski poles are anchored by packs. **B,** Victim is supported by rescuers.

4. *Litter carries.* The victim is unable to sit, or injuries require a horizontal position. Examples would be a femoral fracture or spine immobilization. This type of transport usually requires a minimum of six rescuers. The longer the transport, the more necessary are additional party members. Depending on the terrain, this type of carry may also present significant risk to victim and rescuers.

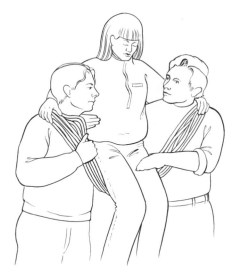

Fig. 41-4. Two-rescuer split-coil seat. Balance could be improved by using a longer coil to carry the victim lower.

Two general types of litters are found on rescues: commercial and improvised.

a. The most common commercial litter is the Stokes litter (wire or plastic), which may be found with or without leg dividers; the latter is preferable because of flexible packaging configuration based on injuries.

b. Another commercial litter is the SKED, which is popular among SAR teams and the military because it is easily carried rolled up in its own backpack, slides easily, and has flotation capability. It is narrower than the Stokes litter and somewhat flexible. A short spine immobilization device is needed with an MOI for spinal injury.

c. Other specialized litters, such as cave-evac litters, may be found in particular environments.

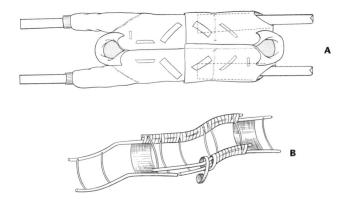

Fig. 41-5. **A,** Parka litter. On right, sleeves are zipped inside to reinforce litter. **B,** Backpack frame litter.

You can construct improvised litters from the external frames of packs, saplings, or ropes (Fig. 41-5).

d. Litter packaging should provide for victim comfort and protection from trauma and environmental impact. This includes securing the victim in the litter by attaching harnesses to siderails, using pretied foot loops hitched to rails, or using torso immobilizing devices (e.g., KED, OSS), which may then be attached to the litter.

e. You must also be able to monitor the victim. Always protect the face from falling objects and passing branches. You can cover the head and face with a Lexan shield or a helmet and goggles or fashion a piece of closed-cell foam (Ensolite) for this if necessary. Package and adequately pad the victim to prevent pressure sores during prolonged transport. Protect the victim from insects with netting, repellent, or a secure outer wrap. Environmental concerns relate primarily to temperature regulation. The goal is warmth without overheating. Immobility reduces heat production. Extra insulation and an external heat source may be needed. In a cold environment a double-vapor barrier system may be needed, with less insulation in a hot environment. A mixed system may be needed in the high desert to allow venting of the package during the day and sealing it at night. You can set up a double-vapor barrier system as follows:

(1) Place the outside vapor barrier on the ground first (e.g., the victim's tent fly or ground cloth).

(2) Place the insulation layer(s), such as a sleeping bag or a number of blankets, on top.

(3) Strip the victim down to a Polypro layer (or just skin), dry off, and place any instrumentation (e.g., blood pressure cuff, stethoscope, Foley catheter) properly.

(4) Cover the victim and seal him or her in an inner vapor barrier (two garbage bags).

(5) Place the victim in the insulation layer.

(6) Wrap the victim like a burrito with the outer vapor barrier.

f. Because the litter carry is strenuous and requires great focus, you should designate a route finder to find the most efficient trail. Choose a medical leader to direct victim monitoring and communication. Litter carries are best performed by at least six persons. Make sure the victim is level (head or feet up as indicated by injuries) and is being transported feet first. On level terrain with few obstructions, position any extra rescuers behind the litter. Rotate the carriers through the three litter-carrying positions on one side until they have finished their forwardmost carry. Then have them rotate to the rear of the line on the opposite side. This allows for a change in sides to limit rescuer fatigue (Fig. 41-6).

(1) On terrain with short drops or obstructions, have extra rescuers place themselves in the direction of travel. This allows for a litter pass with rescuers in a stable, non-moving position. When a rescuer has finished a pass, have the person move to the front of the line, in the direction of travel, on the opposite side.

(2) On steeper terrain, set up a simple belay using a tree wrap as the lowering device or an anchored lowering device such as a Muenter hitch attached to a rock. Leave an extra length of rope, or "tag" line, at the head of the litter to tie off the litter and rescuers during belay transfers. Remind rescuers to lean downhill so that their legs are perpendicular to the hillside. Trying to stand upright usually results in feet slipping out from under the rescuer and dropping the litter.

Victim Evaluation and Treatment During Transport: General Principles for Remote and Long-term Victim Care

1. Victim communication and monitoring can be accomplished as follows:

   a. Minimize the number of rescuers who are directly over the victim's head. Similarly, limit the number of rescuers who communicate directly with the victim. This reduces perceived chaos and helps keep the victim oriented and calm during the evacuation.

   b. Monitor pulses at the temporal or carotid artery with a packaged victim. Unless the pulse's character changes significantly, blood pressure probably does not have to be measured.

   c. Monitor blood pressure by placing a cuff over a

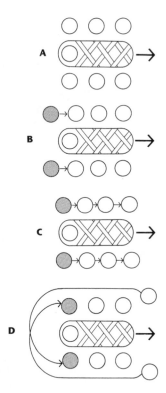

Fig. 41-6. Litter-carrying sequence. **A,** Six rescuers are usually required to carry a litter but may need relief over long distances (farther than ¼ mile). **B,** Relief rescuers can rotate into position while the litter is in motion by approaching from the rear. As relief rescuers move forward **(C),** the forwardmost rescuers can release the litter (peel out) and move to the rear **(D).** Rescuers in the rear can rotate sides so that they can alternate carrying arms. Carrying straps (webbing) can also be used to distribute the load over the rescuers' shoulders. In most cases the litter is carried feet first with a medical attendant at the head monitoring airway, breathing, level of consciousness, and so forth.

flat-diaphragm stethoscope that is taped to the victim's upper arm. Run the cuff bulb, gauge, and stethoscope ear pieces through a hole in the vapor barriers to the outside for easy access. Reseal access holes with duct tape after placement.

d. Monitor respirations using a small pocket mirror or noting condensation on the face mask or in the endotracheal tube.

e. Obtain rectal temperature using an indoor/outdoor remote thermometer (purchased at an electronics outlet). Insert the "outdoor" probe into the rectum after covering with a lubricated finger cot, latex glove finger, or condom. The "indoor" reading reflects the victim's local environment. During the preplanning phase, test the thermometer's accuracy against glass thermometers in water of varying temperatures. Thermometry is an essential component of a double-vapor barrier system because of the potential for raising the victim's core temperature.

f. Be aware that skin color, temperature, and moisture are difficult to monitor in a litter-packaged victim. Other vital signs, especially pulse rate, are used more frequently.

g. Mental status is extremely sensitive to perfusion changes. If the rescuers continue to interact with a conscious victim, they will perceive subtle changes.

2. The respiratory system guidelines are as follows:

a. Protection of the airway is essential.

(1) Oropharyngeal and nasopharyngeal airways are good airway adjuncts, but neither protects the trachea from upper airway bleeding or vomitus. The definitive airway is an endotracheal (ET) tube.

(2) Improvise suction devices using a turkey baster or a 60-ml irrigating syringe with 1.5-cm (⅝-inch) surgical tubing or an inverted nasal airway. A commercial device (V-Vac

hand-powered suction unit) is compact and works well. Remember that gravity is readily available. A well-packaged victim can be quickly rolled to the side or downward without compromise of spinal alignment.

b. With regard to a remote ventilation system, mouth-to-mask ventilation or even a bag-valve-mask may be difficult to manipulate when a victim is packaged in a litter, being carried over steep or rough terrain, or transported in a confined space. For a victim needing ventilation, consider the following system:

  (1) Mask or ET tube (preferable). A mask can be taped to the face (with quick-release capability), or an anesthesia mask and rubber spider strapping may be used (airway must be constantly monitored).

  (2) One-way valve. This is placed in-line near the face mask to limit dead space. In cold weather, this may freeze from condensation, so always carry a spare valve inside your coat or pack.

  (3) Oxygen

  (4) Ventilator tube

  (5) Bag-valve-mask

c. One-way valves purchased through MDI, Respironics, Life Support Products (LSP), or their distributors may be taped to the ventilator tubing, which can be purchased from most hospital respiratory therapy departments. Dan White (Independence, Mo) manufactures the White Pulmonary Resuscitator (WPR), which is a version of the improvised system. LSP makes a Bag Refill-Valve that is a demand valve for the bag-valve-mask, delivers 100% oxygen, and shuts off the flow once the bag is filled. This prolongs a 30-minute E cylinder for up to 1½ hours at high flow.

3. In dealing with the circulatory system, because of weight and space restrictions, IV fluid therapy in the field is usually reserved for SAR teams or large expe-

ditions. IV fluids are typically infused by bolus during stops or when needed. Do not leave any lines hanging during transport. They get in the way and are pulled out too easily. Blood pressure cuff and body weight methods of pressure infusion are usually inadequate for high-volume fluid replacement. In a cold environment, placing the line inside a strip of Ensolite is probably a waste of time. Prewarm IV bags by carrying them inside your coat, and then protect lines from freezing by placing the fluids inside the litter package or your coat. To set up a non–gravity-feed field IV system, proceed through the following steps:

    a. Invert the bag and squeeze out the air.

    b. Start the IV line using a saline lock and a large-bore catheter.

    c. Run in the amount of fluid desired using a pressure IV sleeve, with the quantity measured with the bag.

    d. Disconnect the IV tubing from the saline lock and cap the needle.

    e. Package the remaining fluids with the victim.

4. In evaluating the nervous system, keep the following in mind:

    a. Vomiting is a classic sign of head injury. Remember to monitor the airway carefully.

    b. Compartment syndrome may be a problem with inadequate padding. Pad the system wherever possible (without compromising spine immobilization).

5. Skin and soft tissues may develop pressure sores with inadequate padding.

6. In evaluating the musculoskeletal system, remember the following:

    a. Compartment syndrome from tissue edema is often overlooked because of the intensity of the evacuation. Perform ongoing assessment of injured extremities.

    b. When packaging for a long evacuation, place the

victim's knees and elbows in slight flexion to achieve maximum comfort.

7. Gastrointestinal and genitourinary considerations include the following:

 a. Although the fasting status of victims who may require surgery is a consideration, hydration of the victim during the extended evacuation is important. Persuade victims whose injuries or illness do not preclude fluids by mouth to take small sips of water. Encourage them to eat and drink regularly.

 b. With proper double–vapor barrier packaging and long transport delays unlikely, allow the victim to defecate or urinate freely inside the litter packaging. An improvised diaper helps to reduce discomfort.

 (1) For the unconscious victim, insert a Foley catheter and use a leg bag to allow for the assessment of urine output. In a conscious male, you may use a "condom catheter."

 (2) For the conscious victim, the litter can be inverted or stood on end for urination if the packaging arrangement allows. A bedpan or urinal can also be used.

 (3) Female victims may benefit from an improvised funnel made from an inverted pocket mask held against the perineum. Attach this to 1.5-cm (⅝-inch) surgical tubing and drain it outside the litter. The Lady J is a manufactured device that may also be used.

 (4) For defecation, you can cut a foam pad into a toilet seat (donut shaped) and place the pad over a hole dug into the ground or snow (this method assumes the victim can be moved out of the litter). Constipation and fecal impaction may become problematic in the immobile and dehydrated victim. Adequate hydration is the best prevention.

TERMINATION CRITERIA

Termination criteria should be identified and in place before the start of a rescue. Criteria should center on the probability of success weighed against the risk to rescuers.

GENERAL CONSIDERATIONS
Communication

1. Fire is probably the most effective signaling method during darkness. The international distress signal is three fires in a triangle or in a straight line with about 25 m (80 feet) between fires. It is better to be able to maintain one signal fire if it is too difficult to keep three going. Using a small campfire for a signal conserves fuel and energy. Keep a good supply of rapid-burning materials to throw on the fire quickly if needed.

2. Make sure that smoke signals contrast with the surrounding area. Dark-colored smoke can be made with oil-soaked rags, rubber, plastic, or electrical insulation. Light-colored smoke can be made with green leaves, moss, ferns, or water sprinkled on the fire.

3. You can make a signal mirror from shiny metal or glass; this is probably the most effective method of signaling on a bright, sunny day. Extend your arm while sighting the reflection between your thumb and forefinger on the outstretched arm. Slowly move your arm direction until an aircraft or vehicle comes into sight between your thumb and forefinger, then move the reflection to signal the vehicle. Do not keep the reflection on the cockpit for an extended period because you may "blind" the pilot.

4. Emergency radio communications usually occur on the following bands:
   a. Common public safety bands
      (1) Very high frequency (VHF), 32 to 50 MHz: good for two-way communication and pag-

ing; follows the terrain; susceptible to man-made and natural interference; uses more power and a longer (45-cm [18-inch]) antenna

(2) VHF highband, 140 to 170 MHz: less distance; more line of sight; short (15-cm [6-inch]) antenna

(3) Ultra high frequency (UHF), 460 to 470 MHz or higher: least distance, more penetration of buildings, almost always needs repeaters, shortest (5-cm [2-inch]) antenna

b. Civilian radio bands

(1) Ham (amateur): many bands used; high power and good distance; phone patch and relay possible (IMARS); emergency nets already in place (RACES); worldwide

(2) CB (citizens band): crowded high-frequency (HF) band with poor distance; heavy interference; common and inexpensive

c. The basic parts for all mobile, hand-held, and fixed (base) radios are as follows:

(1) PTT (push-to-talk). Push the key, then talk.

(2) Volume/on-off. Adjust the volume so that the speaker does not distort an incoming broadcast.

(3) Squelch (signal sensitivity). Turn the squelch until the noise just stops for optimum, nonirritating sensitivity. You may need to turn sensitivity up to be able to hear a poor transmission.

d. The protocol for use is as follows:

(1) Turn off transmitter locator beacons because they may interfere with the radio broadcast.

(2) Use normal "clear" speech. Code signal meanings vary from location to location.

(3) Identify the receiver (Rx) first and the transmitter (Tx) second.

(4) Be aware that battery life is limited. Keep batteries warm and as dry as possible. Keep transmissions limited to short periods on a

regular basis rather than transmitting continuously. Transmit energy consumption is much greater than receive consumption.

    (5) Speak from written notes.

5. With cellular phones, it is important to know your location. The actual cell picking up your call may be many miles from your location, particularly if your location is at high altitude. Keep this in mind when placing a 911 call.

Helicopter Operations

General Safety Rules (Fig. 41-7)

1. Approach the helicopter from the front, where the pilot can see and direct you, not from the rear.
2. If on a slope, approach from the downhill side; if the rear is the downhill side, approach from the right or left in view of the pilot.
3. The main and tail rotors are invisible when in operation. Stay clear of the tail rotor area. The main rotor on some helicopters is not fixed and can rise or dip. Keep your head low.

Personnel Safety

1. Remove unsecured hats or helmets and secure any loose or lightweight equipment. Unless directing the actual landing or takeoff, stay at least 30 m (100 feet) from the landing zone (LZ).
2. Wear eye protection.
3. In cold weather, cover any exposed skin during takeoff and landing. **Do the same for the victim.**

Setting Up the Landing Zone

1. Most helicopters require a square area for touchdown of 30 m (100 feet) per side. Make sure that this area is free of hazards such as trees, wires, and poles and of loose objects that can blow into the rotor system.
2. Position the guide (rescuer) for the landing helicopter far enough from the touchdown point for the pi-

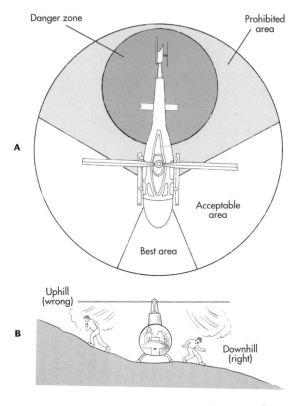

Fig. 41-7. Helicopter safety. **A,** Safe approach zones. **B,** Proper way to approach or depart a helicopter.

lot to stay in eye contact. Have this individual wear eye protection and keep his or her back to the wind because helicopters take off and land into the wind.

3. Be aware that night landings should have the corners of the LZ illuminated with one light indicating wind direction. Red lighting is best because it does not have the blinding effect of white lights on the pilot. If automobile lights are used, use one vehicle to indicate wind direction, aiming low beams at the center

of the LZ and taillights in the direction from which the wind is coming. Use any other vehicles to illuminate hazards such as trees.

4. If you have a radio and know your frequency, let the helicopter pilot know this at the time of dispatch. You can more easily direct them into the LZ (see *back azimuth* in Land Navigation, next) and warn of potential hazards. Wires are almost impossible to see during the daytime and virtually invisible at night.

Land Navigation

Map

1. Basic information
   a. Obtain topographic maps from the U.S. Geological Survey (USGS), U.S. Forest Service, college bookstores, outfitters, sporting goods stores, or engineers.
   b. Topographic maps are available from 1:250,000 (1 degree latitude or 60 minutes) to 1:24,000 (7.5 minutes). For navigation, the 7.5-minute or 15-minute (1:62,500) quads are most convenient. Military topographic maps are 1:25,000.
2. Margin information: declination, year, grid
   a. *Declination* is the magnetic deviation from true north caused by geographic magnetic loading. An example in the continental United States is Hudson Bay, which has a large magnetic load and therefore reduces your reading of true north if you are east of the bay (and increases your reading if you are west of the bay). Therefore you must add for true north (west declination) if you are east of Hudson Bay and subtract for true north (east declination) if you are west of Hudson Bay. For instance, Denver is 15 degrees east declination; true map north is 15 degrees less magnetic compass north.
   b. *Grid* is measured on an x (longitude) vs. y (latitude) axis, using longitude and latitude lines. Extrapolation to find your location on a map is essential to give a helicopter or rescue party your

exact location. A helicopter can input longitude and latitude and fly directly to the location.

Compass

1. Simple travel by map and compass
   a. Orient the map to the terrain, with the magnetic north arrow of the map pointing in the same direction as the magnetic needle of the compass.
   b. Place the straight edge of the base plate along a line between the starting and destination points on the map (the direction-of-travel arrow pointing to the point of destination).
   c. Holding the base plate firmly, rotate the housing so the orienting needle arrow is in line with north on the compass needle.
   d. Look at the terrain and see where the direction-of-travel arrow is pointing. Use a landmark in direct line with the direction of travel.
   e. Hike in that direction. Leapfrog with a companion if necessary. Repeat.
2. Terminology
   a. *Azimuth:* compass bearing (direction from north) to a target.
   b. *Back azimuth:* 180 degrees plus or minus azimuth (opposite direction). *Bringing in a helicopter using back azimuth:* Line your north sign or your declination tick mark up with the direction-of-travel arrow. Turn the compass around until the direction-of-travel arrow is pointing at you. Point the rear of the compass toward the sighted or heard helicopter. The number noted at the direction-of-travel arrow is the back azimuth to the aircraft, but it is the pilot's azimuth to you. Tell the pilot, "we are at X degrees from your location." Updates will bring him directly to your location quickly.
   c. *Pacing:* number of steps per distance per individual
   d. *Timing:* time per distance; this changes with terrain and elevation (group on a trail travels about 2 mph plus 1 hour per 300 m (1000 feet) gain, 1

half-hour per 1000 feet loss; multiply by 2 to 4 for "bushwhacking")
e. *Triangulation:* plotting compass bearings to multiple landmarks on the map to pinpoint an exact map location (Location can also be determined by intersecting a plot with a known line, such as a road or stream.)

Altimeter
1. Knowledge of weather patterns and cloud types is helpful. A falling barometric pressure may mean an incoming storm, not just a rise in altitude because a 150- to 300-m (500- to 1000-foot) change occurs with a large storm.
2. An altimeter can be extremely useful for navigation. To use an altimeter for pinpointing or narrowing down a map location, use known geographic features, then determine where they intersect with a contour line of measured altitude.

Global Positioning System
The global positioning system (GPS) may give you the exact longitude and latitude of your position. It is battery dependent and can be dropped and broken, so you should also have other means of navigation.

NOTE: A good map reader can navigate without a compass. The ability to read terrain features on topographic maps is essential.

Rope and Knot Review
Rope Construction, Strength, and Terminology
1. *Laid rope* is easily abraded, has great stretch, and spins when loaded.
2. *Braided and plaited rope* is used for lighter loads, is pliable, and is easily abraded.
3. *Kernmantle rope* has a braided mantle that covers and protects the core (kern) strands. Kernmantle ropes have variable stretch:
   a. *Static:* low stretch (1% to 5% for 75-kg [165-pound] load, <20% at failure); used for rescue, top roping

b. *Dynamic:* high stretch (5% to 15% for 75-kg load, 20% to 60% at failure); used for lead climbing
4. *Working strength* is about 15% of static (tested) strength (relates to working load).
5. *Fall factor* is a measure of fall severity and is found by dividing the distance fallen by the length of rope used to control the fall.
6. *Impact force* is the amount of force transmitted to the load when the rope stops the fall.

Webbing

1. The two types of webbing are tubular and flat.
2. Webbing is easily abraded and is slippery for knot tying.

Rope and Web Fibers

1. *Nylon* is strong and heavy and has low stretch.
2. *Spectra* is a hybrid nylon with extreme strength; it is very slippery for knotting.
3. *Polypro fiber* is lightweight and floats; it has low strength, high stretch, is easily abraded, and has a low melting temperature.
4. *Kevlar* has extreme strength in line and is very stiff; some debate surrounds its large strength loss when knotted or bent.

Maintenance

1. Rope running on hardware and rope running across a stationary rope can produce melt and weld abrasion. Avoid rapid descents or lowers with sudden stops. However, two ropes running across each other (as with the Muenter hitch) do not generate damaging heat at any single spot along either rope.
2. Store rope in a cool, dry place with no exposure to chemicals or sun.
3. Clean with cold water without detergent, followed by air drying.
4. Inspect ropes before and after use, checking for lumpiness, 50% or more of the sheath fibers broken, stiff spots, a gap under tension, or visible strains.

5. Consider rope retirement when appropriate. The decision to retire the rope is usually subjective, based on hours of service, number of falls vs. fall rating, written rope logs, and manual inspection.

Knots

1. Good knots are easy to tie and untie after loading and have a minimal loss of rope strength during use. Become so familiar with any knot that you use during a rescue that you can tie it either in front of or behind you or with your eyes closed. When a knot is needed, weather and visibility are generally poor and you are out of position. Secure loose ends with a simple overhand knot or grapevine.
2. Family of figure-8 knots
   a. *On-a-bight knot* (and follow-through) is used for anchoring to a fixed object (harness, tree).
   b. *Double figure-8 knot* gives double security on anchors and harnesses.
   c. *Flemish bend knot* (rewoven figure-8 knot) is used for tying two ropes together.
3. Overhand family
   a. *Double fisherman's knot* is used to tie ends of a rope together. An example is a Prusik loop.
   b. *Grapevine knot* is half of a double fisherman's knot and is used as a safety finish for other knots.
   c. *Water knot* ties the ends of webbing together, as for a runner.
4. Bowlines
   a. *Simple bowline knot* attaches a loop to a fixed point.
   b. *Bowline-on-a-coil* knot may be used on litter rigs or for short roping.
5. Miscellaneous knots and hitches
   a. *Clove hitch* is used to anchor to a fixed point when tension changes may be needed (e.g., shoulder support strap for litter carriers).
   b. *Muenter hitch* is used as a belay device on low-angle rescues and can be used to assist with lowering a litter and rescuers as a friction device.

It is used for a rappel device to enable a rescuer to gain access to a victim.

c. *Girth hitch* is used to anchor to a fixed object; it is also used to begin an improvised harness or as the base for the pack carry of a victim.

d. *Prusik knot* is a bidirectional fixed knot when under tension, but it is movable when unweighted. It can be used as an ascender, a moving self-belay, or a mobile midline loop.

CHAPTER 42

Avalanche Rescue

The factors that contribute to avalanche release are terrain, weather, and snow pack. Terrain factors are fixed; however, the state of the weather and snow pack changes daily, even hourly. Precipitation, wind, temperature, snow depth, snow surface, weak layers, and settlement are all factors determining whether an avalanche will occur. Anyone venturing into avalanche terrain must be familiar with proper avalanche hazard evaluation and appropriate route selection.

SAFETY EQUIPMENT

Proper equipment is essential for maintaining safety. This safety equipment should include the following:

1. Snow shovel.
2. Collapsible probe pole or ski pole probe. This is used to pinpoint a victim following a transceiver (rescue beacon) search and is essential for a probe search if a transceiver is not available. A tent pole, the tail of a ski, a ski pole with the basket removed, or an appropriately sized branch can substitute for this piece of equipment.
3. Avalanche rescue transceivers (rescue beacon). Transceivers act as transmitters that emit signals on a frequency of 457 kHz (or in the past, 2.275 kHz). A buried victim's unit/beacon/transceiver

emits the signal, and the rescuer's unit is set to receive the signal. The signal carries about 30 m (100 feet) and, when used properly, can guide searchers to the buried unit. *It is essential to confirm that all members of the party are on the same frequency and have their transceivers set to "transmit" before travel.* In 1986 the International Commission for Avalanche Alpine Rescue (ICAR) adopted a new standard for an avalanche beacon frequency of 457 kHz. As of Aug. 15, 1993, an American National Standard was established concurring with this frequency change and making the 457 kHz frequency mandatory in all devices. This new frequency has a much greater range and effectiveness than any other single- or dual-frequency beacon. The sale and use of 2.275 kHz beacons ceased on Dec. 1, 1995. Be certain that all beacons are either dual-frequency 2.275 kHz and 457 kHz or single-frequency 457 kHz. A single-frequency 2.275 kHz beacon will be incompatible with 457 kHz beacons. It is recommended that all users replace their older transceivers with single-frequency 457 kHz units as soon as possible.

CROSSING AN AVALANCHE SLOPE

Travel through avalanche terrain always involves risk. However, certain travel techniques can minimize this risk and possibly improve the odds of survival. Before crossing a potential avalanche slope, take the following precautions:

1. Tighten up clothing, fasten zippers, and wear hat, gloves, and goggles.
2. If wearing a heavy mountaineering pack, loosen it before crossing so that it can be jettisoned if necessary. A heavy pack makes "swimming" in the snow more difficult.
3. Remove ski pole straps and ski runaway straps because attached poles and skis can make

"swimming" on snow nearly impossible and can greatly add to your trauma.

4. Be sure that all rescue transceivers are set to "transmit."

5. Cross well below the slope if possible. Avalanches can be triggered from the flats below, but this is generally a safe route.

6. If the slope must be crossed at a high point, stay as high as possible. The person highest on a slope runs the least risk of being buried should the slope slide.

7. Cross potential avalanche slopes as quickly as possible. *Never stop moving in the middle of an avalanche slope.*

8. When climbing or descending an avalanche path, stay close to the sides. This makes it easier to escape to the side should the slope begin to slide.

9. *Only allow one member of the group to cross at a time.* This only exposes one person at a time to danger, and it puts less weight on the snow.

10. Try to move toward natural islands of safety such as rock outcroppings or trees.

11. Do not drop your guard. Even the tenth person traveling or skiing a slope can trigger a slide.

12. *Anticipate an avalanche.* Plan your escape route ahead of time.

VICTIM SURVIVAL

1. **Escape to the side.** The moment the snow begins to move, try to escape by moving quickly to the side of the avalanche, similar to the method a swimmer uses to ferry to the side of a river. Turning skis or a snow machine downhill in an effort to outrun the avalanche invariably fails because the avalanche will outrun you.

2. **Shout, then close your mouth.** Shouting alerts companions, and closing the mouth may help prevent snow inhalation.

3. **Swim.** If knocked off your feet, attempt to "swim" with the avalanche. Use whatever motion it takes to stay on the surface. Kick your skis off and toss ski poles away. A lightweight mountaineering pack is probably protective; however, if you are wearing a heavy multiday mountaineering pack, jettison it because it will drag you down rather than allowing you to stay near the surface.

4. **Reach for the surface.** As the avalanche slows down, you may have a second or two to thrust upward with a swimming motion to reach the surface. When the avalanche comes to a halt, use all possible strength to get the head, an arm, or a hand above the surface, which will greatly improve the odds of survival. Also, use your hand to create a breathing space around your mouth and nose.

RESCUE

Although it is usually safe to move onto the bed surface of an avalanche that has just completed its run, beware when the fracture has occurred at midslope, leaving a large mass of snow hanging above the fracture.

1. **Marking the last-seen location.** Mark the victim's last-seen location with a piece of equipment, clothing, or anything that can be seen from a distance down the slope.

2. **Searching for clues.** Search the fall line below the victim's last-seen location for clues. Make shallow probes at likely burial spots with an avalanche probe, ski pole, or tree limb. Likely burial spots are the uphill sides of trees and rocks and benches or bends in the slope where snow avalanche debris is concentrated. The "toe" of the debris is also a place where many victims come to rest.

3. **Using rescue transceivers.** If the group was using transceivers, have all survivors immediately switch their units to "receive." When a signal is

received, the search can be quickly narrowed and the victim pinpointed within a few minutes.

4. **Posting an avalanche guard.** If enough rescuers are available and conditions remain unstable, post one person in a safe place and have him or her shout a warning should a second avalanche slide begin. This also allows rescuers to switch their transceivers back to "transmit."

5. **Going for help.** If the accident occurs in a ski area and several rescuers are available, send one person immediately to notify the ski patrol. If only one rescuer is present, search the surface for clues before leaving to notify the ski patrol. If the avalanche occurs in backcountry terrain, expedient recovery is so essential to the victim's survival that all rescuers should search for the victim. By the time organized rescue personnel return to search, it is unlikely those buried will be alive.

6. **Keeping rescue gear organized.** It is important to keep all rescue gear organized; either keep it with you or put it in a safe location.

AVALANCHE TRANSCEIVER SEARCH
Initial Search

1. Have everyone switch their transceivers to "receive" and turn the volume to "high."
2. If enough people are available, post a lookout to warn others of further slides.
3. Should a second slide occur, have rescuers immediately switch their transceivers to "transmit."
4. Have rescuers space themselves no more than 30 m (100 feet) apart and walk along the slope parallel to one another.
5. For a single rescuer searching within a wide path, zigzag across the rescue zone. Limit the distance between crossings to 30 m.
6. For multiple victims, when a signal is picked up, have one or two rescuers continue to locate the vic-

tim while the remainder of the group carries out the search for additional victims.

7. For a single victim, when a signal is picked up, have one or two rescuers continue to locate the victim while the remainder of the group prepares shovels, probes, and medical supplies for the rescue.

Locating the Victim

With practice, the induction line search is more efficient than the conventional grid search. An induction line search requires a 457 kHz transceiver.

Induction Line Search (Preferred Method)

When an induction line search is used, the rescuer may initially follow a line that leads away from the victim (Fig. 42-1). Remember to lower transceiver volume if it is too loud because the ear detects signal strength variations better at lower volume settings.

1. After picking up a signal during the initial search, hold the transceiver horizontally (parallel with the ground) with the front of the transceiver pointing forward (see Fig. 42-1, *A*).

2. Holding the transceiver in this position, turn until the signal is maximal (maximum volume), then walk five steps (about 5 m [16 feet]), stop, and turn again to locate the maximum signal (see Fig. 42-1, *B*). When locating the maximum signal, do not turn yourself (or the transceiver) more than 90 degrees in either direction. If you rotate more than 90 degrees to locate the maximum signal, you will become turned around and follow the induction line in the reverse direction.

3. Walk another five steps, as described above, and then stop and orient the transceiver toward the maximum signal. Reduce the volume.

4. Continue repeating the above steps. You should be walking in a curved path along the "induction line" toward the victim (see Fig. 42-1, *C*).

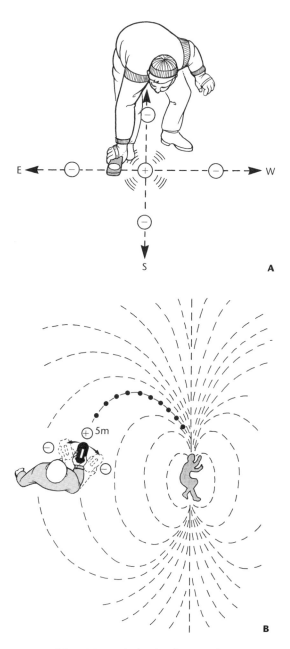

Fig. 42-1. Induction line search.

Continued

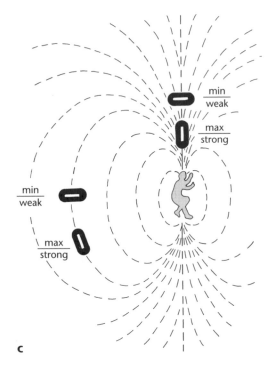

Fig. 42-1—cont'd For legend see p. 489.

5. When the signal is loud at minimum volume setting, you should be very close to the victim and can begin the pinpoint search (see below).

Grid Search

1. When a signal is picked up, stand and rotate the transceiver, which is held horizontally (parallel with the ground), to obtain the maximum signal (loudest volume). Maintain the transceiver in this orientation during the remainder of the search.

2. Turn the volume control down until you can just hear the signal. Walk in a straight line, down the fall line

from the victim's last-seen location, until the signal fades.

3. When the signal starts to fade, turn 180 degrees and walk back toward the starting position. The signal will increase in volume and then fade again. Walk back to the point of loudest volume/maximum signal, which should be in the middle of the two fade points.

4. At this point, turn 90 degrees in one direction or the other. From that position, reorient the transceiver (held parallel with the ground) to locate the maximum signal. After orienting the transceiver to the maximum signal, reduce the volume, and begin walking forward. If the signal fades, turn around 180 degrees and begin walking again.

5. As the signal volume increases, repeat steps 3 and 4 until you have reached the lowest volume control setting on the transceiver. This time, when you return to the middle of the fade points (maximum signal strength), you should be very close to the buried victim and can now begin **pinpointing** him or her.

   a. While stationary, orient the transceiver to receive the maximum signal (loudest volume). At this point, turn the volume control all the way down.

   b. Maintain the transceiver in this orientation and sweep the transceiver from side to side and back and forth just above the surface of the snow.

   c. Find the signal position halfway between fade points (i.e., the loudest signal). At this point, you should be very close to the victim's position and can begin to mechanically probe. Speed is essential.

Probe Search
Spot probe

1. Look for areas likely to contain the victim, such as places where snow is piled up against trees or boulders, where the slope decreases, benches or bends in

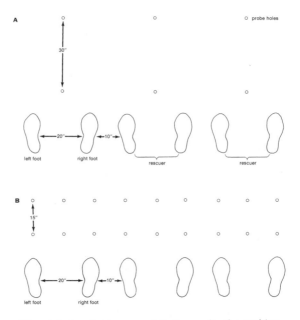

Fig. 42-2. **A,** Coarse and **B,** fine avalanche probing.

the slope, at the "toe" of the avalanche, or anywhere the avalanche deposition is built up.

2. Randomly probe these areas for the victim. Do not "jam" the probe into the ground; rather, push the probe steadily downward.

Coarse probe. If there are no clues to the victim's location, no likely areas for a spot probe, or the spot probe has been unsuccessful, begin a coarse probe (Fig. 42-2, *A*). Coarse probing is 4 to 5 times faster than the more thorough technique of fine probing. Coarse probing is a compromise between thoroughness and speed (70% to 80% chance of finding the victim on the first pass).

1. Spaced with elbows touching and hands on hips, have rescuers line up across the avalanche path at the base of the deposition.
2. Have rescuers probe the space directly in front of them, moving the probe first, then stepping up to meet it. Allow rescuers to advance 70 cm (30 inches) with each probe. Moving uphill is easier on the rescuers' backs and helps keep each advancement uniform.
3. When terrain is steep or rescuers are few, use an alternative and stand "fingertip to fingertip." For this, rescuers first probe on one side of their body, then on the other. This method yields a lower probability of finding the victim.

Fine probe. If several passes of coarse probing yield no results, perform a fine probe (Fig. 42-2, *B*). By this time, the objective is usually to recover the body. On average, 20 searchers can fine-probe an area 100 m by 100 m (330 feet by 330 feet) in 16 to 20 hours.

1. Start the fine probe with the same arrangement as for the coarse probe.
2. Instruct each rescuer to probe in front of the left foot, in the center, and in front of the right foot.
3. Allow rescuers to advance 70 cm (30 inches) and repeat the three probes.
4. When performed correctly, this method is 100% successful in locating the victim.

THE AVALANCHE VICTIM

Avalanches kill in the following two ways:

1. Asphyxiation secondary to airway blockade by snow, pressure of snow on the thorax, and formation of an ice mask around the nose and mouth after burial
2. Trauma secondary to the wrenching action of

snow in motion and the potential for impact with trees, rocks, loose equipment, and cliffs

Prognostic features for low survival potential include the following:

1. *Complete burial of victim.* Survival probabilities greatly diminish with increasing burial depth. No avalanche victim in the United States has survived a burial deeper than 2 m (6½ feet), unless protected by a structure.
2. *Prolonged burial time.* In the first 15 minutes after the avalanche, more persons are found alive than dead. Within 15 to 30 minutes, an equal number of people are found dead and alive. After 30 minutes, more people are found dead than alive, and the survival rate rapidly diminishes thereafter. Trained search dogs can locate buried victims very quickly, but they are typically brought to the scene after victims have been buried for an extended period. Consequently, very few live rescues have been done using search dogs.

CARE OF THE VICTIM

Although speed is essential when digging out the victim, have rescuers begin working from the side and avoid standing on top of the victim, which may collapse the victim's air space. Also instruct rescuers to take care not to injure the victim with their shovels.

Treatment
1. Manage the airway.
2. Immobilize the spine if needed.
3. Stabilize any fractures or other injuries.
4. Provide thermal stabilization (to control heat loss; see Chapter 2).
5. Handle the victim gently in anticipation of hypothermia.
6. Provide for evacuation.

CHAPTER 43

Wilderness Medical Kits

When designing a wilderness medical kit, you must consider certain prerequisites and variables, including the following:

1. Medical expertise of the intended user
2. Environmental extremes
3. Endemic diseases
4. Duration of travel
5. Distance from definitive medical care and availability of rescue
6. Number of persons the kit will need to support
7. Preexisting illnesses
8. Weight and space limitations

Make sure that the wilderness medical kit is well organized in a protective and convenient carrying case or pouch. For backpacking, trekking, or hiking, a nylon or Cordura organizer bag is optimal. Newer-generation bags with clear, vinyl compartments have proved superior to mesh-covered pockets for protecting the components from the environment. The vinyl protects the components from dirt, moisture, and insects and keeps the items from falling out when the kit is turned on its side or upside down.

For aquatic environments, store the kit in a waterproof dry bag or watertight container, such as a Pelican Box. Inside, seal items in resealable plastic bags because moisture will invariably make its way into any container.

Some medicines may need to be stored outside of the main kit to ensure protection from extreme temperatures. Capsules and suppositories melt when exposed to temperatures above 37° C (99° F), and many liquid medicines (e.g., insulin) become useless after freezing.

BASIC SUPPLIES
Wound Management Items
- 10- to 20-ml irrigation syringe with an 18-gauge catheter tip
- Povidone-iodine solution USP 10% (Betadine) to disinfect backcountry water and sterilize wound edges; when diluted tenfold, can be used for wound irrigation
- ¼ × 4-inch wound closure strips
- Tincture of benzoin
- Polysporin or double-antibiotic ointment
- Forceps or tweezers
- First-aid cleansing pads with lidocaine; textured surface ideal for scrubbing dirt and embedded objects out of abrasions
- Antiseptic towelettes with benzalkonium chloride
- Surgical scrub brush, a sterile brush for cleaning embedded objects and dirt from abrasions
- Aloe vera gel, a topical antiinflammatory gel for treating burns, frostbite, and poison oak/ivy dermatitis
- Cyanoacrylate glue ("super glue")
- Scalpel with no. 11 blade
- Surgical gloves

Bandage Material
- 8 × 10-inch or 5 × 9-inch sterile trauma pads
- 4 × 4-inch sterile dressings
- Nonadherent sterile dressings, such as Aquaphor,

Xeroform, Adaptic, or Telfa; Spenco 2nd Skin is an excellent alternative and provides an ideal covering for burns, blisters, abrasions, and cuts (This is a polyethylene oxide gel laminate composed of 96% water that cools and soothes on contact and can be left in place for up to 48 hours.)

✤ Gauze rolled bandages or Kling bandages
✤ Elastic rolled bandage
✤ Assortment of strip and knuckle adhesive bandages
✤ Stockinet bandage, a net-style bandage particularly useful for holding dressings in place over joints
✤ Molefoam, a thick, padded adhesive material for protecting blisters
✤ Moleskin, a thin, padded adhesive material for protecting skin from developing blisters
✤ Assorted widths of adhesive tape

Nonprescription Medications

✤ Acetaminophen (Tylenol)
✤ Ibuprofen
✤ Diphenhydramine (Benadryl)
✤ Calcium carbonate and magnesium hydroxide (Mylanta) or one of the H_2-adrenergic blocking medications
✤ Tolnaftate (Tinactin) or Nystatin Antifungal Cream
✤ Hydrocortisone cream USP 1%
✤ Glutose paste
✤ Loperamide (Imodium)
✤ Oral rehydration salts

Equipment

✤ SAM splint, a malleable, foam-padded splint that can be adapted for use on almost any part of the body; can be fashioned as a cervical collar, arm, leg, or ankle splint
✤ Hyperthermia/hypothermia thermometer, which ideally should be able to read temperatures down to 29.4° C (85° F) and up to 41.6° C (107° F)
✤ CPR Microshield, a compact, easy-to-use, clear, flex-

ible barrier with a one-way air valve for performing mouth-to-mouth rescue breathing; prevents physical contact with a victim's secretions
✤ Bandage scissors, which are designed with a blunt tip to protect the victim while cutting through clothes, boots, or bandages
✤ Cotton-tipped applicators, which may be used to remove insects or other foreign material from the eye; also useful to roll fluid out from beneath a blister or to evert an eyelid in searching for a foreign body
✤ Otoscope
✤ Plastic resealable (Zip-Lock) bags
✤ Safety pins
✤ Duct tape
✤ Accident Report Form
✤ Pencil
✤ Epinephrine 1:1000 solution, or EpiPen Auto Injector

Basic Dental Kit
✤ Mouth mirror
✤ Dental floss
✤ Cavit temporary filling material
✤ Cotton rolls
✤ Zinc oxide
✤ Eugenol (oil of cloves)
✤ Cotton pellets

ENVIRONMENT-SPECIFIC SUPPLIES
High Risk of Venomous Snakes
✤ Sawyer Extractor, a vacuum pump device that provides 1 atmosphere of negative pressure for removing venom from poisonous snakebites
✤ Elastic rolled bandage to apply the pressure immobilization technique for venom sequestration

High Risk of Altitude Illness
✤ Oxygen
✤ Portable hyperbaric bag (Gamow Bag)

✤ Acetazolamide (Diamox) 125 mg for prophylaxis, 250 mg for treatment of altitude illness
✤ Dexamethasone 4 mg
✤ Nifedipine 10 to 25 mg

High Risk of Snowblindness

✤ Ophthalmic anesthetic (e.g., proparacaine or tetracaine 0.5%) to facilitate eye examination and to provide short-term analgesia
✤ Fluorescein stain
✤ Ophthalmic cycloplegic (e.g., cyclopentolate 1%)
✤ Ophthalmic corticosteroid-antibiotic combination (e.g., Maxitrol)
✤ Ophthalmic antibiotic drops

High Risk of Heat Illness

✤ Hyperthermia thermometer
✤ Intravenous normal saline solutions and administration supplies
✤ Chemical ice packs

High Risk of Marine Envenomation

✤ 5% acetic acid (vinegar)
✤ Prednisone

Tropical, Jungle, or Third World Travel

✤ Ciprofloxacin 500 mg, azithromycin 250 mg, and loperamide 2 mg for "traveler's diarrhea"
✤ Clotrimazole or betamethasone dipropionate cream
✤ Lotrisone cream
✤ Permethrin 5% cream and 1% shampoo
✤ Sunscreen and insect repellent

For Expeditions and Medically Trained Members

✤ Stethoscope
✤ Chest tubes (sizes 28 to 36 French)
✤ Foley catheter

✣ Airway supplies (oral and nasal airways, laryngoscope, endotracheal and cricothyrotomy tubes)
✣ Advanced wound management supplies

1. Suture instruments and material
2. Surgical staples
3. 1% lidocaine for anesthesia

✣ Intravenous solutions and tubing
✣ Needles and syringes
✣ Antibiotics (oral, ophthalmic, otic, and parenteral)
✣ Beta-agonist metered-dose inhaler and spacer (for asthma and other allergic reactions)
✣ Analgesics and sedatives

1. Ketorolac (Toradol) 60 mg for injection
2. Acetaminophen with oxycodone (Vicodin)
3. Morphine sulfate for injection
4. Diazepam or midazolam for injection or oral use
5. Fentanyl for injection or oralets
6. Stadol (butorphanol) nasal spray

✣ Gastrointestinal and genitourinary supplies

1. Urine chemstrips
2. Urine pregnancy test
3. Miconazole nitrate 200-mg suppository (Monistat) daily at bedtime for 3 consecutive days for local treatment of vulvovaginal candidiasis
4. Hydrocortisone acetate (Anusol-HC 25-mg suppositories) for inflamed hemorrhoids, one suppository placed in rectum morning and night for 2 weeks
5. Bisacodyl 10-mg suppositories (Dulcolax); one suppository once daily for relief of constipation and irregularity
6. Prochlorperazine 25-mg suppositories (Compazine) or promethazine 25-mg suppositories

(Phenergan) for severe nausea and vomiting; one suppository q8h

✤ Diphenhydramine for injection

1. Allergic reactions or motion sickness: 25 to 50 mg IM q6h
2. Substitute for lidocaine (Xylocaine) for local anesthesia: a 50-mg (1-cc) vial diluted in syringe with 4 cc of normal saline to produce 1% solution; local infiltration carried out as usual

✤ Nitroglycerin tablets or spray
✤ Sumatriptan (Imitrex) for migraine headache

APPENDIX A

Glasgow Coma Scale

This scale evaluates the degree of coma by determining the best motor, verbal, and eye-opening response to standardized stimuli.

EYE OPENING	
Spontaneous	4
To voice	3
To pain	2
None	1
VERBAL RESPONSE	
Oriented	5
Confused	4
Inappropriate words	3
Incomprehensible words	2
None	1
MOTOR RESPONSE	
Obeys command	6
Localizes pain	5
Withdraw (pain)	4
Flexion (pain)	3
Extension (pain)	2
None	1
TOTAL:	

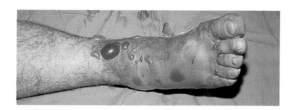

Plate 1. Edema and blister formation 24 hours after frostbite injury occurring in an area covered by a tightly fitted boot.

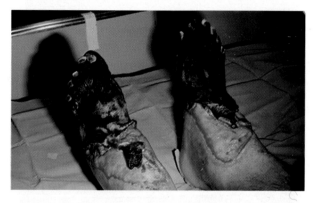

Plate 2. Gangrenous necrosis 6 weeks after frostbite injury shown in Plate 1. *(Plates 1 and 2 courtesy Cameron Bangs, MD.)*

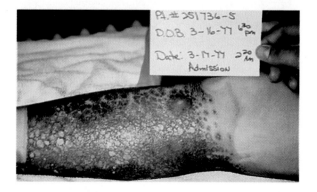

Plate 3. Punctate burns from lightning injury. *(Courtesy Arthur Kahn, MD.)*

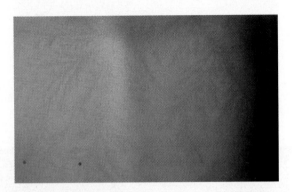

Plate 4. Feathering burns from lightning injury. *(Courtesy Mary Ann Cooper, MD.)*

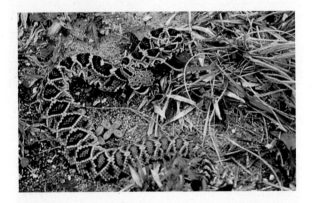

Plate 5. Eastern diamondback rattlesnake *(Crotalus adamanteus).* This is the largest U.S. rattlesnake, which sometimes attains a length of 7.5 feet. Note the definitive diamond-shaped pattern on the dorsum of the animal. *(Courtesy Sherman Minton, MD.)*

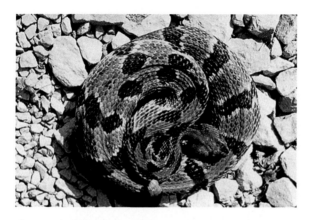

Plate 6. Timber rattlesnake *(Crotalus horridus)*. This is a widely distributed large rattlesnake of the eastern United States. *(Courtesy Sherman Minton, MD.)*

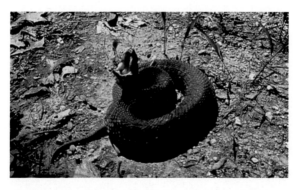

Plate 7. Cottonmouth *(Agkistrodon piscivoris)*. The open-mouthed threat gesture is characteristic of this semiaquatic pit viper. *(Courtesy Sherman Minton, MD.)*

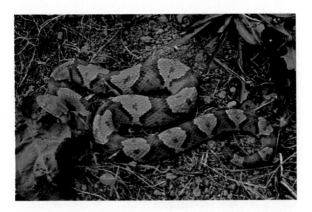

Plate 8. Copperhead *(Agkistrodon contortrix mokasen)*. Copperheads are probably the leading cause of snakebites in the United States, but fatalities from their bites are extremely rare. This specimen is typical of the northeastern variety. *(Courtesy Sherman Minton, MD.)*

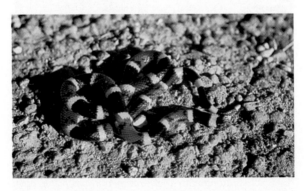

Plate 9. North American coral snake *(Micrurus fulvius)*. Northernmost representative of a tropical American group. *(Courtesy Sherman Minton, MD.)*

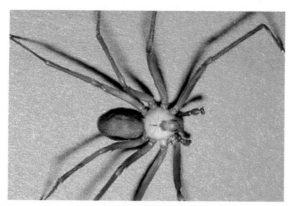

Plate 10. Brown recluse spider *(Loxosceles reclusa)*. The most important member of the genus in the United States. Dark violin-shaped mark on cephalothorax is seen in most North American species. *(Courtesy Indiana University Medical Center.)*

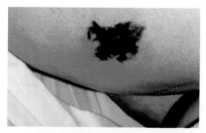

Plate 11. Cutaneous presentation of brown recluse bite after 24 hours, with central ischemia, rapidly advancing cellulitis.

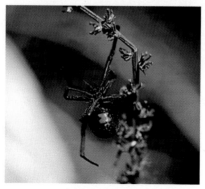

Plate 12. North American black widow spider *(Latrodectus mactans)*.

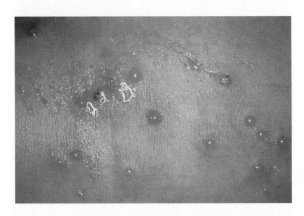

Plate 13. Vesicles produced by fire ant stings approximately 2 hours after the injury. These subsequently became sterile pustules. *(Courtesy Cameron Smith.)*

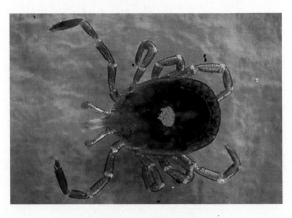

Plate 14. Lone star tick *(Amblyomma americanum)*. This tick has been implicated in cases of tick paralysis in North America. *(Courtesy Sherman Minton, MD.)*

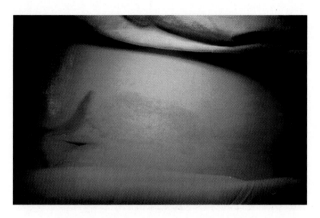

Plate 15. Erythema migrans rash of Lyme disease in a pregnant female.

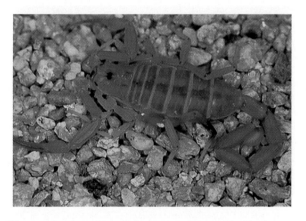

Plate 16. Scorpion of the genus *Centruroides* (bark scorpion). *(Courtesy William Banner, MD.)*

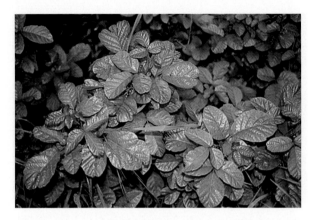

Plate 17. Poison oak.

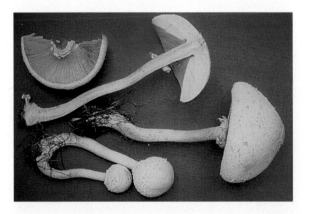

Plate 18. *Chlorophyllum molybdites.* A gastrointestinal irritant. *(From Phillips R:* Mushrooms of North America, *Boston, 1991, Little, Brown.)*

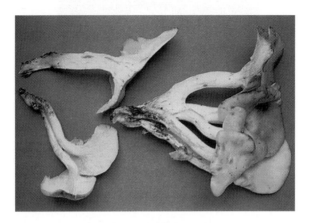

Plate 19. *Omphalotus olearius* (jack o'lantern mushroom). A gastrointestinal irritant. *(From Phillips R:* Mushrooms of North America, *Boston, 1991, Little, Brown.)*

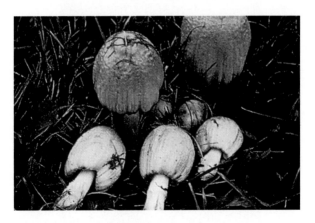

Plate 20. Inky cap *(Coprinus atramentarius). (Courtesy Orson J. Miller, PhD.)*

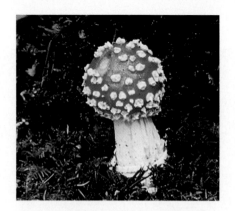

Plate 21. *Amanita muscaria.*

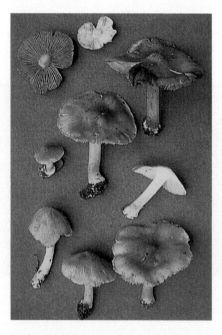

Plate 22. *Inocybe cookei.* Contains muscarinic toxins. *(From Phillips R:* Mushrooms of North America, *Boston, 1991, Little, Brown.)*

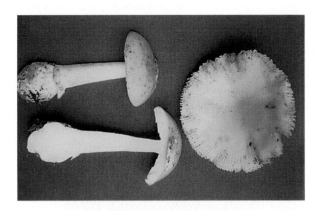

Plate 23. *Amanita pantherina.* Contains the neurotoxins ibotenic acid and isoxazole derivatives. *(From Phillips R:* Mushrooms of North America, *Boston, 1991, Little, Brown.)*

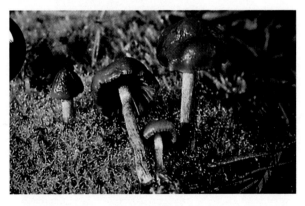

Plate 24. *Psilocybe caerulipes.*

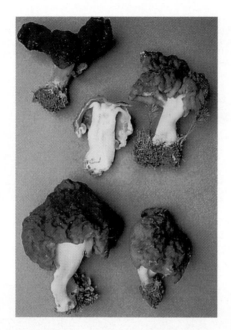

Plate 25. *Gyromitra esculenta.* Contains the hepatotoxin gyromitrin. *(From Phillips R: Mushrooms of North America, Boston, 1991, Little, Brown.)*

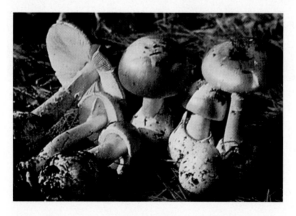

Plate 26. Death cap *(Amanita phalloides).*

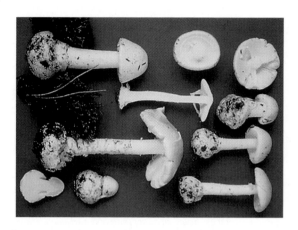

Plate 27. *Amanita virosa.* Causes delayed hepatotoxicity. *(From Phillips R:* Mushrooms of North America, *Boston, 1991, Little, Brown.)*

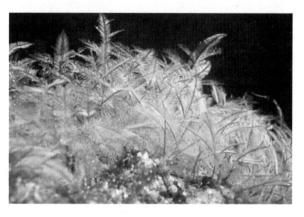

Plate 28. Coelentrate hydroid.

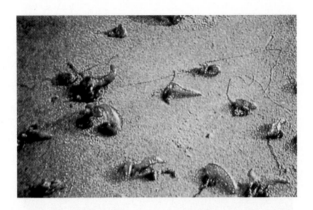

Plate 29. Pacific man of war *(Physalia utriculus)* washed ashore may retain their stinging potency for weeks. *(Courtesy Bruce Halstead, MD.)*

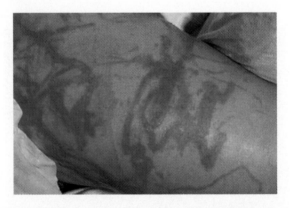

Plate 30. Early intense necrosis is typical of a severe box jellyfish *(Chironex fleckeri)* sting. *(Courtesy Mike Shacter.)*

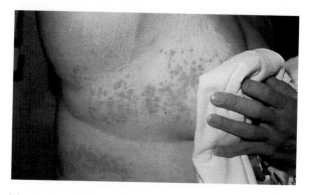

Plate 31.   Seabather's eruption. *(From Wong DE, et al: J Am Acad Dermatol 30(3):399-406, 1994.)*

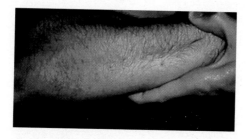

Plate 32.   Forearm immediately after multiple punctures by the spines of black sea urchins. In 24 hours, the darkened discolorations were absent, indicative of spine dye without residual spines. *(Courtesy Kenneth W. Kizer, MD.)*

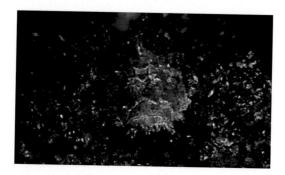

Plate 33.   The Galapagos scorpionfish conceals itself to await passing prey.

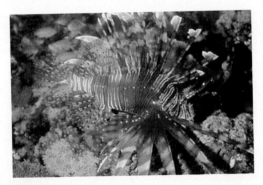

Plate 34. The ornate lionfish is the most extravagantly plumed of the venomous scorpionfishes.

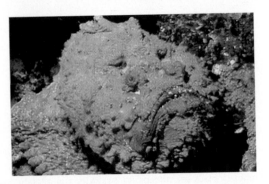

Plate 35. The deadly stonefish *(Synanceia horrida)*. *(Courtesy Carl Roessler.)*

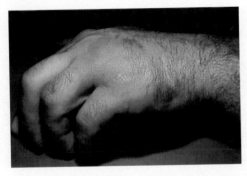

Plate 36. Typical appearance of *Erysipelothrix rhusopathiae* skin eruption.

Pediatric Wilderness Medical Kit: Basic Supplies

Assorted adhesive bandages
Butterfly bandages or Steri-Strips
Gauze pads
Cotton-tipped applicators
Gauze roll
Nonadherent dressings
Tape
Moleskin or Spenco 2nd Skin
Eye patches
Triangular bandage or sling
Elastic bandage
Povidone-iodine solution 10% (use to cleanse wounds and disinfect water)
Antiseptic wipes (benzalkonium chloride)
Antibacterial soap
Tincture of benzoin
Alcohol wipes
Lightweight malleable splint (SAM splint)
Needles
Safety pins
Syringe, 20 to 35 cc (for wound irrigation)
Plastic catheter or irrigation tip, 18-gauge (for wound irrigation)
Bulb syringe
Digital thermometer
Scissors
Tweezers
Sunscreen waterproof cream, SPF of at least 15
Insect repellent (no more than 35% DEET)
First-aid book

APPENDIX C

Contigency Supplies for Wilderness Travel

ITEM	DESCRIPTION, QUANTITY (NO., WEIGHT)*	COMMENT
1. Whistle	Nonmetal, shrill (1 oz)	Emergency signal (bursts of three)
2. Knives	A sturdy folding or straight knife plus a multitool knife	e.g., Swiss Army knife
3. Maps	Trail and topographic (1 oz) (some per group)	Plastic coated or with cover
4. Compass, fluid-filled	≤2° gradations (1-2 oz)	Know area declination
5. Flashlight	Two C cell most efficient; lithium or alkaline No. 1 (6-8 oz)	Headlamp attachment desirable

*Quantity is per person per trip, unless otherwise specified; weight given is per individual item, in ounces (35 oz = 1 kg = 2.2 lb).

Continued

ITEM	DESCRIPTION, QUANTITY (NO., WEIGHT)	COMMENT
6. Sunglasses	With side and nose blocks; polycarbonate or glass lens (1-3 oz)	>98% UVB filtering; >85% light absorption
7. Rescue and survival guide	Condensed (3-6 oz) (per group)	Learn basic air-to-ground signals
8. Pencil and paper	Waterproof paper preferred (2 oz)	
9. Quarters	Two (1 oz)	Phone calls; wrap in plastic and tape inside kit
10. Accident report forms	Waterproof preferred, two (1 oz) (per group)	
11. Spare sunglasses	(1-3 oz) (per group)	May improvise—make slits in cardboard, cloth
12. Toilet paper, small roll	One (1 oz)	Store in plastic bag
13. Matches, waterproof	"Strike-anywhere" type, 12	Store in plastic bag
14. Spare bulb, batteries	(1-3 oz)	Store in plastic bag

Continued

ITEM	DESCRIPTION, QUANTITY (NO., WEIGHT)	COMMENT
15. Closed-cell foam pads	1 × 1 ft sections; one to three (3 oz)	e.g., Ensolite; to insulate stove, seats, use as cervical collar or splint pads
16. Avalanche cord	Red; metal arrows (2 oz)	Attach to body
17. "Space" blanket	56 × 84 inches, two or three (1 oz)	Emergency insulation (replace every 3 yr)
18. Surveyor's trail tape	Bright color, 50 ft (1 oz) (per group)	Trail, avalanche site markers
19. Utility cord	Nylon 25-50 ft (2 oz)	Shelter; utility
20. Heat source	Candle; fuel tabs, one or two (2 oz)	
21. Emergency toboggan kit	Variable (per 2-3 persons)	Convert skis and poles; e.g., NSP
22. Goggles	Rose or amber (4 oz)	Double lens, polarized preferred
23. Radio beacon	(8 oz); e.g., Pieps, Skadi, Ortovox	Use in avalanche terrain
24. Scraper	Metal edged (1 oz)	Ice and wax removal
25. Shovel	Lexan or aluminum (16-32 oz) (per 1-3 persons)	e.g., REI

Continued

ITEM	DESCRIPTION, QUANTITY (NO., WEIGHT)	COMMENT
26. Face mask	Leather, silk, or synthetic (1 oz)	
27. Aerial flares; ground smoke bombs	Red smoke, two to four (1oz) (per group)	Rescue signal
28. "Bungie" elastic cords with hooks	6-12 inch #1-2 (1 oz)	Pack compression; lash equipment to pack
29. Swami belt	1-inch webbing 10-20 ft (4-8 oz)	Waist, seat harness
30. Carabiner, locking type	Aluminum, two or three (3 oz)	Climbing or rappel harness; rope brake; Prusik handle
31. Rescue pulley	Small one or two (2 oz)	Cliff, crevasse rescue
32. Rope, Perlon or Goldline	5.5-9 mm 50-75 ft (8-16 oz) (per group)	Rescue, evacuation
33. Magnifying lens	8-15× (1 oz) (per group)	Snow crystal examination; map reading; splinter removal; fire starter
34. Altimeter	≤20-ft accuracy (2 oz) (per group)	Altitude orienteering; barometric changes

Continued

ITEM	DESCRIPTION, QUANTITY (NO., WEIGHT)	COMMENT
35. Saw	Wire or blade (2-15 oz) (per 1-4 persons)	Fuel or shelter (cuts wood, snow, ice)
36. Extra food and candy	1-day supply (8-16 oz)	Prevent hypo-thermia
37. Extra cloth-ing	Wool preferred	Sock doubles as mitten
38. Signal mirror	Unbreakable preferred (1 oz)	
39. Road flare	5-minute, one or two (3 oz)	Rescue signal; emergency fire starter
40. Extra ski wax	Klister or two-wax system (3 oz)	
41. Emergency shelter	"Tube" tent, tarp, or bivvy sack (3-16 oz)	May improvise with large plastic bags
42. Extra water	1 pint, metal preferred (18 oz)	Metal canteen can be heated directly
43. Thermom-eter, outdoor	In protective case (0.5 oz) (per group)	Snow, water, air temperature
44. Lens anti-fogger	Liquid or stick (1 oz)	For glasses, goggles
45. Climbing skins, adhe-sive	"Skinny" type (11-16 oz)	Urgent snow climbing, or slowing descent

Repair Supplies for Wilderness Travel

ITEM	DESCRIPTION, QUANTITY, WEIGHT*	COMMENT
1. Needle or sewing awl	With heavy thread (1 oz)	Clothing, pack repair
2. Screwdrivers	Flat and Phillips No. 2 (3-6 oz)	For skis, No. 3 "posidrive" (or filed-down No. 2 Phillips)
3. Tape, duct or reinforced strapping	1-2 inches wide, 5 yards (2 oz) (per person per trip)	
4. Wire	Braided steel, 3-6 ft (2 oz)	Repair of binding, boot, snowshoe, and pack

*Quantity is per group unless specified; weight given is per individual item, in ounces (35 oz = 1 kg = 2.2 lb). *Continued*

ITEM	DESCRIPTION, QUANTITY (NO., WEIGHT)*	COMMENT
5. Awl	On multifunction knife (2 oz) (per person per trip)	Repair of clothing, pack, shelter
6. Visegrip pliers	5-inch (5-8 oz)	
7. Glue	Two-component epoxy, or meltable nylon glue stick (1 oz)	
8. Spare bale and screws	Two	Repair of ski binding
9. "P-tex" ski base stick	Meltable No. 1 (1 oz)	Repair of plastic ski base
10. Spare ski tip	Plastic or aluminum (3-5 oz)	
11. Spare crampon wrench	No. 1 (one)	
12. Knife sharpener	Diamond-bar, ceramic, or stone (2-3 oz)	

Priority First-Aid Equipment

Most Useful

Airways
Alcohol sponges
Arm or hand splint (wire, SAM splint)
Dressings, bandages, Kling, tape, cravats, Ace wrap
Extrication collar (can use SAM splint)
Flashlight
Germicidal soap
Heat-generating device (heat pads, Heatpak, Heat Treat)
Light traction splint (Sager or Kendrick Traction Device)
Litter
Long leg air splint
Lubricant for thermometer
Notebook and pencil, tags
Pain medications
Plastic bags (for snow, sprain and contusion treatment)
Pocket mask

Useful but Heavy, Expensive, or Needing Special Expertise

Bag-mask
Chest tube set (Heimlich valve, McSwain dart)
Cricothyrotomy set
Foley catheter, gloves, lubricant, clamp, and plug
For allergic reactions and anaphylaxis: bee sting kit, EpiPen, Benadryl
For high altitude: Diamox, Decadron, Lasix
For pneumonia and other infections: antibiotics
IV solutions, sets, needles
Military antishock trousers (MAST)
Oxygen
Suction device (mechanical)

Continued

Most Useful

Portable, short backboard
  (KED, Oregon Spine Splint)
Safety pins
Scissors
Seam ripper
Sterile irrigation solution (IV
  bag of 0.9% solution)
Suction device (bulb or
  syringe)
Syringe (20 cc) for irrigating
Thermometer (low-reading
  for cold weather and high
  altitude; regular for hot
  weather)
Urinal or pee bottle
Vaseline gauze

Less Useful

Defibrillator
Instant glucose
Cardiac monitor
Short leg air splint

Recuer's Personal Gear

Extra clothing
Food and hot drinks
Ice ax, ice hammer, ski poles,
  Ensolite, Therm-a-Rest (use
  for splint improvisation)
Poncho
Stove, gas, cooking pot
Tent, bivouac set

Medicines Specific to Women's Health

MEDICATION	INDICATION	DOSE	LENGTH OF TRIP (HR)
Acetamino-phen 325 mg	Dysmenor-rhea	1-2 q3-4h	>24
Trimethoprim/ sulfameth-oxazole* double strength	Urinary infec-tion	bid for 3 days	>72
Ampicillin* 250 mg	Urinary infec-tion	qid for 7 days	>72
Metronida-zole† 250 mg	Nonyeast vaginitis	tid for 7 days	>72

*Trimethoprim-sulfamethoxazole is contraindicated in individuals with sulfa allergy, and ampicillin is contraindicated in individuals allergic to penicillin.

†Metronidazole (Flagyl) has not been shown to be safe in pregnancy. The other medications suggested may be used in both pregnant and nonpregnant patients.

Continued

MEDICATION	INDICATION	DOSE	LENGTH OF TRIP (HR)
Miconazole cream	Yeast vaginitis	Nightly for 3 nights	>24
Estrogen 2.5 mg	Nonpregnant irregular vaginal bleeding	bid	>48
Pregnancy test kit	Irregular vaginal bleeding	As needed	>48

Antibiotics

Amoxicillin: adult dose 250 to 500 mg q8h; pediatric dose 10 to 15 mg/kg (2.2 lb) body weight q8h (tid).

Amoxicillin/clavulanate (Augmentin): adult dose 500 to 875 mg bid; pediatric dose 25 to 45 mg/kg body weight in 2 divided doses per day. For otitis media in children, use the higher dose.

Ampicillin: same dose as phenoxymethyl penicillin (see below).

Azithromycin (Zithromax): adult dose 500 mg day one, then 250 mg per day for 4 additional days; pediatric dose 10 mg/kg body weight day one, then 5 mg/kg body weight for 4 additional days.

Cefadroxil (Duricef): adult dose 500 mg to 1 g bid. For pharyngitis, to eradicate the Group A streptococcus, an acceptable dose is 1 g once a day for 10 days. Pediatric dose: for skin infections, 30 mg/kg body weight per day in 2 divided doses; for pharyngitis, administer in a single dose or 2 divided doses for 10 days.

Cefixime: adult dose 400 mg per day; pediatric dose 8 mg/kg once per day; no refrigeration needed—discard 14 days after the dry powder is reconstituted with water.

Cefuroxime axetil: adult dose 500 mg bid; pediatric dose 30 mg/kg body weight in 2 divided doses a day.

Cefpodoxime (Vantin): adult dose 200 to 400 mg bid for pneumonia.

Cephalexin (Keflex): adult dose 250 mg q4-6h or 500 mg q12h; pediatric dose the same as for phenoxymethyl penicillin. *Avoid use in a person with penicillin allergy* because 5% to 10% of persons allergic to penicillin are allergic to cephalosporins.

Ciprofloxacin (Cipro): adult dose 500 mg bid for 3 days to treat infectious diarrhea. *This drug should not be given to pregnant women or children under age 18.*

Clarithromycin (Biaxin): adult dose 500 mg bid; pediatric dose 15 mg/kg body weight in 2 divided doses per day.

Dicloxacillin: same dose as phenoxymethyl penicillin (below).

Doxycycline (Vibramycin): adult dose 100 mg bid for treatment or once a day for prevention of infectious diarrhea. *Do not give to pregnant women or children up to age 7* because this drug may cause permanent dark discoloration of the teeth.

Erythromycin: same dose as phenoxymethyl penicillin (see below). A common side effect is stomach upset and diarrhea. This drug is the first alternative for penicillin in penicillin-allergic individuals.

Erythromycin/sulfisoxazole (Gantrisin): pediatric dose 50 mg/kg body weight based on the erythromycin component in 4 divided doses a day.

Fleroxacin: adult dose 400 mg once a day for 3 days for the treatment of infectious diarrhea.

Metronidazole (Flagyl): adult dose 250 mg tid. *Do not drink alcohol when taking this medication and for 3 days afterwards. The interaction would cause severe abdominal pain, nausea, and vomiting.*

Noroxin: adult dose 400 mg q12h.

Ofloxacin: adult dose 300 to 400 mg q12h.

Phenoxymethyl penicillin (Penicillin Vee K): adult dose 250 to 500 mg q4-6h; pediatric dose: 2 to 6 years, 125 mg q6-8h, 6 to 10 years, 250 mg q6-8h. For pharyngitis, to eradicate the Group A streptococcus, an acceptable adult dose is 1 g bid for 10 days.

Tetracycline: adult dose 500 mg 4 qid. *Do not give to pregnant women or children up to age 7* because this drug may cause permanent dark discoloration of the teeth.

Trimethoprim with sulfamethoxazole (Bactrim or Septra double strength): adult dose 1 pill (80 mg TMP with 400 mg SMX) bid for infectious diarrhea or bladder infection; 1 pill once a day for prevention of traveler's diarrhea. The pediatric dose for an ear infection or severe infectious diarrhea (caused by *Shigella* bacteria) is 1 tsp of the pediatric suspension per 10 kg body weight q12h (bid), not to exceed 4 tsp (the adult dose) per dose. More precisely, the pediatric dose is 4 mg/kg/dose TMP with 20 mg/kg/dose SMX.

Wilderness Eye Kit

OPHTHALMIC ANTIBIOTIC SOLUTIONS
Quinolone
Ciprofloxacin (Ciloxan) 0.3% ophthalmic solution

Ciprofloxacin provides excellent coverage for serious corneal infections. This drug should be considered for remote expeditions with potential for prolonged evacuation times.

Other Topical Antibiotic Solutions
Gentamicin (Garamycin) 3 mg/ml ophthalmic solution
Tobramycin (Tobrex) 0.3% ophthalmic solution

Topical Antiseptic/Antibiotic Ointments
Bacitracin (AK-Tracin) 500 U/g ophthalmic ointment
Erythromycin (Ilotycin) 5 mg/g ophthalmic ointment
Gentamicin (Garamycin) 3 mg/g ophthalmic ointment
Tobramycin (Tobrex) 0.3% ophthalmic ointment

Antiviral Agent
Trifluridine (Viroptic) 1% ophthalmic solution

Systemic Antibiotics

Although not specific to ocular infection, quinolones are ideal because of their high intraocular tissue penetration; for example, ciprofloxacin (Cipro) 500-mg or 750-mg tablets.

TOPICAL ANESTHETIC AGENT

Proparacaine hydrochloride (Ophthaine) 0.5% ophthalmic solution. The ocular examination is better tolerated after administration of a topical anesthetic agent. Do not use a topical anesthetic agent repeatedly because it can delay corneal reepithelialization. A few drops of a topical anesthetic can help differentiate a superficial (corneal or conjunctival) process from a deeper intraocular cause of pain. Do not use a topical anesthetic with a suspected open globe injury.

MYDRIATIC-CYCLOPLEGIC

Cyclopentolate hydrochloride (Cyclogyl) 1% ophthalmic solution, intermediate duration, or homatropine (Isopto homatropine) 5% ophthalmic solution, longer duration (approximately 1 to 2 days). Homatropine has greater efficacy than cyclopentolate, but there are times when the longer duration of homatropine may be excessive (e.g., when the victim needs to negotiate difficult terrain the next morning). Ciliary muscle spasm is thought to play a role in the pain of many ocular conditions. A mydriatic paralyzes the pupillary constrictor muscle (sphincter), causing pupillary dilation. A cycloplegic relaxes the ciliary muscles.

TOPICAL STEROID

Prednisolone acetate (Pred Forte) 1% ophthalmic solution

Prolonged use of an ocular steroid may cause exacerbation of infectious keratitis (herpes simplex), increasing intraocular pressure, and cataract formation. A topical steroid will probably not cause significant side effects if given to a victim **with a fluorescein-negative eye disorder** for no more than 2 to 3 days.

TOPICAL VASOCONSTRICTOR AND DECONGESTANT

0.3% pheniramine maleate plus 0.025% naphazoline ophthalmic solution (Naphcon-A)

This combination helps control the inflammatory symptoms of conjunctivitis. It is most useful for the treatment of allergic symptoms.

FLUORESCEIN STRIPS OR DROPS

Strips are lighter in weight and avoid the potential for contamination. When examining an eye with a possible infectious process, always use a separate fluorescein strip for each eye to avoid gross contamination.

ARTIFICIAL TEARS

Polyvinyl alcohol 1% (HypoTears) ophthalmic solution
Hypertonic ophthalmic saline solution (Muro 128) solution
This is used for corneal erosion (relatively rare but difficult to treat; see below).

COTTON-TIPPED APPLICATORS
PREDNISONE 20-MG TABLETS
OPTIONAL AGENTS FOR TREATMENT OF ANGLE-CLOSURE GLAUCOMA

(this is an unlikely presentation)
Timolol 0.5% (Timoptic) ophthalmic solution
Pilocarpine hydrochloride (Pilocar) 2% ophthalmic solution
Acetazolamide (Diamox) 250-mg tablets

HEADLAMP OR FLASHLIGHT
SMALL MAGNIFYING LENS

Small, very lightweight, Fresnel-type hand lenses can be purchased at many office supply stores.

APPENDIX I

Recommended Oral Antibiotics for Bite Wounds

DRUG	CHILD	ADULT
ORGANISMS KNOWN		
Treat according to specific antibiotic sensitivities of cultured organism.		
ORGANISMS UNKNOWN*†		
Dog and most other bites:		
Dicloxacillin (least expensive) or cephalexin	50-100 mg/kg/day in 4 divided doses	500 mg PO qid
Cefuroxime (best coverage, not needed in most cases)	250 mg PO bid	500 mg PO bid
If penicillin allergic:		
Erythromycin *or*	30-50 mg/kg/day in 4 divided doses	500 mg PO qid

Continued

DRUG	CHILD	ADULT
Trimethoprim/ sulfamethox- azole	40 mg/200 mg per 10 kg bid	160 mg/ 800 mg (DS) bid

Cat bites (high likelihood of *Pasteurella multo-cida*)‡

DRUG	CHILD	ADULT
Penicillin plus di- cloxacillin (least expensive)	50-100 mg/kg/day in 4 divided doses	500 mg PO qid
Cefuroxime (best coverage)	250 mg PO bid	500 mg PO bid
If penicillin allergic:		
Trimethoprim/ sulfamethox- azole	40 mg/200 mg per 10 kg bid	160 mg/ 800 mg (DS) bid
or		
Ciprofloxacin (nonpregnant adults only)	Contraindicated	500 mg bid

Listed are antibiotics chosen for efficacy against most likely organisms at lowest cost.

Which antibiotic is the cheapest varies greatly over time and by local-ity. The difference between lowest and moderately priced antibiotics typically averages $25 and $35 cost to the patient, which is not war-ranted in low-risk cases but in high-risk cases may be cost-effective if the antibiotic prevents infection and additional physician visits.

*This regimen is effective for most potential pathogens. No one antibi-otic covers all.

†Most patients can take an oral cephalosporin such as cephalexin without adverse effect. Erythromycin is not effective against *Staphylo-coccus*.

‡Penicillin is excellent for *Pasteurella* but is not optimal for many other significant pathogens; dicloxacillin has a much broader spectrum but slightly less efficacy against *Pasteurella*.   *Continued*

DRUG	CHILD	ADULT
Human bites of hand (organisms of concern include *Streptococcus, Staphylococcus,* and *Eikenella corrodens*)		
Dicloxacillin plus ampicillin (least expensive) *or*	50-100 mg/kg/day in 4 divided doses	500 mg PO qid
Cefuroxime (best coverage)	250 mg PO bid	500 mg PO bid
If penicillin allergic: Ciprofloxacin plus erythromycin	Contraindicated	500 mg bid

APPENDIX J

Therapy for Parasitic Infections

ETIOLOGIC AGENT	INDICATION	DRUG AND DURATION
Giardia lamblia	Proven disease	Quinacrine* 100 mg tid for 7 days for adults, 7 mg/kg/day in 3 divided doses for 7 days for children
	Infants	Furazolidone 1.5 mg/kg qid for 7 days
	Empirical (unproven)	Metronidazole 250 mg tid for 7 days for adults, 15 mg/kg/day in 3 divided doses for children

*If available; otherwise, use metronidazole or tinidazole.

Continued

ETIOLOGIC AGENT	INDICATION	DRUG AND DURATION
Entamoeba histolytica	Carrier/no symptoms	Diiodohydroxyquin 650 mg tid for 10 days for adults and 40 mg/kg/day in 3 divided doses for 7 days for children or diloxanide furoate (unlicensed)
	Intestinal disease	Metronidazole 750 mg tid for 5-10 days plus diiodohydroxyquin 650 mg tid for 21 days for adults or metronidazole 50 mg/kg/day in 3 divided doses for 10 days plus diiodohydroxyquin 40 mg/kg/day in 3 divided doses for 21 days

Continued

ETIOLOGIC AGENT	INDICATION	DRUG AND DURATION
Dientamoeba fragilis or *Balantidium coli*	Intestinal disease	Tetracycline 250-500 mg qid for 7 to 10 days or di-iodohydroxyquin 650 mg tid for 20 days for adults
Entamoeba polecki	Intestinal disease	Metronidazole 750 mg tid for 10 days followed by diloxanide furoate 500 mg tid for 10 days for adults
Blastocystis hominis	Intestinal disease	Diiodohydroxyquin 650 mg tid for 20 days or metronidazole 750 mg tid for 10 days for adults
Cryptosporidium parvum	Intestinal disease	Paromomycin 500 mg tid for 5 to 7 days for adults
Isospora belli	Intestinal disease	TMP/SMX 160 mg/800 mg bid for 3 to 4 weeks
Cyclospora or *Sarcocystis*	Intestinal disease	Uncertain

Index

Death cap mushroom, 311, plate
26
Débridement, wound, 154-155
Declination, 477
Decompression, pleural,
performing, 74, 75-78
Decompression sickness,
406-408
Decongestant, ophthalmic, 521
Deep fascial space infection,
248-249
Deep partial-thickness burns, 33
Deep-sea slickheads, 435
DEET, 293
to prevent malaria, 379
"Deformity, dinner fork," 103
Dehydration, 457
Dengue virus, 361-362
Dental emergencies, 245-252
Dental floss to hold wound
closed, 160
Dental kit, basic, 498
Dermatitis, 297-303, 442-446
Dermatome pattern, 59-60
Deterioration, high-altitude, 2
Diabetes mellitus, 199-203
Diabetic emergencies, 199-203
Diamondback rattlesnake,
Eastern, plate 5
Diamox (acetazolamide), 521
Diarrhea, 330, 331
traveler's; see Traveler's
diarrhea
Dicloxacillin, dose of, 517
Dientamoeba fragilis, 345, 527
"Dinner fork deformity," 103
Diphtheria and tetanus
immunization, 381, 382,
384
Discharge from upstream
towns, 356
Disease
cat-scratch, 319-320
diarrheal, 330
Lyme, 285-287
erythema migrans rash of,
plate 15
meningococcal, 367-369
pelvic inflammatory, 219-221
tick-borne, 292-294
Disinfection of water, 347-359

Dislocation; *see also*
Fracture/dislocation
ankle, 147-148
calcaneal, 148-149
distal interphalangeal joint of
hand, 121-123
elbow, 116-117
glenohumeral joint, 111-113
hindfoot, 148-149
hip, 144-145
evacuation decisions with,
91
reduction of, 146
of interphalangeal joints of
foot, 149-150
knee, 145-146
evacuation decisions with,
91
kneecap, 146-147
Lisfranc's, 149
lower extremity, 144-150
metacarpophalangeal joint,
118-119
metatarsophalangeal joint, of
toe, 149-150
midfoot, 149
patellar, 146-147
posterior ring, of pelvis, 123
posterior shoulder, 113-115
proximal interphalangeal
joint of hand, 119-121
shoulder, 111-113
shoulder harness for
support after, 114
sternoclavicular joint, 108-109
tibia, 145-146
upper extremity, 108-123
volar, 121
wrist, 117-118
Distal femur and patella
fracture, 130-132
Distal interphalangeal joint of
hand, dislocation of,
121-123
Disulfiram-like mushroom
toxins, 306
Diuretics, 22
Divers Alert Network, 405, 408
Diving equipment, 449
Dog bites, 315, 522-523
Dolphin, Hawaiian, 436
Domoic acid intoxication, 441
Double figure-8 knot, 481